Animals and Environments

Animals and Environments

Proceedings of the Third International Conference of Comparative Physiology and Biochemistry held in KwaZulu-Natal, South Africa, between 7 and 13 August 2004

Editors:

Dr. Steve Morris
University of Bristol
School of Biological Sciences
Bristol
UNITED KINGDOM

and

Dr. André Vosloo
North-West University
School of Environmental Science & Development
Potchefstroom Campus
Potchefstroom
SOUTH AFRICA

ELSEVIER

2005

ELSEVIER B.V.
Sara Burgerhartstraat 25
P.O. Box 211, 1000 AE Amsterdam
The Netherlands

ELSEVIER Inc.
525 B Street, Suite 1900
San Diego, CA 92101-4495
USA

ELSEVIER Ltd
The Boulevard, Langford Lane
Kidlington, Oxford OX5 1GB
UK

ELSEVIER Ltd
84 Theobalds Road
London WC1X 8RR
UK

First edition 2005

Library of Congress Cataloging in Publication Data
A catalog record is available from the Library of Congress.

British Library Cataloguing in Publication Data
A catalogue record is available from the British Library.

International Congress Series No. ICS 1275
ISBN: 0-444-51763-4
ISSN: 0531-5131

⊗ The paper used in this publication meets the requirements of ANSI/NISO Z39.48-1992 (Permanence of Paper).
Printed in The Netherlands.

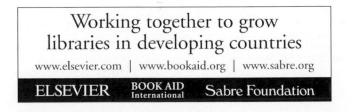

International Congress Series 1275 (2004) v–vii

ELSEVIER

www.ics-elsevier.com

Preface

Introduction 'Animals and environments' 3rd ICCPB in Africa: Ithala 2004 Ithala Game Reserve, KwaZulu-Natal, South Africa

André Vosloo[a],*, Steve Morris[b],*

[a]School of Environmental Science and Development North-West University, Potchefstroom Campus,
Potchefstroom, South Africa
[b]Morlab, School of Biological Sciences, University of Bristol, Bristol, U.K.

Keywords: Physiology; Biochemistry; Environment; Africa; Molecular; Adaptation

The third International Conference on Comparative Physiology and Biochemistry in Africa was held in the Ithala Game Reserve, in the highlands of Zululand in South Africa. At Ntshondwe Camp, situated at the foot of the "Ngotshe" plateau ("*a place to which when a man is gone there he can no longer be seen!*"), the conference followed on the ethos of the first meeting held in Kruger National Park [1] which has been embodied in subsequent ICCPB in Africa meetings [2]. The objective was to bring together International Delegates in a special and secluded corner of Africa for a week of relaxed and contemplative discussion of adaptive animal physiology and biochemistry, and to view it first hand!

The ICCPB in Africa meetings were conceived to bring delegates into Africa, and to expose them to Africa, to African problems and to promote interaction with their African research colleagues. Most importantly, the meetings continue to provide unique opportunities for indigenous African researchers, and all involved in biological research in southern Africa, to present and showcase their work and their institutions.

The Ithala 2004 meeting had a special structure. With predawn starts to sessions but with the afternoons and evenings held free for informal business, the format provided for

* Corresponding authors. André Vosloo is to be contacted at School for Environmental Sciences and Development, North-West University, Potchefstroom Campus, Private Bag X6001, Potchefstroom, 2520, South Africa. Tel.: +27 18 299 2375; fax: +27 18 299 2503. Steve Morris, Morlab, School of Biological Sciences, University of Bristol, Woodland Road, Bristol BS8 1UG, UK. Tel.: +44 117 928 9181; fax: +44 117 928 8520.
E-mail addresses: drkav@puk.ac.za (A. Vosloo), Steve.Morris@bris.ac.uk (S. Morris).

0531-5131/ © 2004 Elsevier B.V. All rights reserved.
doi:10.1016/j.ics.2004.09.042

the opportunity to discuss physiological and biochemical adaptation of animals while actually touring the majestic Ithala Game Reserve. Where else would it be possible, for example, to discuss red cell metabolism of rhinoceros in a scientific session and then step outside and view them in their natural habitat! To enjoy conversations with new and old colleagues while gazing to the far horizons of the Pongola River Valley and the hills of Zululand, uninterrupted by email and cellular telephones. Two delegates were reported in heated discussion of animal locomotion after viewing the hartebeest, the fastest antelope in Africa!

The Science program and the resultant papers were constructed to cross the entire gamut from unicellular organisms to whole animals in their environment, and what was required for them to succeed in those environments. The meeting was attended by 185 people, with 111 oral and 30 poster papers presented, from which the papers presented in this volume were selected. Unlike the sectional structure of many international meetings, Ithala 2004 was organised to encourage delegates to attend the entire range of papers from a variety of fields and to meet colleagues not previously encountered.

'Animals and environments' was selected as the umbrella title to promote wide discussion but most importantly to encourage an integrated discussion of how animals persist and succeed in the normal habitats. Most importantly, the meeting sought to bring together molecular, cellular, biochemical, physiological, and ecological approaches, and to foster synergistic interactions between them, with the view to improving our appreciation of the interaction with, and response to, environmental circumstances.

This volume begins by considering the genetic and molecular basis of some physiological responses most especially in response to hypoxia and the role of hypoxia inducible factors. Crustaceans are an important component of the freshwater and marine African macroinvertebrate fauna and papers included here consider the molecular and adaptive mechanisms of ion homeostasis in these animals. Insects are similarly considered with regard to cell signalling and respiration. Heavy metal contamination is of acute concern at specific localities within South Africa and elsewhere within southern Africa; this volume collects papers which address this issue, ranging from the genetics of biomining bacteria through to the morphological damage caused to fish. Extremes of temperature and limited water availability are important environmental factors influencing the distribution of species and their access to different habitats. These factors were discussed firstly in a series of papers outlining the thermal and developmental biology of reptiles, and then in a more diverse series of papers including frogs, birds, and mammals. The theme of 'animals and environments' was further developed by considering foraging and predation, the acquisition of food, and the quality and utilization of this resource in the light of specific environmental demands in both terrestrial and aquatic habitats.

In a time of persistent reductionism in biological studies [3,4], the meeting created a special environment with time to discuss both breadth and depth of adaptive animal biology from more holistic perspectives. A number of new and fertile collaborations and career opportunities resulted.

The sponsorship of indigenous delegates allowed the attendance of nationals from Botswana, Ethiopia, Sudan, and South Africa; almost all of whom presented papers. In addition, the conference provided an injection into the local economy of a remote corner of South Africa, as well as supporting the wildlife conservation efforts in KwaZulu-Natal. In this regard our thanks go to Ezemvelo KZN Wildlife, to Ithala Game Reserve, and to the staff at Ntshondwe Camp. Outside of delegates from southern Africa, the meeting was attended by delegates from almost 20 other countries. Special travel arrangements, including a number of the weeklong overland trips to and from the meeting, brought together delegates who have gone on to establish joint projects and new friendships. Importantly, many of the delegates came to see aspects and parts of southern Africa unseen by the casual observer and fulfilled one goal of the meeting—to promote a long and enduring attachment to southern Africa, to the biology, and to the people of the area.

Biological, molecular, and biochemical research in southern Africa is now burgeoning within a climate of political change and evolution which strongly influences research opportunities and directions within the University systems [5]. The biological and wildlife wealth of the region is an important economic asset, and, under circumstances of increasing social change, the continued and increased investment in biological research seems increasingly important in maintaining global biodiversity [6,7]. It is our hope that Ithala 2004 and the ICCPB in Africa meetings contribute to this is some small way and that they will continue to do so in future.

Acknowledgement

Special thanks go to all at Natural Events http://www.natural-events.com.

References

[1] S. Afr. J. Zool. 33 (1998) 53–140 (Collected papers).
[2] Comp. Biochem. Physiol., A 133 (2002) 419–899 (Collected papers).
[3] H. Andersen, The history of reductionism versus holistic approaches to scientific research, Endeavour 25 (2001) 153–156.
[4] P.J.M. Verschuren, Holism versus reductionism in modern social science research, Qual. Quant. 35 (4) (2001) 389–405.
[5] P. Ingwersen, D. Jacobs, South African research in selected scientific areas: status 1981–2000, Scientometrics 59 (2004) 405–423.
[6] A.S.L. Rodrigues, et al., Effectiveness of the global protected area network in representing species diversity, Nature 428 (6983) (2004) 640–643.
[7] E. Meir, S. Andelman, H.P. Possingham, Does conservation planning matter in a dynamic and uncertain world? Ecol. Lett. 7 (2004) 615–622.

Contents

Preface

International Congress Series 1275 (2004) 1–13

ELSEVIER

www.ics-elsevier.com

Gene regulation in physiological stress

Kenneth B. Storey*

Institute of Biochemistry, Carleton University, 1125 Colonel By Drive, Ottawa, Ontario, Canada K1S5B6

Abstract. A range of new tools in molecular biology are now available to allow the comparative biochemist to explore animal responses to environmental stress at multiple levels. In particular, new techniques of gene discovery, such as cDNA array screening, allow broad assessment of the responses of thousands of genes to a stress. This approach frequently identifies genes (and their associated metabolic functions) that have never before been associated with the stress under study and allows coordinated patterns of gene responses (e.g., by families of genes or by genes encoding multiple proteins in a metabolic pathway or a signal transduction cascade, etc.) to be elucidated. New methods for mRNA (e.g., quantitative PCR) and protein (e.g., peptide antibodies, phospho-specific antibodies) analysis, coupled with major advances in bioinformatics, also simplify the exploration of gene/protein regulation. Techniques and approaches for gene/protein discovery and regulatory analysis are discussed and illustrated with examples drawn from new studies of the responses to anoxia by the marine gastropod, *Littorina littorea*. © 2004 Elsevier B.V. All rights reserved.

Keywords: Gene expression; Anoxia tolerance; Marine mollusc; cDNA array, Polysome profiles

1. Introduction

For many years, studies of biochemical adaptation to environmental stress centered primarily at the level of protein/enzyme function [1]. However, new molecular tools are now providing a huge range of opportunities for the comparative biochemist to examine adaptive responses at most, if not all, levels of metabolic organization including signal transduction, transcription, translation, kinetic and allosteric controls, post-translational modification, subcellular localization, and protein degradation [2]. Within the last decade, major advances have been made in the technology for gene screening and in our understanding of the mechanisms of gene regulation. Furthermore, the methods for gene

* Tel.: +1 613 520 3678; fax: +1 613 520 2569.
E-mail address: kenneth_storey@carleton.ca.

0531-5131/ © 2004 Elsevier B.V. All rights reserved.
doi:10.1016/j.ics.2004.09.031

and protein expression studies are no longer cumbersome and difficult technologies but have become relatively simple tools that can be put to excellent use in comparative biochemistry. Gene discovery techniques such as cDNA array screening are providing amazing opportunities for identifying the genes that are turned on in animals under different environmental stresses, frequently highlighting previously unsuspected genes and proteins (and their cell functions) that participate in adaptive response. Easy entry into the study of virtually any gene/protein found in GenBank is available by using consensus sequences to design gene primers that are then synthesized commercially and used with automated polymerase chain reaction (PCR) technology to "pluck" the mRNA for almost any identified gene from an organism. This mRNA can then be used as the starting point for studies in several directions. For example, after sequencing, species-specific primers can be made and used to quantify changes in tissue transcript levels using quantitative PCR (Q-PCR) or Northern blotting and full-length sequences can be retrieved using 5′ or 3′ RACE (rapid amplification of cDNA ends) to assess species-specific changes in gene/protein sequence. The cDNA sequences can also be used to screen genomic libraries to find complete gene sequences (introns plus exons) as well as promotor (5′ untranslated) regions. Knowledge of promotor sequences—those sites where transcription factors bind—can then unlock regulatory aspects of gene function. Bioinformatics programs can be applied to either cDNA or genomic sequences to detect regulatory motifs in both gene and protein to give hints about the signal transduction pathways that are involved in their regulation or to analyze species-specific differences in amino acid sequence that may be adaptive (e.g., amino acid substitutions that could aid stress resistance such as optimizing proteins for low-temperature function). Species-specific cDNA sequences can also be used to design peptides for antibody production to follow stress-induced changes in protein levels and phospho-specific antibodies can be used to assess the changes in relative activity of the many proteins that are modified by reversible phosphorylation. Use of phospho-specific antibodies is especially key for tracing multicomponent signal transduction cascades leading from cell surface to nuclear gene activation. Hence, we now have the molecular tools to evaluate almost any metabolic system and to search for the breadth and depth of biochemical adaptations that define the differences between stress-tolerant and stress-intolerant organisms.

Recent studies in my lab have used the technologies described above to analyze stress-responsive gene and protein expression underlying animal adaptive strategies such as anoxia tolerance, freeze tolerance, hibernation and estivation as well as to identify the universal mechanisms of metabolic rate depression (MRD) that are a part of each of these strategies [2–5]. In the remainder of this article, I will review the main mechanisms of gene/protein regulation, highlight some advances in our understanding of the role of these mechanisms in MRD, and illustrate some of these mechanisms from recent studies by my lab of anoxia tolerance in the marine gastropod, *Littorina littorea*.

2. Review of transcriptional and translational control

For most cellular proteins, the initiation of gene transcription is the principle point at which their expression is regulated [6]. Hence, many regulatory controls, both positive and negative, global and specific, are applied to transcription. Global controls include regulation of the assembly and binding of RNA polymerase II and a group of general transcription factors at the gene promoter as well as mechanisms of chromatin remodelling and histone modification to allow polymerase to gain access to the DNA template. Such controls often alter overall transcriptional activity in cells in response to factors such as environmental stress, growth and developmental timetables, and nutrient availability. Global activation of transcription has been extensively studied whereas global repression is less well understood [6] but is an area of active interest in my lab due to the obvious need to suppress this energy-expensive activity in animals that exhibit stress-induced MRD [2]. More specific controls on individual genes or groups of genes are applied via the actions of gene-specific transcription factors and their cofactors that bind at more distant sites (generally in the 5' untranslated region) to stimulate or repress transcription in response to specific signals [7]. Activation of transcription factors is often a result of protein phosphorylation mediated by protein kinases that are often at the terminus of long signal transduction cascades [8]. Identification of the transcription factor response elements present in different genes as well as of the protein kinases that phosphorylate each transcription factor provide the clues to the signal transduction cascades that regulate different genes. In addition, by using phospho-specific antibodies, the relative levels of active kinases and transcription factors can be quantified to help confirm the signal transduction cascade operating in each situation of stress-responsive gene expression. Other controls also regulate transcript elongation, capping and splicing, polyadenylation and export of the completed mRNA to the ribosomes [6,7].

The stability of mRNA transcripts, both pre-translation and during translation, is another level at which control can be exerted. Most mRNA transcripts proceed directly to the ribosomes where they are translated a variable number of times with half-lives for transcript stability ranging from seconds to hours. However, transcripts of some genes are not immediately translated but are maintained in an untranslatable state by bound inhibitor proteins that are only released by the binding of specific ligands. Hence, primary control over the expression of these genes is actually at the translational level. Other layers of regulatory controls are applied to translation. Because protein synthesis is energy-expensive (needing ~5 ATP equivalents per peptide bond formed), the rate of protein synthesis must be closely matched with the cell's ability to generate ATP. Not surprisingly, then, protein synthesis is a main target of MRD; strong global suppression of translation occurs with only a few stress responsive genes that are up-regulated and translated [2]. Two main mechanisms of global protein synthesis control are (a) the state of ribosome assembly, and (b) reversible phosphorylation that modifies the activities of multiple ribosomal initiation and elongation factors. Active translation takes place on polysomes whereas monosomes are translationally silent. The proportion of ribosomes in polysomes can vary widely depending on the cellular demand for protein biosynthesis and/or the availability of ATP and amino acids. Tight regulation is required and the dissociation of polysomes and sequestering of mRNA into monosome and ribonuclear protein fractions is one of the major events in cells entering hypometabolic states [2]. Phosphorylation of key ribosomal proteins also modifies global translational activity. Inhibitory controls on translation include phosphorylation of the alpha subunit of eukaryotic initiation factor 2 (eIF2α), which halts delivery of the initiating methionine residue to the ribosome and several types of inhibitory and fragmentation events affect subunits of eIF4 to block the entry of m^{7}G-capped mRNAs (the majority of transcripts) onto the 40S ribosomal subunit [9]. However, some transcripts can circumvent this mode of transcription initiation due to the presence in their mRNA sequence of an internal ribosome entry signal (IRES). This provides the means for selected translation of stress-responsive proteins under conditions where global translation is strongly suppressed. For example, this is how the alpha subunit of the hypoxia-inducible factor 1 (HIF-1α) can be translated under low oxygen conditions [10]. Similar methods using an IRES or other novel method of translation initiation may be involved in the selective up-regulation of the stress-responsive genes that support animal adaptation to other challenges (e.g., high or low temperature, freezing, dehydration, heavy metals, etc.). Other controls target the elongation stage of peptide synthesis. For example, signals acting through a variety of protein kinases regulate the eukaryotic elongation factor 2 (eEF2), another key site for global inhibition of translation during hypometabolism [2].

Once synthesized, proteins are then subject to multiple controls on their actions and activities within cells. This is a massive subject of its own and such controls include substrate/ligand availability, allosteric regulation, binding with regulatory proteins, subcellular compartmentation, and many kinds of covalent modification [1,11]. A final set of controls on the overall expression level of proteins is at the level of proteolysis. Global controls can be exerted by inhibition of the proteasome or by inhibition of the ubiquitination reactions that target proteins for recognition by the proteasome. Both can participate in MRD [2]. Selected proteins are also regulated at the level of degradation via specifically tailored mechanisms. For example, the oxygen-dependent hydroxylation of two proline residues on HIF-1α targets the protein for attack by an E3 ubiquitin-protein ligase and subsequent rapid degradation by the proteasome under aerobic conditions. However, under hypoxia, hydroxylation is inhibited and HIF-1α is stabilized.

3. Transcriptional and translational control in a model of anoxia tolerance

A primary interest of my laboratory is anoxia tolerance—mechanisms and adaptations used by animals to survive long-term oxygen deprivation. We study both vertebrate [5] and invertebrate models, the latter focused mainly on marine molluscs [12,13]. Studies have examined different aspects of biochemical control including alternative routes of anaerobic energy production, regulation of glycolytic enzymes by multiple mechanisms (e.g., allosteric regulation, reversible phosphorylation, subcellular enzyme binding), and antioxidant defenses that aid recovery when oxygen is reintroduced [12–15]. Our recent work [16–26] has focused on the periwinkle, *L. littorea*, an inhabitant of the intertidal zone around the north Atlantic, examining both anoxia tolerance and freezing survival.

A key component of anoxia tolerance in all systems where it has been studied is MRD; for marine molluscs, metabolic rate under anoxia is typically <10% of the aerobic rate [2]. The strong reduction in ATP turnover results from coordinated repression of ATP-utilizing and ATP-producing reactions so that vital processes can be supported over the long-term by the ATP output of fermentative metabolism. A critical mechanism of MRD is reversible protein phosphorylation that produces major changes in the activity states of many enzymes and functional proteins with consequences for all areas of metabolism. As in other anoxia-tolerant molluscs, reversible phosphorylation of selected enzymes of glycolysis in *L. littorea* is critical for redirecting carbon flow into anaerobic routes of fermentative metabolism as well as suppression of glycolytic rate [2,14]. For example, changes in the properties of phosphofructokinase and pyruvate kinase were consistent with a conversion of the enzymes to less active forms under anoxia [16,20]. Anoxia also reduced the percentage of cAMP-dependent protein kinase (PKA) present as the active catalytic subunit from ~30% in normoxia to just 1–3% in anoxia [19]. Hence, metabolic functions that are PKA-stimulated would be suppressed during anaerobiosis; indeed, general suppression of signal transduction cascades seems to be a part of MRD [2].

It is estimated that gene transcription consumes 1–10% of a cell's ATP budget whereas protein synthesis can utilize as much as 40% [2]. Not surprisingly, studies have shown that both are crucial targets of MRD during anaerobiosis. We used the nuclear run-on technique to evaluate transcription in *L. littorea*; this method measures the rate of mRNA elongation in isolated nuclei and we found that the overall rate of ^{32}P-UTP incorporation into nascent mRNAs in hepatopancreas nuclei fell to less than one-third of the normoxic rate [13]. Similarly, the rate of ^{3}H-leucine incorporation into protein in hepatopancreas extracts was reduced by 50% within 30 min of anoxic exposure and remained low over a 48 h anoxia exposure [23]. Interestingly, these events occurred without signs of energy stress in the snails (ATP levels remain high for several days

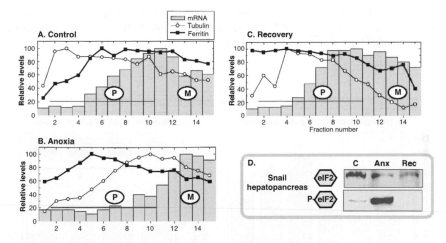

Fig. 1. Controls on protein synthesis in hepatopancreas of marine snails *L. littorea*. Panels A through C show the distribution of rRNA and of mRNA transcripts of alpha-tubulin (a constitutive gene) and ferritin (an anoxia up-regulated gene) in hepatopancreas of (A) control, (B) 72 h anoxic, and (C) 6 h aerobic recovered snails. Ribosomes were separated on a 15–30% continuous sucrose gradient and fractions were collected with highest sucrose (30%) in fraction 1 and lowest sucrose (15%) in fraction 15. Each fraction was assessed for rRNA content by absorbance at 254 nm and mRNA levels via Northern blotting. Data are expressed relative to the fraction containing the highest rRNA or mRNA content. The horizontal line running between fractions 2 and 10 shows the general position of polysome fractions (labeled with a P), whereas the higher fractions contained monosomes (labeled with an M). (D) Western blots show the relative levels of eukaryotic initiation factor 2 alpha (eIF2α) in hepatopancreas from control, anoxic and recovered snails. The upper panel shows total eIF2α protein whereas the lower panel shows the amount of phosphorylated eIF2α that is the inactive form. Data are reworked from Larade and Storey [23,25].

under anoxia) [17] showing that suppression of transcription and translation are actively regulated components of MRD, not reactions to energy limitation. The mechanisms of translational regulation were those mentioned earlier: polysome dissociation and phosphorylation of ribosomal proteins (Fig. 1). The latter was documented by Western blotting, which found no change in total eIF2α protein during anoxia/recovery whereas the use of phospho-specific antibodies revealed that the amount of phosphorylated eIF2α rose by ~15-fold in hepatopancreas of anoxic *L. littorea*, compared with aerobic controls (Fig. 1D) [23].

Changes in polysome content were revealed by separating polysomes and monosomes on a sucrose gradient and tracking the distribution of rRNA, the mRNA for α-tubulin (a constitutively active gene) and the mRNA for ferritin heavy chain (an anoxia-responsive gene) [23–25]. Under aerobic conditions, rRNA distribution showed

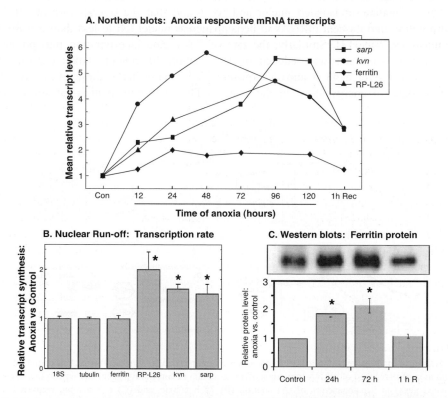

Fig. 2. Anoxia responsive gene expression in hepatopancreas of marine snails *L. littorea*. (A) Northern blots show changes in mRNA transcript levels over a time course of anoxia exposure followed by 1 h of aerobic recovery for four genes identified as anoxia responsive from cDNA library screening. Con-aerobic control; RP-L26-ribosomal protein L26. (B) The nuclear run-off technique monitored ^{32}P-UTP incorporation into mRNA in vitro to measure the rate of transcription in isolated nuclei from aerobic control versus 48 h anoxic snails. Transcription rates of two housekeeping genes, 18S ribosomal RNA and alpha-tubulin, were also measured. (C) Western blotting shows ferritin heavy chain protein levels in hepatopancreas during anoxia and after 1 h of aerobic recovery. Upper panel shows a representative blot. Histograms in both B and C show means±S.E.M. for n=3 independent trials. *Significantly different from the control value, $P<0.05$. Data are reworked from Refs. [22,24–26].

that most ribosomes were in the high-density polysome fractions (Fig. 1A). The mRNA for α-tubulin was also found predominantly with the polysomes; both results are consistent with a state of active translation in the control state. However, after 24 h of anoxia, rRNA began to shift towards lower densities indicating polysome disaggregation [23] and by 72 h there was little evidence of polysomes remaining in hepatopancreas (Fig. 1B); α-tubulin transcripts also moved into monosome fractions. These data are consistent with the idea that most mRNA species are maintained and but not translated in the hypometabolism state. However, within 6 h of the return to oxygenated conditions, both parameters indicated reassembly of polysomes and the return of mRNA for the constitutively active gene to the polysome fractions (Fig. 1C) [23]. The mRNA transcripts of anoxia up-regulated genes, *kvn* and ferritin, behaved very differently [24,25]. Fig. 2C illustrates this for ferritin showing that a higher proportion of ferritin transcripts were found in the polysome fractions under anoxia than in the aerobic control situation. This suggests preferred translation of ferritin by the remaining polysomes during anoxia. This result was supported by a measured ~2-fold increase in ferritin protein in hepatopancreas of anoxic snails (Fig. 2C) [25].

4. Anoxia-induced gene expression in the marine gastropod *L. littorea*

A variety of modern techniques can be used for gene discovery and recent studies in our lab have used two of these (cDNA library screening, cDNA microarrays) to reveal anoxia responsive genes in *L. littorea* [13,21–26]. We constructed and screened cDNA libraries from both foot [21] and hepatopancreas [22]. This method is time-consuming and expensive and favors the discovery of mRNA species that are in abundant supply but its key advantage is the ability to find novel species-specific transcripts that have no homologues in gene banks. We found two such genes in periwinkle hepatopancreas [24,26] that may have novel functions in anaerobiosis (see below). For the comparative biochemist, this ability to seek out novel genes/proteins that may be species- or stress-specific is of great importance for understanding biochemical adaptation. In the past, stress-specific genes and proteins were generally detected by an obvious functional footprint, such as the action of the antifreeze proteins of cold-water fishes in creating a thermal hysteresis between freezing and melting points of blood plasma. However, many important stress-specific proteins may, in fact, have no easily detectable physiological action. Hence, species-specific gene screening is invaluable.

Giant advances in gene discovery are also coming from the use of cDNA array screening, which allows simultaneous screening of the expression of thousands of named genes for their responses to an imposed stress or treatment. To date, arrays are available for only a few species but we have had excellent results using human 19,000 cDNA arrays (from the Ontario Cancer Institute, Toronto) for heterologous probing for stress-responsive genes in frozen frogs [3], hibernating ground squirrels and bats [4], and anoxic turtles [5]. The percentage of genes that cross-react falls off with phylogenetic distance but, nonetheless, can still provide dozens or even hundreds of "hits" for follow-up studies. We used the human arrays to search for anoxia-responsive gene expression in *L. littorea* hepatopancreas. Not unexpectedly, cross-reactivity was low, only 18.35%, and of the genes that did cross-react, most showed no change in transcript levels in anoxia (88.8%)

whereas 0.6% showed reduced transcripts in anoxia. This finding is consistent with the idea that most transcripts are simply maintained/sequestered during anoxia so that they are available when the reintroduction of oxygen allows MRD to be lifted and normal translational activity to be resumed. However, 10.6% of the cross-reacting genes were putatively up-regulated by twofold or more in anoxia and this represented over 300 genes. These included protein kinases and phosphatases, mitogen-activated protein kinase interacting factors, translation factors, antioxidant enzymes, and nuclear receptors [13]. Virtually all of these are proteins that have never before been implicated in anoxia tolerance and, hence, we now have a much broader view of the potential gene expression responses that may play significant roles in anaerobiosis. Results from heterologous array screening must be confirmed by other methods and we are analyzing several of these candidate genes. The current methods for follow-up with any given gene are: (1) design of DNA primers based on a consensus sequence put together from available sequences for the gene in GenBank; (2) use of the primers to retrieve the species-specific cDNA via PCR; (3) nucleotide sequencing of the retrieved cDNA for confirmation of identity and then synthesis of species-specific probe to evaluate organ-, time-, and stress-specific gene expression via Q-PCR; (4) as needed, use of 3′ or 5′ RACE to retrieve the full sequence for analysis of possible adaptive changes in amino acid sequence compared with other species; and (5) use of the putative amino acid sequence to design and synthesize peptide antibodies for quantifying patterns of protein expression in anoxia.

Our first studies using cDNA library screening revealed several anoxia-responsive genes. Libraries were constructed from *L. littorea* foot and hepatopancreas using equal amounts of mRNA from snails given 1, 12, or 24 h N_2 gas exposure. By combining mRNA from multiple stress points, the screening (against normoxic controls) can detect genes that are up-regulated at any point in the anoxic time course. Later, the time-dependent expression of individual genes can be characterized using methods such as Northern blotting or Q-PCR to quantify mRNA levels at each sampling time. Screening revealed several genes that were putatively up-regulated in anoxia; these included metallothionein (MT) from the foot library [21] and ferritin, the L26 ribosomal protein, and two novel genes from the hepatopancreas library [22,24–26]. Each showed independent patterns of transcript elevation over a time course of anoxia exposure and transcripts of all four genes were significantly reduced again within 1 h of the return to aerobic conditions (Fig. 2A).

The novel genes are particularly intriguing and were named *kvn* and *sarp-19* [24,26]. The clone *kvn* contained 525 bp with a full open reading frame that encoded 99 residues of the KVN protein. The predicted molecular weight of KVN was 12 kDa and it showed an N-terminal hydrophobic signal sequence. Such sequences typically direct proteins to the endoplasmic reticulum where they are processed and secreted to a final destination; this suggests that KVN has an extracellular function. Features of its sequence such as the spacing of cysteine clusters suggest that KVN may be an iron–sulfur protein that binds iron and is related to the ferredoxin family [24]. It may function similar to other ferredoxin-like proteins, possibly mediating electron transfer reactions during anoxia or recovery. *Sarp-19* (snail anoxia-responsive protein 19 kDa) codes for a different protein type [26]. The open reading frame encoded 168 amino acids with an N-terminal signal sequence and two putative EF-hand domains. The common function of EF-hand domains is calcium binding, typically inducing a conformational change causing activation (or inactivation) of target proteins [27]. The function of SARP-19 in anaerobiosis may include calcium-activated signaling or calcium sequestering. The latter might be a key physiological function for SARP-19 in extracellular spaces for the following reason. The shift from aerobic to anaerobic life in shelled molluscs is accompanied by a significant dissolution of the calcium carbonate shell with the bicarbonate released buffering acidic products of fermentative metabolism [28]. Aerial exposure stimulates bivalve molluscs to close their valves and gastropods to "seal themselves in" by covering the shell opening with the operculum. Hence, they become closed systems, a feature that aids water and osmotic balance but means that hemolymph calcium levels rise substantially during anaerobiosis [29]. Calcium is a key signaling molecule and intracellular levels are strictly regulated at very low values in all cells by sarcoplasmic reticulum and plasma membrane Ca^{2+} pumps. Hence, elevated amounts of a Ca^{2+}-binding protein under anoxia could help to minimize free Ca^{2+} levels, particularly under hypometabolic conditions when ATP expenditure on Ca^{2+} pumping should be minimized.

The identifiable genes revealed from screening of L. littorea libraries also revealed prominent up-regulation of ion-binding proteins under anoxia, suggesting that this may be a principle of marine invertebrate anoxia tolerance. Screening of the foot library showed anoxia-responsive up-regulation of MT [21]. Periwinkle MT shared ~50% identity with the copper- and cadmium-binding MT isoforms from the land snail, Helix pomatia and ~45% identity with marine bivalve MTs and contained the mollusc-specific C-terminal motif: Cys-X-Cys-X(3)-Cys-Thr-Gly-X(3)-Cys-X-Cys-X(3)-Cys-X-Cys-Lys [30]. Northern blots showed up-regulation of MT within 1 h and transcripts rose by 3–3.5-fold in foot and 5–6-fold in hepatopancreas within 12–24 h of either anoxia or freezing exposure [21]. Hence, MT responds to changing oxygen levels within the time frame of normal tidal cycles and that adds support to the idea that variation in MT protein aids anoxia tolerance in the natural environment. Although MTs are typically thought of as metal-binding proteins and are widely used as bioindicators of heavy metal pollution in the marine environment [31], recent evidence from both mammalian and marine invertebrate systems suggests that MTs also function in antioxidant defense. In mammals, ischemia–reperfusion injury was lessened by MT overexpression but enhanced by MT knock-out [32,33]. In molluscs, MT induction via pre-exposure to cadmium greatly increased the survival of mussels that were then exposed to iron in an anoxic environment [34]. Although MT could contribute to antioxidant defense by binding copper and thereby limit copper-induced reactive oxygen species (ROS) generation via the Fenton reaction, MT is poor at binding iron, the main metal involved in Fenton chemistry. Hence, the antioxidant effect of MT does not appear to derive from iron binding but, instead, there is evidence that MT can scavenge ROS (including hydroxyl radicals and superoxide) via thiolate oxidation of its cysteine residues [35,36].

Another metal-binding protein, ferritin heavy chain, was identified as up-regulated from screening the L. littorea hepatopancreas library [25]. Northern blots showed that transcript levels rose twofold during anoxia exposure and Western blots showed a comparable rise in protein content followed by a return to control levels within 1 hour of normoxic recovery (Fig. 2A,C). However, when nuclear run-off assays were used to evaluate the rate of transcription of anoxia-responsive genes, the results showed that the ferritin gene was not actually transcriptionally activated under anoxia, unlike the L26, *kvn* and *sarp* genes that showed enhanced transcript synthesis under anoxia (Fig. 2B). This result for ferritin concurs with data on the regulation of the protein in other systems. Ferritin transcripts contain *cis*-acting nucleotide sequences in the 5′-UTR called iron regulatory elements (IREs) that are recognized by cytosolic RNA-binding iron-regulatory proteins (IRPs). When bound, IRPs prevent the transcript from associating with ribosomes but, when iron levels are high, iron binds to the IRPs and triggers their dissociation from ferritin transcripts [37]. Hence, ferritin protein levels are controlled at the transcript level. Oxygen is another of several signals that regulates the system; in mammals, hypoxia reduces the RNA binding activity of IRPs and this is reversed by reoxygenation [38]. Anoxia exposure in littorines may similarly reduce the number of IRP-blocked ferritin transcripts and, thereby, promote translation of ferritin mRNA. Furthermore, as noted earlier, ferritin mRNA transcripts remain associated with polysomes during anoxia, another factor that would promote their translation [25].

5. Regulation of anoxia-induced gene expression

The signal transduction pathways that regulate anoxia-induced gene expression in *L. littorea* are another area of great interest. We have begun to explore this by incubating hepatopancreas explants in vitro with various second messengers and stimulators including dibutyryl cAMP, calcium ionophore A23187, phorbol 12 myristate 13 acetate (PMA), and dibutyryl cGMP to stimulate protein kinases A, B, C and G, respectively [22,24–26]. Transcript levels of ferritin, L26 ribosomal protein, *kvn* and *sarp 19* all increased when tissues were incubated in a medium bubbled with nitrogen gas as compared with aerobic control samples; this confirmed that anoxia exposure stimulated gene up-regulation both in vivo and in vitro. Tissue samples were then incubated under aerobic conditions with each of the protein kinase stimulators. Analysis via Northern blotting showed that transcript levels of the four anoxia responsive genes all increased by 1.5–2.5-fold when aerobic tissues were incubated with dibutyryl cGMP. However, the genes did not respond to dibutyryl cAMP. Transcripts of *sarp-19* also rose in response to calcium ionophore and PMA which suggests that the gene responds to Ca^{2+} levels, in line with the structural information that indicates that SARP-19 is a Ca^{2+} binding protein, as discussed earlier [26]. The common response by all four genes to cGMP suggests a central role for cGMP and protein kinase G (PKG) in the regulation of gene expression responses to anoxia in *L. littorea*. Indeed, previous studies have implicated PKG in the control of intermediary metabolism during anaerobiosis in other marine molluscs. For example, PKG mediates the anoxia-induced phosphorylation of enzymes (in particular, pyruvate kinase) as part of glycolytic rate depression [39]. Incubation with cGMP also mimicked the effect of anoxia on the kinetic properties of phosphofructo-kinase from the anterior byssus retractor muscle of *Mytilus edulis* whereas cAMP incubation had the opposite effect [40]. A well-known activator of guanylyl cyclases is the diffusible signal molecule, nitric oxide (NO) [41]. Recent studies have shown that NO is involved in low oxygen signaling in *Drosophila melanogaster* [42] and this, coupled with the evidence cited above of cGMP mediation of anoxia-induced events in molluscs, suggests that the NO/cGMP signaling pathway may be central in the response to oxygen deprivation in anoxia-tolerant invertebrates, coordinating both metabolic and gene expression responses to anoxia. In line with this, NO up-regulates herritin transcripts in land snail neurons [43].

Much remains to be determined about the mechanisms of oxygen sensing, the signal transduction cascade(s) involved in transmitting low oxygen signals, and the metabolic and gene expression responses to low oxygen by anoxia tolerant species. Continuing explorations will not only solve the mysteries of life without oxygen but will help to highlight the key differences in sensing, signaling and responding to low oxygen that differentiate anoxia tolerant and intolerant species, and aid in the search for applied treatments in medicine that can prevent or correct hypoxic/ischemic damage. New technologies for screening and analyzing gene expression will play a primary role in this search, allowing researchers to view broad patterns of response by hundreds of genes across a broad spectrum of species, using the power of comparative biochemistry to identify the critical gene/protein responses that impart stress tolerance on organisms.

Acknowledgements

Thanks to J.M. Storey for editorial review of the manuscript. K.B.S. holds the Canada Research Chair in Molecular Physiology and research is supported by a Discovery grant from the Natural Sciences and Engineering Research Council of Canada. To learn more about gene regulation in physiological stress, visit http://www.carleton.ca/~kbstorey.

References

[1] P.W. Hochachka, G.N. Somero, Biochemical Adaptation: Mechanism and Process in Physiological Evolution, Oxford University Press, Oxford, 2002.
[2] K.B. Storey, J.M. Storey, Metabolic rate depression in animals: transcriptional and translational controls, Biol. Rev. Camb. Philos. Soc. 79 (2004) 207–233.
[3] K.B. Storey, Strategies for exploration of freeze responsive gene expression: advances in vertebrate freeze tolerance, Cryobiology 48 (2004) 134–145.
[4] K.B. Storey, Mammalian hibernation: transcriptional and translational controls, Adv. Exp. Med. Biol. 543 (2003) 21–38.
[5] K.B. Storey, Molecular mechanisms of anoxia tolerance, In: XXXXXX, (Ed.) XXXXX, Elsevier, Amsterdam, 2004, in press (this volume).
[6] K. Gaston, P.S. Jayaraman, Transcriptional repression in eukaryotes: repressors and repression mechanisms, Cell. Mol. Life Sci. 60 (2003) 721–741.
[7] W.G. Willmore, Control of transcription in eukaryotic cells, in: K.B. Storey (Ed.), Functional Metabolism: Regulation and Adaptation, Wiley, New York, 2004, pp. 153–187.
[8] J.A. MacDonald, Tyrosine phosphorylation and the control of cellular information, in: K.B. Storey (Ed.), Functional Metabolism: Regulation and Adaptation, Wiley, New York, 2004, pp. 125–151.
[9] D.J. DeGracia, et al., Molecular pathways of protein synthesis inhibition during brain reperfusion: implications for neuronal survival or death, J. Cereb. Blood Flow Metab. 22 (2002) 127–141.
[10] K.J.D. Lang, A. Kappel, G.J. Goodall, Hypoxia-inducible factor-1α mRNA contains an internal ribosome entry site that allows efficient translation during hypoxia, Mol. Biol. Cell 13 (2002) 1792–1801.
[11] K.B. Storey, Biochemical adaptation, in: K.B. Storey (Ed.), Functional Metabolism: Regulation and Adaptation, Wiley, New York, 2004, pp. 383–413.
[12] S.P.J. Brooks, K.B. Storey, Glycolytic controls in estivation and anoxia: a comparison of metabolic arrest in land and marine molluscs, Comp. Biochem. Physiol., A 118 (1997) 1103–1114.

[13] K. Larade, K.B. Storey, A profile of the metabolic responses to anoxia in marine molluscs, in: K.B. Storey, J.M. Storey (Eds.), Cell and Molecular Responses to Stress, vol. 3, Elsevier, Amsterdam, 2002, pp. 27–46.

[14] K.B. Storey, J.M. Storey, Oxygen limitation and metabolic rate depression, in: K.B. Storey (Ed.), Functional Metabolism: Regulation and Adaptation, Wiley, New York, 2004, pp. 415–442.

[15] M. Hermes-Lima, J.M. Storey, K.B. Storey, Antioxidant defenses and animal adaptation to oxygen availability during environmental stress, in: K.B. Storey, J.M. Storey (Eds.), Cell and Molecular Responses to Stress, vol. 2, Elsevier, Amsterdam, 2001, pp. 263–287.

[16] E.L. Russell, K.B. Storey, Anoxia and freezing exposures stimulate covalent modification of enzymes of carbohydrate metabolism in *Littorina littorea*, J. Comp. Physiol., B 165 (1995) 132–142.

[17] T.A. Churchill, K.B. Storey, Metabolic responses to freezing and anoxia by the periwinkle, *Littorina littorea*, J. Therm. Biol. 21 (1996) 57–63.

[18] T.M. Pannunzio, K.B. Storey, Antioxidant defenses and lipid peroxidation during anoxia stress and aerobic recovery in the marine gastropod, *Littorina littorea*, J. Exp. Mar. Biol. Ecol. 221 (1998) 277–292.

[19] J.A. MacDonald, K.B. Storey, Cyclic AMP-dependent protein kinase: role in anoxia and freezing tolerance of the marine periwinkle, *Littorina littorea*, Mar. Biol. 133 (1999) 193–203.

[20] S.C. Greenway, K.B. Storey, The effect of seasonal change and prolonged anoxia on metabolic enzymes of *Littorina littorea*, Can. J. Zool. 79 (2001) 907–915.

[21] T.E. English, K.B. Storey, Freezing and anoxia stresses induce expression of metallothionein in the foot muscle and hepatopancreas of the marine gastropod, *Littorina littorea*, J. Exp. Biol. 206 (2003) 2517–2524.

[22] K. Larade, A. Nimigan, K.B. Storey, Transcription pattern of ribosomal protein L26 during anoxia exposure in *Littorina littorea*, J. Exp. Zool. 290 (2001) 759–768.

[23] K. Larade, K.B. Storey, Reversible suppression of protein synthesis in concert with polysome disaggregation during anoxia exposure in *Littorina littorea*, Mol. Cell. Biochem. 232 (2002) 121–127.

[24] K. Larade, K.B. Storey, Characterization of a novel gene up-regulated during anoxia exposure in the marine snail *Littorina littorea*, Gene 283 (2002) 145–154.

[25] K. Larade, K.B. Storey, Accumulation and translation of ferritin heavy chain transcripts following anoxia exposure in a marine invertebrate, J. Exp. Biol. 207 (2004) 1353–1360.

[26] K. Larade, K.B. Storey, Anoxia-induced transcriptional up-regulation of sarp-19: cloning and characterization of a novel EF-hand containing gene expressed in hepatopancreas of *Littorina littorea*, Biochem. Cell. Biol. 82 (2004) 285–293.

[27] S. Weinman, Calcium-binding proteins: an overview, J. Biol. Buccale 19 (1991) 90–98.

[28] R.A. Byrne, T.H. Dietz, Ion transport and acid–base balance in freshwater bivalves, J. Exp. Biol. 200 (1997) 457–465.

[29] H.B. Akberali, K.R.M. Marriott, E.R. Trueman, Calcium utilization during anaerobiosis induced by osmotic shock in a bivalve mollusc, Nature 266 (1977) 852–853.

[30] P.A. Binz, J.H.R. Kagi, Metallothionein: molecular evolution and classification, in: C. Klaassen (Ed.), Metallothionein, vol. 4, Birkhauser, Basel, 1999, pp. 7–13.

[31] I. Boutet, et al., Immunochemical quantification of metallothioneins in marine molluscs: characterization of a metal exposure bioindicator, Environ. Toxicol. Chem. 21 (2002) 1009–1014.

[32] M.L. Campagne, et al., Evidence for a protective role of metallothionein-1 in focal cerebral ischemia, Proc. Natl. Acad. Sci. U. S. A. 96 (1999) 12870–12875.

[33] J.S. Lazo, et al., Enhanced sensitivity to oxidative stress in cultured embryonic cells from transgenic mice deficient in MT I and II genes, J. Biol. Chem. 27 (1995) 5506–5510.

[34] A. Viarengo, et al., Role of metallothionein against oxidative stress in the mussel *Mytilus galloprovincialis*, Am. J. Physiol. 277 (1999) R1612–R1619.

[35] P. Thornalley, M. Vâsàk, Possible role for metallothionein in protection against radiation-induced oxidative stress. Kinetics and mechanism of its reaction with superoxide and hydroxyl radicals, Biochim. Biophys. Acta 827 (1985) 36–44.

[36] P. Irato, et al., Oxidative burst and metallothionein as a scavenger in macrophages, Immunol. Cell Biol. 79 (2001) 251–254.

[37] E.C. Theil, Targeting mRNA to regulate iron and oxygen metabolism, Biochem. Pharmacol. 59 (2000) 87–93.

[38] B.D. Schneider, E.A. Leibold, Effects of iron regulatory protein regulation on iron homeostasis during hypoxia, Blood 102 (2003) 3404–3411.

[39] K.B. Storey, Molecular mechanisms of metabolic arrest in mollusks, in: P.W. Hochachka, P.L. Lutz, T.J. Sick, M. Rosenthal, G. van den Thillart (Eds.), Surviving Hypoxia: Mechanisms of Control and Adaptation, CRC Press, Boca Raton, 1993, pp. 253–269.

[40] B. Michaelidis, K.B. Storey, Phosphofructokinase from the anterior byssus retractor muscle of *Mytilus edulis*: modification of the enzyme in anoxia and by endogenous protein kinases, Int. J. Biochem. 22 (1990) 759–765.

[41] J. Stamler, D. Singel, J. Loscalzo, Biochemistry of nitric oxide and its redox activated forms, Science 258 (1992) 1898–1902.

[42] J. Wingrove, P. O'Farrell, Nitric oxide contributes to behavioural, cellular, and developmental responses to low oxygen in *Drosophila*, Cell 98 (1999) 105–114.

[43] M. Xie, et al., Nitric oxide up-regulates ferritin mRNA level in snail neurons, Eur. J. Neurosci. 13 (2001) 1479–1486.

International Congress Series 1275 (2004) 14–21

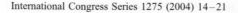

www.ics-elsevier.com

Analyzing biological function with emerging proteomic technologies

Justin A. MacDonald*, Meredith A. Borman

University of Calgary, Smooth Muscle Research Group, Canada

Abstract. Strong evidence exists that many adaptive processes are associated with quantitative, post-translational and functional changes in protein complement. While the acquisition of large bodies of genomic sequence is facilitating the use of global techniques to analyze cellular function, much of the regulation of physiological processes happens at a post-translational level. The emerging field of 'proteomics' is being used to identify the sources and extent of biological variation at the protein level. This review will present a general overview of the currently available proteomic tools including two-dimensional gel electrophoresis and mass spectrometry as well as more advanced technologies under development. Particular attention will be paid to technologies and methodologies being used to analyze signal transduction networks (i.e. protein phosphorylation and the regulation of biological function). The advantages and limitations of proteomic technologies and their suitability for use in the study of diverse organisms will be discussed. © 2004 Elsevier B.V. All rights reserved.

Keywords: Proteomics; Signal transduction; Phosphorylation; Mass spectrometry

1. Introduction

The scientific field has been moving beyond genomics towards proteomics research for a number of years. While DNA is the information archive of the cell, the proteins are the main functional output of the cell and ultimately dictate the biological processes and cellular fates. The term proteomics is defined as the analysis of the entire protein complement of a given cell, tissue, or organism at a given point in time [1, 2]. Proteomic analysis involves both the qualitative alterations in proteins along with the quantitative

* Corresponding author. Department of Biochemistry and Molecular Biology, University of Calgary, 3330 Hospital Drive N.W., Calgary, AB, Canada T2N 4N1. Tel.: +1 403 210 8433; fax: +1 403 270 2211.
 E-mail address: jmacdo@ucalgary.ca (J.A. MacDonald).

0531-5131/ © 2004 Elsevier B.V. All rights reserved.
doi:10.1016/j.ics.2004.08.060

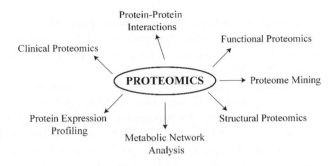

Fig. 1. Areas of study within the field of proteomics.

changes in protein expression levels that occur in response to a given set of conditions [3]. However, proteomics is much more than just developing exhaustive lists of all the proteins within an organism. The true scientific goal of proteomics is to characterize the information flow. The analysis of proteomes is significantly more challenging than that of genomes. In particular, the proteome is a dynamic entity, both spatially and temporally, and will reflect the immediate environment in which it is studied. In response to internal or external cues, proteins can be modified by post-translational modification, undergo translocation within the cell, or be degraded or synthesized [4]. As such it is possible for a single genome to give rise to an infinite number of proteomes. Furthermore, proteomic analysis is substrate-limited as there are no methods available for protein amplification.

The field of proteomics encompasses a number of different areas of study (Fig. 1). The main areas of this field are functional proteomics and protein expression profiling. Functional proteomics is a broad term used to describe many specific, directed proteomics approaches. In general, functional proteomic studies characterize protein activity, protein interactions, and the presence of post-translational modifications. In some cases a specific sub-proteome is isolated for further study thereby allowing the characterization of a select group of proteins. Protein expression proteomics is the differential measurement of protein expression levels between cells or conditions.

The execution of a proteomics-based study involves the integration of a number of technologies. These technologies span the fields of molecular biology, biochemistry, physiology, statistics, and bioinformatics. The key steps in proteomics are the separation of complex mixtures of proteins, followed by protein identification. The success of any proteomics study is directly linked to performing each aspect in a consistent and reproducible fashion, and to minimizing the incorporation of artefacts.

2. Protein separation

2.1. Two-dimensional gel electrophoresis

The most widely used method for protein separation is two-dimensional polyacrylamide gel electrophoresis (2D-PAGE). In 2D-PAGE, proteins are separated according to their net charge in the first dimension and according to their molecular mass in the second dimension. A separation resolution far exceeding that obtained by one-dimensional PAGE alone can be achieved. One of the greatest benefits of 2D-PAGE is the ability to resolve proteins that have undergone post-translational modification. This resolution is made possible by the fact that many protein modifications confer a difference in both charge and mass. For example, the phosphorylated form of a protein can be resolved from the non-phosphorylated form by 2D-PAGE [5].

The primary application of 2D-PAGE is protein expression profiling. Using this approach, the protein expression of any two samples can be qualitatively and quantitatively compared by evaluating the appearance or disappearance of protein spots as well as any changes in protein intensity. This technique has been used to compare healthy and diseased tissues [6], to compare the protein complement of muscle tissues from high and low altitude dwellers [7], and to compare proteins specific to bacterial growth at 4 versus 23 °C [8]. This technique is currently the only proven method to simultaneously separate proteins and to quantitatively compare changes in their profiles within cells, tissues, or organisms [9].

Although 2D-PAGE has been used extensively for the separation of complex protein mixtures, certain limitations still exist. The detection of proteins that occur in low copy number remains a major limitation. In addition, certain key classes of proteins are not efficiently represented on 2D-PAGE. These include: very high or very low molecular weight proteins, extremely acidic or basic proteins, and very hydrophobic proteins [10].

2.2. Two-dimensional liquid chromatography

The drawbacks of 2D gel methodology have led to the development of alternative methods for protein profiling such as 2D liquid chromatography. This 2D liquid separation involves the use of isoelectric focusing (IEF) in a liquid phase followed by a nonporous silica-reversed-phase HPLC separation as the second dimension [11]. Proteins that elute from the second dimension can be detected directly on-line using electrospray ionization (ESI)-mass spectrometry or off-line using matrix-assisted laser desorption ionization-mass spectrometry (MALDI-MS). Multidimensional protein identification technology, referred to as MudPIT, has been used to identify 1484 proteins in the large-scale analysis of the yeast proteome [12]. This method potentially offers higher throughput and faster sample resolution than 2D-PAGE.

2.3. Isotope-coded affinity tags (ICAT)

ICAT has emerged as a powerful alternative to protein electrophoresis. This technique allows the measurement of quantitative differences in protein abundance between two samples regardless of the source of the sample [13]. The ICAT reagent introduces stable isotope tags into proteins via the selective alkylation of the side chains of reduced cysteines with either a deuterium-labelled heavy isoform (d8) or a hydrogen-labelled light isoform (d0) [14]. A reduced protein sample from one specimen is derivitized with the d8 version of the ICAT reagent while the other protein sample is derivitized with the d0 isoform. The two samples are combined and digested, and the cysteine-containing peptides are isolated through avidin affinity chromatography. Identification and quantification is then determined by liquid chromatography and tandem MS [14].

The principal advantage of this method is the elimination of 2D gels for protein quantification. Consequently, an increased amount of sample can be used to enrich for low abundance proteins. One of the primary limitations of the current ICAT method is the relatively rare occurrence of cysteine residues in proteins. The result is poor sequence coverage using this method. Consequently, the ICAT method is not well suited to the analysis of post-translational modifications or the analysis of protein isoforms generated by alternative mRNA splicing [10].

3. Mass spectrometry

Mass spectrometry is now the dominant tool for protein identification [15], with mass spectrometry methods routinely capable of identifying proteins in the femtomolar range. Mass spectrometers are made up of three primary components: the ionization source, the mass analyzer, and the detector. Typically, two types of ionization techniques are used to deliver peptide ions to the mass analyzer: matrix-assisted laser desorption/ionization (MALDI) or electrospray ionization (ESI). Both ionization types can convert polar molecules into gas-phase ions without degradation or fragmentation. Peptide ions are then separated in a mass analyzer (i.e. a linear flight tube) on the basis of mass to charge (m/z) ratio. Ion flight in the mass analyzer is directed by magnetic-quadrupoles to direct ions to a detector in an m/z dependent manner.

3.1. MALDI-Time of Flight (MALDI-TOF)

The primary application of the MALDI-TOF mass spectrometer is in generating Peptide Mass Fingerprints (PMFs) for enzymatically digested proteins. Excised protein spots are proteolytically digested, typically with trypsin, yielding a mixture of peptides. The masses of the peptides are then measured to produce a characteristic mass profile or "fingerprint" of that protein. The mass profile is then compared with peptide masses predicted from theoretical digestion of known protein sequences contained within databases. Because of its speed and ability to be completely automated, MALDI-TOF MS is the method of choice for large-scale proteomics [16]. However, not all proteins can be identified through PMF's alone. Furthermore, MALDI-TOF is typically less effective for analyzing complex protein mixtures as only the most abundant proteins tend to be identified. Similarly small proteins, less than 20 kDa, are generally difficult to analyze as they tend to produce fewer appropriately sized tryptic peptides. A variation on the MALDI technique, surface enhanced laser desorption/ionization (SELDI)-TOF employs a variety of selective chips onto which complex protein mixtures can be spotted. Each of the different chip surfaces will retain a subset of proteins that are subsequently analyzed by a mass spectrometer to look for pattern changes amongst samples [17]. This methodology has become increasingly popular in clinical proteomics where the principle goal is the identification of diagnostic bio-markers.

3.2. Tandem mass spectrometry (MS/MS)

Data related to the primary amino acid sequence of the peptide can be highly desirable. So called tandem mass spectrometers have been developed to select a particular peptide ion of specific mass, fragment it in a collision chamber, and then measure the m/z ratio of the resulting fragment ions. The actual amino acid sequence or de novo sequence is reconstructed from the fragmentation pattern with computer software. The primary advantage of tandem mass spectrometry is the ability to select a particular peptide ion from a mixture, allowing for the identification of components of complex mixtures.

3.3. Fourier transform ion cyclotron resonance mass spectrometry (FT-ICR)

FT-ICR mass spectrometers are ion-trap instruments capable of making mass measurements with a combination of resolution and accuracy that is higher than any other type of mass spectrometer [18]. Its high resolution makes FT-ICR especially well suited for the analysis of complex protein mixtures. However, the procurement and operational costs tend to limit the use of FT-ICR.

4. Data base searching

4.1. Peptide mass fingerprinting (PMF)

Using this approach, peptide masses obtained from MALDI-MS are compared against theoretical spectra obtained from primary-sequence databases. Because the protein analysis and database searching can be fully automated, the primary advantage of PMF is speed. However, PMF is only effective in the analysis of proteins from organisms whose genome is small, completely sequenced, and well annotated [19]. In addition, the presence of post-translational modifications leads to peptides that may not match the unmodified protein in the database making PMF unsuitable for analysis of extensively modified proteins. Furthermore, PMF is not suitable for analysis of protein mixtures. There are a number of search programs used for PMF including: PepSea [20]; PeptIdent/MultiIdent [21]; and ProFound [22].

4.2. Peptide mass tag searching

In this method, a partial amino acid sequence is obtained from the MS/MS spectrum (the sequence tag) and this information is combined with the mass of the peptide and the masses of the peptide on either side of the sequence tag where the sequence is not known. Peptide mass tag searching is a more specific tool for protein identification than PMF [23]. In addition, one of the primary advantages to utilizing MS/MS to obtain primary amino acid sequence is that it is compatible with protein mixtures [24]. The major disadvantage however is that this process is not easily automated.

4.3. De novo sequence searching

An alternative approach to protein identification is to obtain de novo sequence data from peptides by MS/MS and then search appropriate databases with all of the peptide sequences. Using the FASTS program [25], multiple peptide sequences can be used for protein identification. The result is the capability of searching peptide information across both DNA and protein databases. This method is useful for organisms that do not have well-annotated databases [24]. However, because this method requires that several peptides be sequenced, it is time consuming and not generally the first method of choice.

5. Cell signaling

Signal transduction pathways have traditionally been elucidated by identifying all of the signaling molecules (receptors, kinases, phosphatases, and substrates) one by one and then individually verifying the connections between them [26]. In recent years, developments in mass spectrometric techniques and instrumentation have dramatically improved our ability to analyze the cellular proteome on a large-scale basis.

The apparent information gap between a genome and the cellular processes resulting from its gene products can be largely attributed to post-translational modifications such as phosphorylation and glycosylation [27]. These modifications, which cannot be monitored through the use of genomic data, have been shown to be involved in an enormous number of regulatory processes. For example, virtually all known cellular signaling pathways are largely mediated through a complex cascade of reversible protein phosphorylation [28].

5.1. Affinity chromatography

In cell signaling, experiments are often designed to activate or inhibit specific pathways in order to elucidate the components and mechanisms of regulation of the pathway of interest. The primary challenge involved in studying cellular signaling lies in reducing the complexity of the sample. Because the signaling architecture makes up such a small percentage of total cellular protein, enrichment strategies are often used to select for a specific sub-proteome. In this method, affinity chromatography is used to isolate specific types of proteins related to the biological question at hand. The advantage of this strategy is both the reduction of complexity of the analysis and the enrichment of low abundance proteins that would otherwise go undetected.

A number of different affinity resins are available for the isolation of specific sub-proteomes. Of primary interest in the study of signal transduction pathways are γ-phosphate-linked ATP-Sepharose and microcystin (MC)-Sepharose. ATP-Sepharose was designed for favourable binding of protein kinases and has proven to be a valuable tool for cell signaling studies [29–31]. In addition to binding protein kinases, ATP-Sepharose has been shown to bind a large variety of purine-utilizing enzymes, including heat shock proteins, dehydrogenases, DNA-ligases, and various other purine-utilizing enzymes [32]. Microcystin, an irreversible inhibitor of type 1 (PP-1) and type 2A (PP-2A) protein phosphatases has been immobilized on Sepharose beads for the selective capture of protein phosphatase regulatory subunits [33]. This affinity resin has been used to identify a number of PP-1 binding proteins [33–35].

5.2. Phosphoproteome analysis

While most proteomic studies deal with changes in protein expression levels, post-translational modifications often do not coincide with a change in abundance. Protein phosphorylation, one of the most prevalent post-translational modifications, is a critical event in a variety of signaling cascades. Methods have thus been developed for the selective study of the phosphoproteome. Comparison of phosphorylation profiles under different conditions may lead to the identification of relevant targets of signal transduction cascades.

Protein labelling with either inorganic phosphate ($^{32}P_i$) or γ-(^{32}P)-ATP is the classic approach to study protein phosphorylation. Integration of this approach with 2D-PAGE and autoradiography has been used to visualize phosphoproteins in cells following in vivo labelling [36, 37]. Phosphoproteins can then be identified by MS analysis of gel spots. The primary disadvantage of this technique is that proteins that can be visualized by autoradiography may not be present in sufficient amounts to be identified. To overcome this problem, methods to obtain a fraction enriched in phosphoproteins have been developed to facilitate isolation and identification.

5.3. Immobilized metal affinity chromatography (IMAC)

IMAC is a technology that has been used to purify phosphorylated peptides [38], and when combined with mass spectrometry, to identify phosphoproteins from cell lysates [39, 40]. One limitation of IMAC technology is the co-enrichment of peptides containing multiple carboxylic acid groups [41]. However, by converting the carboxylate groups in peptides to their corresponding methyl esters, the binding of non-phosphorylated peptides to the IMAC matrix can be reduced [40]. Recently, a method was described in which peptides were separated by strong anion exchange chromatography prior to IMAC [26]. This additional step both decreased the complexity of IMAC-purified phosphopeptides and yielded a greater coverage of monophosphorylated peptides.

6. Conclusion

The rapidly expanding field of proteomics currently offers unlimited potential for comparative biochemists and physiologists. Proteomic technologies can now provide qualitative, quantitative, and functional information on all proteins present within a biological system. The ability to identify proteins and characterize their differential expression and post-translational modifications will contribute significantly to the understanding of biochemical adaptation to environment. Furthermore, since it is proteins rather than genes that are directly responsible for cellular function under any given condition, proteomic information promises to have a greater impact than could be derived from genomic information alone.

References

[1] M.R. Wilkins, et al., Biotechnol. Genet. Eng. Rev. 13 (1995) 19–50.
[2] V.C. Wasinger, et al., Electrophoresis 16 (7) (1995) 1090–1094.
[3] N.L. Anderson, N.G. Anderson, Electrophoresis 19 (11) (1998) 1853–1861.
[4] J.A. MacDonald, T.A. Haystead, Recent applications of functional proteomics: investigations in smooth muscle cell physiology, in: J.E. Van Eyk, M.J. Dunn (Eds.), Proteomic and Genomic Analysis of Cardiovascular Disease: Wiley-VCH, 2003.
[5] T.S. Lewis, et al., Mol. Cell 6 (6) (2000) 1343–1354.
[6] M.J. Dunn, Drug Discov. Today 5 (2) (2000) 76–84.
[7] C. Gelfi, et al., FASEB J. 18 (3) (2004) 612–614.
[8] A. Goodchild, et al., Mol. Microbiol. 53 1 (2004) 309–321.
[9] M. Quadroni, P. James, Electrophoresis 20 (4–5) (1999) 664–677.
[10] W.F. Patton, B. Schulenberg, T.H. Steinberg, Curr. Opin. Biotechnol. 13 (4) (2002) 321–328.
[11] D.B. Wall, et al., Anal. Chem. 72 (6) (2000) 1099–1111.
[12] M.P. Washburn, D. Wolters, J.R. Yates 3rd, Nat. Biotechnol. 19 (3) (2001) 242–247.
[13] M.E. Wright, R. Aebersold, Differential expression proteomic analysis using isotope coded affinity tags, in: J.E. Van Eyk, M.J. Dunn (Eds.), Proteomic and Genomic Analysis of Cardiovascular Disease: Wiley-VCH, 2003.
[14] S.P. Gygi, et al., Nat. Biotechnol. 17 (10) (1999) 994–999.
[15] A. Pandey, M. Mann, Nature 405 (6788) (2000) 837–846.
[16] S. Ekstrom, et al., Anal. Chem. 72 (2) (2000) 286–293.
[17] K.E. Wilson, et al., J. Neurol. Neurosurg. Psychiatry 75 (4) (2004) 529–538.
[18] J. Amster, J. Mass Spectrom. 31 (1996) 1325–1337.
[19] J. Qin, et al., Anal. Chem. 69 (19) (1997) 3995–4001.
[20] M. Mann, P. Hojrup, P. Roepstorff, Biol. Mass Spectrom. 22 (6) (1993) 338–345.

[21] M.R. Wilkins, et al., Methods Mol. Biol. 112 (1999) 531–552.
[22] W. Zhang, B.T. Chait, Anal. Chem. 72 (11) (2000) 2482–2489.
[23] M. Mann, M. Wilm, Anal. Chem. 66 (24) (1994) 4390–4399.
[24] P.R. Graves, T.A. Haystead, Microbiol. Mol. Biol. Rev. 66 (1) (2002) 39–63.
[25] A.J. Mackey, T.A. Haystead, W.R. Pearson, Mol. Cell. Proteomics 1 (2) (2002) 139–147.
[26] T.S. Nuhse, et al., Mol. Cell. Proteomics 2 (11) (2003) 1234–1243.
[27] J. Macri, S.T. Rapundalo, Trends Cardiovasc. Med. 11 (2) (2001) 66–75.
[28] D.W. Meek, Cell. Signal. 10 (3) (1998) 159–166.
[29] M.A. Borman, et al., J. Biol. Chem. 277 (26) (2002) 23441–23446.
[30] J.A. MacDonald, et al., Proc. Natl. Acad. Sci. U. S. A. 98 (5) (2001) 2419–2424.
[31] C.M. Haystead, et al., Eur. J. Biochem. 214 (2) (1993) 459–467.
[32] P.R. Graves, et al., Mol. Pharmacol. 62 (6) (2002) 1364–1372.
[33] G. Moorhead, et al., FEBS Lett. 356 (1) (1994) 46–50.
[34] M. Campos, et al., J. Biol. Chem. 271 (45) (1996) 28478–28484.
[35] C.K. Damer, et al., J. Biol. Chem. 273 (38) (1998) 24396–24405.
[36] G.R. Alms, et al., EMBO J. 18 (15) (1999) 4157–4168.
[37] E.E. Corcoran, et al., J. Biol. Chem. 278 (12) (2003) 10516–10522.
[38] L. Andersson, J. Porath, Anal. Biochem. 154 (1) (1986) 250–254.
[39] M.C. Posewitz, P. Tempst, Anal. Chem. 71 (14) (1999) 2883–2892.
[40] S.B. Ficarro, et al., Nat. Biotechnol. 20 (3) (2002) 301–305.
[41] P.R. Graves, T.A. Haystead, Recent Prog. Horm. Res. 58 (2003) 1–24.

International Congress Series 1275 (2004) 22–31

www.ics-elsevier.com

Oxidative fuel selection: adjusting mix and flux to stay alive

Jean-Michel Weber*, François Haman

Biology Department, University of Ottawa, 30 Marie Curie, Ottawa, Ontario, Canada K1N 6N5

Abstract. To be able to match ATP supply with demand, animals must ensure adequate delivery of metabolic fuels and oxygen to tissue mitochondria. Therefore, the mixture of fuels provided and their individual flux must be tightly orchestrated to cope with changing physiological needs. In exercising mammals, metabolic rate—expressed relatively to the aerobic maximum: $\%VO_2$ max—determines what mixture of oxidative fuels is being used. This simple model of fuel selection accurately predicts the relative contributions of lipids and carbohydrates to total metabolism, and it applies widely across body sizes, aerobic capacities, and even to exercise in hypoxic environments. However, it is also becoming obvious that significant exceptions to this pattern exist in other vertebrates that rely more heavily on lipids (e.g., migrating birds) or proteins (e.g., migrating salmonids), or for stresses other than exercise (e.g., cold exposure in mammals). Instantaneous fuel use is determined by multiple interacting mechanisms involving fuel availability, storage location, muscle recruitment, fiber recruitment within each muscle, and metabolic pathway selection within each fiber. These various mechanisms are being characterized in more detail to try designing a general model of fuel selection applicable to a wider range of animals and physiological stresses. © 2004 Elsevier B.V. All rights reserved.

Keywords: Animal energetics; Energy metabolism; Metabolic substrate; Exercise; Shivering thermogenesis; Migration; Hibernation; Metabolic depression; Lipid; Carbohydrate; Protein

1. Introduction

The ability to adjust energy expenditure to cope with changing physiological circumstances is a key feature of organismal survival, and a lot of research has focused on understanding the fundamental mechanisms involved in the upregulation

---

* Corresponding author. Tel.: +1 613 562 5800 6007; fax: +1 613 562 5486.
E-mail address: jmweber@science.uottawa.ca (J.-M. Weber).

(exercise, cold exposure, lactation) or depression of metabolism (fasting, hypoxia, torpor, hibernation, estivation). However, merely changing total flux of O_2 and substrates to mitochondria is not sufficient to ensure long-term survival because internal fuel sources are extremely diverse in size, chemical properties, and storage locations. Therefore, the capacity to select an adequate mixture of metabolic fuels (change in mix) and to modulate this blend (change in flux) is another essential requirement for survival. This paper examines the strategies used by animals to alter their pattern of fuel selection together with the supply rate of each individual substrate to mitochondria. The tight regulation of mix and flux is necessary to balance rates of ATP production with prevailing rates of ATP utilization. Locomotion, thermogenesis, and metabolic depression are perhaps the most striking examples of functional needs that critically depend on modulating the quality and quantity of oxidative fuel supply.

2. Oxidative fuel diversity

To produce ATP for long-term activities, animals must rely on the oxidation of lipids, carbohydrates, and proteins stored within their tissues. These metabolic fuel reserves are obtained from the diet and are usually replenished during periods of rest, recovery from exercise, or seasonal preparation for prolonged fasting associated with long-distance migration or hibernation. The oxidation of each fuel presents clear advantages and disadvantages for any particular physiological situation. To illustrate the convenience and constraints afforded by such diversity, different criteria can be used for comparing the various sources of energy, and, in this context, key characteristics of the fuels available are summarized in Table 1.

Lipids represent the most concentrated source of energy in living organisms for two important reasons: (i) they are the most chemically reduced of all fuels and (ii) they can be stored without water. Therefore, animals favour lipids for energy storage, and most land species could simply not afford to transport the additional weight associated with alternative fuels. Despite their enormous "weight handicap", carbohydrates are essential when ATP must be produced at high rates, without delay, or, possibly, when O_2 availability is compromised. For many aquatic animals, weight is not an issue because fuel reserves do not have to be carried against gravity. Unlike lipids, carbohydrates and

Table 1
Comparison of the different oxidative fuels available for ATP synthesis

	Unit	Lipids	Carbohydrates	Proteins
Isocaloric weight	g fuel MJ^{-1}	26	239	55
Percent total energy reserves	%	85	1	14
Maximal rate of ATP production	μmol ATP g^{-1} min^{-1}	20	30	
Time to reach maximal rates	min	>30	<2	
Energy per volume O_2	kJ l O_2^{-1}	19.8	21.1	18.7

Adapted from Refs. [1–4]. Lipid values are based on triacylglycerol with an average mammalian fatty acid composition. Carbohydrate values were calculated for natural glycogen with an average level of hydration. For proteins, values were calculated for ureotelic animals and only for the mobilizable fraction of total proteins.

proteins are soluble in aqueous biological fluids and do not depend on carrier molecules like serum albumin and fatty acid-binding proteins (FABP) for circulatory and cytoplasmic transport. The complete oxidation of all fuels produces CO_2 and H_2O, two end-products that can usually be managed without problems. However, protein oxidation presents a unique metabolic limitation because it also yields noxious ammonia that must be eliminated or detoxified.

The size of fuel reserves may be altered drastically in preparation for specific physiological challenges. As an extreme example, lipid stores can be increased to reach up to 50% of total body mass before hibernation in small mammals [5] or long-distance migration in birds [6]. To a lesser extent, fuel storage is also affected by endurance training [7,8] or large shifts in diet composition [9]. In turn, these changes in internal substrate availability can influence the pattern of fuel selection during exercise, cold exposure, or metabolic depression. In addition to inflating or decreasing the size of specific energy reserves, animals can also change the distribution of each type of fuel among storage sites. During sustained exercise, ATP production of locomotory muscles depends on the oxidation of both, intramuscular fuels (muscle glycogen and muscle triacylglycerol), and circulatory fuels brought to working muscles from remote storage sites (hepatic glucose and adipose tissue lipids) [10]. To be able to reach high rates of oxidative fuel supply to muscle mitochondria, very aerobic mammals (high VO_2 max) rely relatively more on intramuscular fuels, and relatively less on circulatory fuels than sedentary species (low VO_2 max) [11,12]. This strategy is necessary to circumvent significant constraints associated with the multiple *trans*-membrane crossings required to bring fuels from distant storage locations [13–15]. Nowhere is this adaptation made more obvious than in the way intramuscular lipid reserves are organized: all muscle lipid droplets are actually in direct contact with mitochondria [16,17]. With such a spatial arrangement, lipid transport from storage to the enzymatic

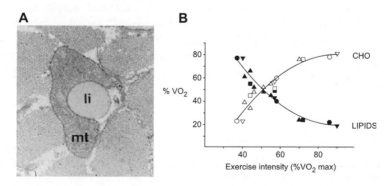

Fig. 1. (A) Transmission electron-micrograph of dog triceps muscle illustrating the close association between intramuscular lipid droplets loaded with triacylglycerol (li) and mitochondria (mt). Adapted from Ref. [17]. (B) Fuel selection pattern for mammalian exercise. Changes in the relative contribution of carbohydrate oxidation (CHO; open symbols) and lipid oxidation (closed symbols) to total oxygen consumption of the whole organism (VO_2) as a function of exercise intensity (%VO_2 max). Values are for dogs (○, ●) [18], goats (▽, ▼) [18], humans (□, ■) [19] and rats (△, ▲) [20,21]. Results include values for trained and untrained rats acclimated to normoxia or to hypoxia.

machinery of energy metabolism is reduced to its simplest form: one single membrane to cross (see Fig. 1A).

3. Exercising mammals: a robust model of fuel selection

Almost all the information available on fuel selection comes from one experimental model: *mammalian exercise*. For this group of animals, the observed pattern is surprisingly simple. Total ATP production can be attributed exclusively to lipid and carbohydrate oxidation because the contribution from proteins is minimal [17,22]. More importantly, exercise intensity, expressed in relation to the aerobic maximum (%VO_2 max), determines the relative importance of lipids and carbohydrates according to the relationship presented in Fig. 1B. The contribution of carbohydrates increases progressively, and that of lipids decreases progressively as exercise intensifies. Therefore, the oxidation of each one of these two fuels is responsible for half the metabolic rate of the whole organism at a work intensity of about 50% VO_2 max (or the work intensity sometimes referred to as the "crossover point"; Ref. [22]).

Different approaches have been used to build this model and to ensure that it could be generalized to all mammals. Because the balance between lipids and carbohydrates originally seemed to depend on %VO_2 max, the robustness of the model was assessed by exploiting various ways to manipulate aerobic capacity. Large adaptive differences in VO_2 max (i.e., genetic differences) exist in nature between very sedentary and highly aerobic species. Dogs and goats of the same size were used in this context because their aerobic capacities differ by more than twofold [18]. Although highly aerobic dogs (geared for endurance exercise) were anticipated to favor the use of the ample lipid reserves available to all animals (see Table 1), results show that both species oxidize the same mixture of fuels when they exercise at the same relative intensity (Fig. 1B) [18]. Because mass-specific VO_2 max varies greatly with body mass, measurements were extended to smaller species (0.3 kg rats) and larger ones (70 kg humans), but without finding significant deviation from the dog-goat pattern (Fig. 1B). Finally, experiments were carried out under low oxygen availability because aerobic capacity is reduced by acclimation to hypoxia. In addition, there is a convincing theoretical reason to think that animals should favor carbohydrates when exercising in hypoxia because this fuel yields 11% more ATP per unit volume of oxygen than lipids (Table 1, but see Ref. [23] for arguments supporting an even greater difference). Again, results show that, individuals acclimated to hypoxia, running under normoxic or hypoxic conditions, follow the same pattern of fuel selection previously observed in all other mammals (Table 1) [20,24,25]. Therefore, the theoretical O_2-saving advantage provided by carbohydrates seems to be outweighed by the potential danger of depleting this small, but critical energy reserve [25]. Although the *relative* partitioning between lipids and carbohydrates is the same for different mammals, it is important to realize that, for each relative exercise intensity, *absolute* rates of lipid and carbohydrate oxidation are scaled directly with VO_2 max (i.e., they are more than two times higher in dogs than in goats). From these observations, we can conclude that the fuel selection model proposed for exercising mammals (Fig. 1B) is extremely robust because it is independent of aerobic capacity when tested for: *adaptive variation* (dog vs. goat), *allometric variation* (0.3 kg rat vs. 70 kg human), and *environmental variation* in O_2 availability (normoxia vs. hypoxia).

4. Alternative fuel selection patterns: swimming fish, flying birds, and shivering humans

Multiplying measurements in more examples of exercising mammals is unlikely to yield further useful insights. Instead, developing a theoretical framework explaining the reasons for the observed pattern appear more promising. To achieve this goal, two interrelated strategies come to mind: uncover clear exceptions to this seemingly general pattern (this section) and characterize the mechanisms available for altering fuel selection (next section). In the last few years, several examples of divergent patterns have emerged, and these exceptions could prove very useful for future research. As more information is accumulating for various animals, it is obvious that the mammalian pattern is far from universal; major differences in fuel metabolism can be found, even among vertebrates. In fish, ignoring the contribution from proteins, as it was done for mammals, could lead to enormous errors because some species are probably able to rely almost exclusively on this source of energy for sustained swimming (e.g., during the late stages of migration in sockeye salmon [3]). In addition, the three to fourfold increments in glucose flux (rate of hepatic glucose production) and fatty acid flux (rates of lypolysis and fatty acid supply) classically reported for all exercising mammals, are completely absent in rainbow trout, even during prolonged swimming [26,27]. Salmonids clearly fail to follow the mammalian model, but more research is needed to determine whether their fuel selection pattern is typical of teleosts in general.

Long-distance migrant birds are another example at variance with mammals because their relative use of lipids is much higher than that predicted in Fig. 1B. They have been able to push conventional energy metabolism well beyond the limits set by the best mammalian athletes. Many bird species migrate at 10–15 times their basal metabolic rate, or twice the VO_2 max of same-size mammals [28]. More importantly, most of the energy used to power long-distance flights is provided by the circulation from adipose lipid reserves [29]. These characteristics are incompatible with the mammalian model, stipulating that, at intensities approaching VO_2 max, over 80% of the energy comes from carbohydrates (mainly muscle glycogen) [15], and that the oxidation of circulating lipids accounts maximally for 10–20% of VO_2 [11,12]. Although limited quantitative information is available on the fuel metabolism of migrant birds, we can deduce from first principles that using glycogen at such high rates is impossible; glycogen reserves of the necessary magnitude do not exist in nature because their weight would prevent movement (see Table 1). During migration flights, rates of circulatory lipid oxidation are therefore at least 10, possibly 20 times higher than the maximal rates ever measured in exercising mammals. Therefore, we can conclude that the mammalian crossover curves presented in Fig. 1B must be strongly shifted to the right for long-distance migrant birds.

Artificially modifying the size of energy reserves can also lead to significant adjustments in substrate use. In humans [30–32] and sled dogs [8], important changes in fuel selection have been elicited by dietary manipulations (high-fat diet or glycogen loading). Therefore, "on-board" availability of each fuel type influences the mixture of metabolic substrates oxidized. Although the exact signals relaying information about the size of energy stores are still poorly understood, major advances have been made in this area. For example, leptin levels signal the size of lipid stores [33], and, on its own, this hormone has significant effects on fuel selection [34,35]. Finally, recent experiments on the effects of cold exposure in humans suggest that the fuel selection patterns of shivering and exercise are different [36]. Detailed measurements of fuel oxidation for thermogenesis show that carbohydrates play a much more important role during shivering than exercise, when these activities are compared at the same metabolic rate [32,36–38]. Therefore, the fuel selection pattern of shivering humans can probably be obtained by shifting the exercise curves of Fig. 1B to the left. The fact that the same muscles use different mixtures of fuels during shivering and exercise when they function at the same metabolic rate is very intriguing. The quest for an explanation of this fascinating difference could provide novel insights on the fundamental mechanisms of fuel selection.

5. Mechanisms for selection

Fuel selection can occur by changing the *supply* rate or the *utilization* rate of the different substrates available. Most of the well-characterized mechanisms of selection operate directly at the level of *fuel utilization*, but a simple (and often overlooked) mechanism acting at the level of *fuel supply* can also play an important role. Experiments on thoroughbred horses have allowed showing that the supply of circulatory fuels to working muscles is regulated in two ways [39,40]. First, the animal can change the supply rate of all the fuels provided through the circulation by adjusting cardiac output and blood flow to target tissues (coarse control of substrate flux acting indiscriminately on all circulatory fuels). Second, the supply rate of individual fuels can be modulated separately by changing their concentration in the blood (fine control of flux acting specifically on each fuel). Together, these two mechanisms allow adjusting the flux of each blood-borne substrate, thereby setting a fuel mixture adequate for present conditions.

The last part of this review deals with the best-characterized selection mechanisms that act at the level of fuel utilization in skeletal muscle. These mechanisms can be divided in three categories based on the level of organization where they exert their effects. Changing the mixture of fuels can be done by selective recruitment of: (i) different muscles, (ii) different fibers within the same muscle, or (iii) different metabolic pathways within the same fiber. The selective recruitment of different muscles was first demonstrated in fish where red muscle (made of slow fibers specialized for lipid oxidation) and white muscle (made of fast fibers specialized for carbohydrate oxidation) are spatially separated (e.g., see Refs. [41,42]). The same mechanism can also regulate fuel selection in exercising mammals and birds, although their muscles are made of mixed fibers. Using blood flow as an index of recruitment, it has been possible to show that muscles with predominantly slow fibers (specialized for fat oxidation) are already active at low work intensities, whereas muscles with predominantly fast fibers (oxidizing carbohydrates) are only recruited at high exercise intensities [43,44].

Similarly, it has been accepted for a long time that fuel metabolism can be regulated within individual muscles through the selective recruitment of different fiber populations specialized for different substrates [18]. Direct proof of this mechanism has only been provided very recently by making simultaneous measurements of fiber recruitment and fuel utilization. Clear enough electromyographic (EMG) signals cannot be obtained during exercise because of the large background noise created by limb movements. Therefore, the problem was eliminated by using an alternative experimental model: shivering muscles of humans exposed to cold. During high-intensity shivering, large differences in fuel selection between individuals (i.e., carbohydrates accounting for 33% to 78% of metabolic rate) are explained by differences in the recruitment of fast (type II) fibers, specialized for carbohydrate oxidation [36]. Interestingly, the alternative mechanism of selection—the recruitment of different metabolic pathways within the same muscle fibers—is used during low-intensity shivering. Detailed EMG analyses reveal that glycogen-depleted and glycogen-loaded individuals can have the same (low) thermogenic rate, but by using widely different fuel mixtures within the same (type I) muscle fibers [32,38]. Biochemical mechanisms of fuel selection have been investigated in mammalian muscles and they continue to be the subject of intense research [19]. Numerous extra- and intracellular signal molecules have been implicated. Since the early sixties, the "glucose–fatty acid cycle" of Randle et al. [45] has often been invoked to explain how the balance between lipids and carbohydrates can be achieved. When fatty acid availability is high, carbohydrate oxidation is reduced and lipid oxidation is stimulated. Randle et al. [45] proposed that high plasma fatty acid concentration caused these changes by suppressing the activation of the pyruvate dehydrogenase complex (PDC; through a rise in the mitochondrial acetyl-CoA/CoA ratio) and by decreasing glycolysis (through inhibition of phosphofructokinase via elevated citrate levels). Although PDC is still considered a significant element in the regulation of fuel selection [46], it has become clear that other mechanisms such as the direct inhibition of glucose transporters (GLUT-4) and of glucose phosphorylation can also play important roles [47].

Over the last few years, malonyl-CoA has also attracted some attention as a possible regulator of fuel selection [48]. The high glycolytic flux associated with intense exercise causes the accumulation of acetyl-CoA, and it has been proposed that this would increase cytosolic malonyl-CoA, thereby causing the inhibition of carnitine palmitoyltransferase I (CPT I) and limiting fatty acid entry into mitochondria. However, direct measurements of malonyl-CoA levels suggest that this probable intramuscular signal does not increase during heavy exercise (at least in rats and humans). Therefore, this mechanism remains doubtful [49]. Ongoing research suggests the involvement of free carnitine levels and intracellular pH that would both inhibit CPT I when low [19,50]. Finally, it has been suggested that fatty acid-binding proteins could play a significant role in fuel selection through their direct regulation of glycolytic enzymes [51].

6. Conclusions

An array of fuels with different properties is available for energy metabolism, and each one (or each mix) is advantageous for a particular physiological situation. Fuel selection strategies are geared to manage energy reserves in a way to avoid the complete depletion of any individual fuel to preserve the capacity to respond adequately to all life challenges. Exercising mammals follow a simple pattern of fuel utilization whereby the balance between lipids and carbohydrates is determined by relative work intensity (%VO_2 max).

This model is very robust because it is independent of aerobic capacity across adaptive, allometric, and environmental variation. In contrast, swimming fish, long-distance migrant birds, and shivering humans follow different patterns of fuel selection whose study will provide important novel insights on fundamental aspects of energy metabolism. The mechanisms responsible for the regulation of fuel selection in working muscles include the selective recruitment of different muscles, of different fibers within the same muscle, and of different metabolic pathways within the same fiber. Reconciling detailed mechanistic information with the fuel selection patterns observed in the whole organism remains a major challenge for future research.

Acknowledgements

This research program is supported by NSERC grants (Canada) to J.-M. Weber.

References

[1] J.M. Berg, J.L. Tymoczko, L. Stryer, Biochemistry, 5th ed., W.H. Freeman, New York, 2002.

[2] R.W. Hill, G.A. Wyse, M. Anderson, Animal Physiology, Sinauer Associates, Sunderland, MA, 2004.

[3] P.W. Hochachka, G.N. Somero, Biochemical Adaptation. Mechanism and Process in Physiological Evolution, Oxford University Press, New York, 2002.

[4] K. Schmidt-Nielsen, Animal Physiology, 4th ed., Cambridge Univerity Press, New York, 1990.

[5] M.M. Humphries, D.W. Thomas, D.L. Kramer, The role of energy availability in mammalian hibernation: a cost–benefit approach, Physiol. Biochem. Zool. 76 (2) (2003) 165–179.

[6] C.R. Blem, Avian energy storage, Curr. Ornithol. 7 (1990) 59–113.

[7] B.F. Hurley, et al., Muscle triglyceride utilization during exercise: effect of training, J. Appl. Physiol. 60 (1986) 562–567.

[8] A.J. Reynolds, et al., Effect of diet and training on muscle glycogen storage and utilization in sled dogs, J. Appl. Physiol. 79 (5) (1995) 1601–1607.

[9] H.W. Goforth, et al., Effects of depletion exercise and light training on muscle glycogen supercompensation in men, Am. J. Physiol. 285 (6) (2003) E1304–E1311.

[10] J.-M. Weber, Pathways for oxidative fuel provision to working muscles: ecological consequences of maximal supply limitations, Experientia 48 (6) (1992) 557–564.

[11] J.-M. Weber, et al., Design of the oxygen and substrate pathways: III. Partitioning energy provision from carbohydrates, J. Exp. Biol. 199 (1996) 1659–1666.

[12] J.-M. Weber, et al., Design of the oxygen and substrate pathways: IV. Partitioning energy provision from fatty acids, J. Exp. Biol. 199 (1996) 1667–1674.

[13] J.-M. Weber, Oxidative metabolism in muscle cells, in: R.G. Crystal, J.B. West, E.R. Weibel, P.J. Barnes (Eds.), The Lung: Scientific Foundations, 2nd ed., Lippincott-Raven, Philadelphia, 1997, pp. 1883–1888, Chap. 139.

[14] J.-M. Weber, Adjusting maximal fuel delivery for differences in demand, in: E.R. Weibel, C.R. Taylor, L.C. Bolis (Eds.), Principles of Animal Design: The Optimization and Symmorphosis Debate, Cambridge University Press, Cambridge, UK, 1998, pp. 249–254, Chap. 9.3.

[15] E.R. Weibel, et al., Design of the oxygen and substrate pathways: VII. Different structural limits for O_2 and substrate supply to muscle mitochondria, J. Exp. Biol. 199 (1996) 1699–1709.

[16] R. Vock, et al., Design of the oxygen and substrate pathways: VI. Structural basis of intracellular substrate supply to mitochondria in muscle cells, J. Exp. Biol. 199 (1996) 1689–1697.

[17] C.R. Taylor, et al., Design of the oxygen and substrate pathways: I. Model and strategy to test symmorphosis in a network structure, J. Exp. Biol. 199 (1996) 1643–1649.

[18] T.J. Roberts, et al., Design of the oxygen and substrate pathways: II. Defining the upper limits of carbohydrate and fat oxidation, J. Exp. Biol. 199 (1996) 1650–1658.

[19] L.J.C. van Loon, et al., The effects of increasing exercise intensity on muscle fuel utilisation in humans, J. Physiol. 536 (1) (2001) 295–304.

[20] G.B. McClelland, et al., High-altitude acclimation increases the triacylglycerol/fatty acid cycle at rest and during exercise, Am. J. Physiol. 281 (2001) E537–E544.

[21] G.A. Brooks, C.M. Donovan, Effect of endurance training on glucose kinetics during exercise, Am. J. Physiol. 244 (1983) E505–E512.

[22] G.A. Brooks, J. Mercier, Balance of carbohydrate and lipid utilization during exercise: the "crossover" concept, J. Appl. Physiol. 76 (6) (1994) 2253–2261.

[23] J.F. Hutter, H.M. Piper, P.G. Spieckermann, Effect of fatty acid oxidation on efficiency of energy production in rat heart, Am. J. Physiol. 249 (1985) H723–H728.

[24] G.B. McClelland, P.W. Hochachka, J.-M. Weber, Effect of high-altitude acclimation on NEFA turnover and lipid utilization during exercise in rats, Am. J. Physiol. 277 (1999) E1095–E1102.

[25] G.B. McClelland, P.W. Hochachka, J.-M. Weber, Carbohydrate utilization during exercise after high-altitude acclimation: a new perspective, Proc. Natl. Acad. Sci. U. S. A. 95 (1998) 10288–10293.

[26] S.F. Bernard, et al., Glycerol and fatty acid kinetics in rainbow trout: effects of endurance swimming, J. Exp. Biol. 202 (1999) 279–288.

[27] D.S. Shanghavi, J.-M. Weber, Effects of sustained swimming on hepatic glucose production of rainbow trout, J. Exp. Biol. 202 (1999) 2161–2166.

[28] P.J. Butler, A.J. Woakes, Fat storage and fat metabolism in relation to migration, in: E. Gwinner (Ed.), Bird Migration: Physiology and Ecophysiology, Springer-Verlag, New York, 1990, pp. 300–318.

[29] L. Jenni, S. Jenni-Eiermann, Fuel supply and metabolic constraints in migrating birds, J. Avian Biol. 29 (1998) 521–528.

[30] J.A. Hawley, F. Brouns, A. Jeukendrup, Strategies to enhance fat utilisation during exercise, Sports Med. 25 (4) (1998) 241–257.

[31] S.D. Phinney, et al., The human metabolic response to chronic ketosis without caloric restriction: preservation of submaximal exercise capability with reduced carbohydrate oxidation, Metabolism 32 (8) (1983) 769–776.

[32] F. Haman, et al., Effects of carbohydrate availability on sustained shivering: I. Oxidation of plasma glucose, muscle glycogen and proteins, J. Appl. Physiol. 96 (1) (2004) 32–40.

[33] R.S. Ahima, J.S. Flier, Leptin, Annu. Rev. Physiol. 62 (2000) 413–437.

[34] S.P. Reidy, J.-M. Weber, Accelerated substrate cycling: a new energy-wasting role for leptin in vivo, Am. J. Physiol. 282 (2002) E312–E317.

[35] S. Reidy, J.-M. Weber, Leptin: an essential regulator of lipid metabolism, Comp. Biochem. Physiol., A 125 (3) (2000) 285–297.

[36] F. Haman, S.R. Legault, J.-M. Weber, Fuel selection during intense shivering in humans: EMG pattern reflects carbohydrate oxidation, J. Physiol. 556 (1) (2004) 305–313.

[37] F. Haman, et al., Effect of cold exposure on fuel utilization in humans: plasma glucose, muscle glycogen and lipids, J. Appl. Physiol. 93 (2002) 77–84.

[38] F. Haman, et al., Effects of carbohydrate availability on sustained shivering: II. Relating muscle recruitment to fuel selection, J. Appl. Physiol. 96 (1) (2004) 41–49.

[39] J.-M. Weber, et al., Cardiac output and oxygen consumption in exercising thoroughbred horses, Am. J. Physiol. 253 (1987) R890–R895.

[40] J.-M. Weber, et al., Lactate kinetics in exercising thoroughbred horses: regulation of turnover rate in plasma, Am. J. Physiol. 253 (1987) R896–R903.

[41] B.C. Jane, G.V. Lauder, How swimming fish use slow and fast muscle fibers: implications for models of vertebrate muscle recruitment, J. Comp. Physiol., A 175 (1) (1994) 123–131.

[42] L.C. Rome, P.T. Loughna, G. Goldspink, Muscle fiber activity in carp as a function of swimming speed and muscle temperature, Am. J. Physiol. 247 (16) (1984) R272–R279.

[43] M.H. Laughlin, R.B. Armstrong, Muscular blood flow distribution patterns as a function of running speed in rats, Am. J. Physiol. 243 (1982) H296–H306.

[44] R.L. Marsh, et al., Partitioning the energetics of walking and running: swinging the limbs is expensive, Science 303 (2004 (2 January)) 80–83.

[45] P.J. Randle, et al., The glucose–fatty acid cycle: its role in insulin sensitivity and the metabolic disturbances of diabetes mellitus, Lancet 1 (1963) 785–789.

[46] M.C. Sugden, K. Bulmer, M.J. Holness, Fuel-sensing mechanisms integrating lipid and carbohydrate utilization, Biochem. Soc. Trans. 29 (2) (2001) 272–278.

[47] M. Roden, How free fatty acids inhibit glucose utilization in human skeletal muscle, News Physiol. Sci. 19 (2004) 92–96.

[48] N.B. Ruderman, et al., Malonyl-CoA, fuel-sensing, and insulin resistance, Am. J. Physiol. 276 (39) (1999) E1–E18.

[49] D. Dean, et al., Exercise diminishes the activity of acetyl-CoA carboxylase in human muscle, Diabetes 49 (2000) 1295–1300.

[50] A.E. Jeukendrup, Regulation of fat metabolism in skeletal muscle, Ann. N.Y. Acad. Sci. 967 (2002) 217–235.

[51] J.M. Stewart, Fatty acid binding proteins as metabolic regulators, in: A.K. Duttaroy, F. Spener (Eds.), Cellular Proteins and Their Fatty Acids in Health and Disease, Wiley-VCHm, Weinheim, 2003, pp. 383–395.

International Congress Series 1275 (2004) 32–46

ELSEVIER

www.ics-elsevier.com

Molecular modalities of insect cold survival: current understanding and future trends

M. Robert Michaud*, D.L. Denlinger

Department of Entomology, Ohio State University, Columbus, OH 43210, USA

Abstract. Insect cold survival has drawn increased attention in recent years, prompting a new classification of survival phenotypes that reflect the ecological and physiological differences in the manner in which insects survive the winter. In addition, more is known about the nature of cold injury and its effects on an insect system from the whole body to the subcellular level, although much remains to be discovered. Other than the detection of misfolded protein by the heat shock response, signal transduction of low temperatures by insects is largely unexplored. Recent advances in *Drosophila* and a few vertebrate systems reveal the potential importance of transient receptor potential ion channels in low temperature signal transduction, and membrane fluidity also possibly plays a role in the detection of low temperatures by insects. Physiological changes that occur in insect cells as a result of low temperatures or in anticipation of low temperatures include the induction of a suite of heat shock proteins, metabolic polyol synthesis, antifreeze protein production, and the induction of extracellular ice nucleation. In addition, a variety of new genes are now known to be induced upon cold exposure, but the roles of these molecules in cold survival are still largely unknown. © 2004 Elsevier B.V. All rights reserved.

Keywords: Insecta; Cold shock; Heat shock protein; Molecular response; Cytoskeleton; Cryobiology

1. Introduction

The field of insect cryobiology advanced considerably in recent years due to its potential applicability in pest control, its contribution to understanding evolutionary trends in adaptation to abiotic stress, and its potential role in understanding effects of global climate change. A number of cold hardiness behavioural strategies, physiological

* Corresponding author. Tel.: +1 614 292 4477; fax: +1 614 292 2180.
E-mail address: michaud.11@osu.edu (M.R. Michaud).

0531-5131/ © 2004 Elsevier B.V. All rights reserved.
doi:10.1016/j.ics.2004.08.059

mechanisms, and phenotypes have been elucidated for the 250+ species studied thus far, weaving a convoluted tapestry that underscores the great variability of insect systems, but these studies also shed light on common cold survival adaptations arising independently over several insect lineages [1].

Cold survival is influenced by a number of abiotic factors. The lowest temperature which the insect experiences, the length of time the environment remains at that temperature, the rate of cooling, and the presence of water all influence survival at the abiotic level and have been proposed to influence certain adaptive strategies, as well [2]. At the biotic level, the insect's physiological reaction to cold is equally as influential to winter survival. The detection of daylength changes with subsequent deployment of cryoprotective mechanisms (e.g., diapause) increases the ability of an insect to survive the upcoming winter when compared to insects that rely solely on direct detection of low temperature. In addition, insects benefit from tracking the temperature in real-time and adjusting their physiology accordingly (e.g., rapid cold hardening). Finally, an insect influences its survival by employing reparative mechanisms that ameliorate the damage sustained from a cold insult when conditions return to normal (e.g., heat shock proteins).

The molecular and biochemical basis of insect cold survival has been studied with considerable detail; however, evidence suggests that there are pathways and molecular species yet undiscovered. In this review, we briefly discuss cold survival phenotypes and the nature of cold injury, and then provide an overview of the molecular aspects of insect cold hardiness.

2. Cold hardiness phenotypes

Insects in temperate and cooler climates employ various mechanisms to survive temperatures of 0 °C or lower. These mechanisms fall into two broad categories: freeze-tolerance and freeze-avoidance [3]. Freeze-tolerant insects are characterized by their ability to raise their supercooling point to freeze extracellular spaces, preventing damage to the cell membranes from encroaching ice crystals [4]. The second category, freeze-avoidance, covers a broad range of insects that survive the cold by preventing the formation of ice crystals, although the cold survival phenotype and the mechanisms employed vary considerably.

Because of this variation, Bale [5,6] has proposed that freeze-avoidance should be further subcategorized into four groups based on the observation that freeze-avoidance falls into four distinct survival phenotypes. The first of these categories, freeze-avoidance (sensu stricto), applies only to insects that do not experience significant mortality until the body begins to freeze. These insects benefit from lowering the supercooling point alone. On a worldwide scale, the number of insect species that fall into freeze tolerance and freeze avoidance (sensu lato) categories is comparatively small [5].

The next three categories are based on the observation that many insects begin to experience mortality long before the supercooling point is reached. The first of these, chill-tolerance, refers to species that experience mortality only after long exposures (days) to temperatures below 0 °C but above the supercooling point. A similar category, chill-susceptibility, describes insects that experience mortality after short (minutes or hours) exposure to temperatures similar to those above. Although the dividing line between these two groups is not clearly defined, acknowledgment of these two categories reflects the physiological distinction between flesh flies (*Sarcophaga crassipalpis*) that are chill-tolerant in the diapause state but chill-susceptible during the remainder of their life cycle [7].

The final category, opportunistic survival, refers to insects that are incapable of employing preventative cold hardening mechanisms. To survive, these insects must avoid low temperatures altogether by seeking thermally favorable microhabitats [5].

This new subcategorization of freeze-avoidance conforms to natural trends [2] and encompasses the entire range of observed responses in species from the tropics to the poles [6].

3. The nature of low-temperature injury

Cold injury is divided into three categories based on the exposure temperature and its relation to the freezing point of water and the freezing point of the insect itself. If the insect suffers damage from positive temperatures at or near 0 °C, usually over a period of time expressed in days, then the insect is injured through indirect chilling [4]. Direct chilling injury, or cold shock, describes damage from temperatures that are below 0 °C but above the supercooling point [8]. Cold shock injury arises from low temperature exposures of minutes, hours, or days, depending on the insect species under study and the intensity of the exposure. Finally, insects that suffer damage because of intracellular ice crystal formation (due to temperature depression below the supercooling point) suffer from freezing injury [9]. For freeze-tolerant insects, freezing injury occurs well below the supercooling point if the insect is physiologically prepared for winter [10], but freeze-avoiding insects experience this injury at their supercooling point [4].

3.1. Injury at the whole-body level

A few studies have concentrated on the effects of cold exposure at the whole-body level. The flesh fly, *S. crassipalpis*, can survive for up to 25 days when exposed to 0 °C [11], but flies that have suffered from indirect chilling injury at 2 °C for 10 days are slow to emerge from the puparium, provided they are capable of opening the puparium at all. Many that fail to emerge after this exposure are also unable to retract the ptilinum if the flies are removed from the puparium artificially. The coordination of muscular movement is preserved in this particular instance, but the amplitude of such movement is reduced to one-third the level of untreated controls, hence the impairment of eclosion. Many flesh flies that successfully emerge have wing abnormalities from failure to properly expand their wings after eclosion [12]. Developmental abnormalities have been reported from indirect chilling injury in other species as well [13,14]. Study of the blood-sucking hemipteran, *Panstrongylus megistus*, revealed that short exposures (1 h) to 5 or 0 °C greatly reduces molting incidence, but survival is only affected by 0 °C exposures, with 96.7% mortality reached after 12 h without induced cryotolerance [15].

Nondiapausing *S. crassipalpis* pupae exposed to a −10 °C cold shock (16 °C above their supercooling point) for 45 min fail to emerge 50% of the time and die soon afterwards. These flies also have disrupted emergence patterns and reduced coordination of extrication movements, although the amplitude of muscular coordination is unaffected [12]. Cold-shocked flesh flies have reduced motor neuron conductivity and decreased activity at the neuromuscular junction [16]. Even more important to overall viability, the fecundity of these flies is also affected, showing a reduction of viable eggs after a 1-h cold shock at $-10\,°C$. Fecundity reduction from cold shock was caused by a dramatic reduction in male mating frequency [17]. In contrast, a study in the house fly, *Musca domestica*, has shown that cold shock reduces total egg production in females, but the effect on males was not measured [18].

By definition, freezing injury often leads to immediate, catastrophic consequences for the survival of freeze-avoiding insects. Often the freezing injury begins in the gut where potential ice nucleators reside; this is one reason why *S. crassipalpis* possesses a lower supercooling point in its nonfeeding stages [7]. Freeze-tolerant species can only withstand low temperatures to a certain point below their SCP, often a few degrees below the SCP in the Southern hemisphere or tens of degrees below the SCP in the Northern hemisphere [1]. When this critical point is reached, the freeze-tolerance mechanism loses its ability to stem the increasing growth of ice crystals, and the cells lethally freeze.

3.2. Injury at the tissue level and below

At the tissue and cellular level, cold injury is poorly understood, although research in this area is beginning to attract more attention. It is generally accepted that damage from cold shock at the cellular level results from the loss of cell function due to denaturation, the formation of insoluble protein aggregates, and the loss of membrane homeostasis from phase transitions [19]. Vital dyes and direct microscopic examination have been applied to insect cells to determine what effects are the most common after cold exposure. In *P. megistus*, exposure to sequential temperatures of 5 and 0 °C leads to a reduction in apoptotic events for Malphigian tubule epithelial cells. Concurrently, the level of necrosis increases when compared to controls, leading to the hypothesis that cold shock injury favors necrosis either through direct apoptotic suppression or indirectly by ATP depletion [15].

Vital dye studies of fat body cells from the freeze-tolerant species, *Eurosta solidaginis*, have demonstrated that after freezing, these cells have much larger lipid droplets but fail to show signs of membrane damage [20]. A subsequent *Eurosta* investigation using fluorescent vital dyes revealed increased freeze injury susceptibility (>50% cell mortality) for integumentary muscle, hemocytes, tracheae, the distal portion of the Malphigian tubules, and the fat body after treatment for 10 days at $-80\,°C$. The tissues least susceptible to damage from this treatment were the gut, proximal portion of the Malphigian tubules, and the salivary gland [9].

Ultrastructural analysis of lethally frozen brain tissues from *Eurosta* larvae demonstrated intermembranous expansions of the nuclear envelope, clumping of chromatin in the brain with associated rough endoplasmic reticulum expansion, and increased presence of autophagic bodies in the cytoplasm. Muscles studied in this manner had missing Z-lines as a result of myofilament breakdown, and the nuclei changed from displaying a structured peripheral array of chromatin to having diffuse organization. Finally, the Malpighian tubules of lethally frozen *Eurosta* had expanded mitochondria with broken cristae and an increased number of autophagic bodies [10].

All of the evidence above reveals tissue vulnerability to cold damage in nervous tissues and muscles, both of which are heavily reliant on membrane integrity, cytoskeletal structure, and energy for normal functioning. To further complicate matters,

ATP production may be hampered by tracheal damage and mitochondrial disruption, although no immediate change in oxygen consumption has been reported from cold shock damage in S. crassipalpis [8]. Changes in nuclear organization also seem to be commonly associated with damage to insects from the cold [10,15]. In future studies of cold damage at the tissue level or below, it would be useful to see the differences between cold injury types for each of the five groups of low-temperature survival phenotypes. Such work may reveal the cellular benefits of the various insect cold survival strategies based on differences in observed tissue damage or intracellular phenomena after low-temperature insult.

4. Detection of low-temperature stimuli

For an insect to initiate protective mechanisms that aid in low-temperature survival without seasonal acclimation, the cell must be able to detect low temperatures directly or to detect subtle changes in the cell's composition that accompany reduction in temperature. This area of research remains largely uncharted for insects, but work in other model systems illuminates potential targets for study.

4.1. Detection of denatured protein

Cold shock damage is thought to lead to the denaturation of many different protein species within the cell [21]. Thus, these proteins often lose their hydrophobic/hydrophilic interactions and become insoluble. When this occurs, the Heat-shock-cognate 70 (Hsc70) protein, which normally is heterodimerized with the Heat-shock transcription factor (HSF), dissociates from HSF in favor of binding to the newly denatured protein [22]. The free HSF molecule then trimerizes with other free HSF molecules and subsequently enters the nucleus to bind with genomic promoters called heat shock elements (HSEs) [23].

By far, the most notable group of molecules to contain HSEs in their promoters are the various heat shock proteins (Hsps), which, upon an HSF trimer binding to the HSE, are then transcribed and translated to protect the cell from further damage and to repair the damage already sustained (Section 5.2). Studies of heat shock in Drosophila melanogaster have not only shown the presence of most of these molecules in the Drosophila genome, but have also drawn functional conclusions for many of these molecules [24], including HSF [25]. The fact that heat shock proteins (including Hsc70) are highly expressed during recovery from cold shock in S. crassipalpis [26–30] is the best indicator that the HSF cascade is involved in cold shock recovery, but this has not been confirmed experimentally.

Although this method of low-temperature detection and repair is highly conserved throughout all kingdoms [22], it is not proactive; it is reactive. Other cellular methods of low-temperature detection may be involved in priming the cell for cold hardiness long before damage is sustained, a response strategy arguably more favorable than a damage-dependent response.

4.2. Transient receptor potential ion channels

When faced with a temperature gradient, insects tend to move to a point in the gradient that is optimal for their physiology. This behavior must be controlled by a reception system that can detect small differences in temperature in order to "know" what temperature is ideal. For adult insects, cold-sensing cells in the antennae called "cold cells" generate action potentials in response to low temperature [31]. Using Ca^{2+} influx as a marker for neural activity, cold-sensing neurons of the terminal organs were identified as the primary cold receptors for *Drosophila* larvae [32]. These neurons, which have the same physiological characteristics of "cold cells" [33], can sense changes in temperature as small as 0.3 °C, beginning at temperatures below 18 °C [34].

Molecular temperature sensors for insects have yet to be convincingly identified, but evidence is emerging that *painless*, a transient receptor potential (TRP) gene, is responsible for detection of supraoptimal temperatures in *Drosophila* larvae [35]. *Painless* is related to vertebrate TRPV1, the protein most responsible for thermoreception in vertebrates [36]. In addition, research in mammals has also uncovered a TRP Ca^{2+} channel that is responsible for the reception of cold as well as menthol [37]. A BLAST search through Genbank reveals a similar gene in both the *D. melanogaster* (3e-76) and *Anopheles gambiae* (8e-77) genome, although both genes await study.

4.3. Membrane fluidity and histidine kinase 33

Changes in membrane fluidity in response to short-term, low-temperature exposure have not been well-studied in insects, although a reduction in saturated fatty acids is typical of winter preparation [38,39]. One study in the arctiid moth, *Cymbalophora pudica*, found extensive lipid composition changes in the brain and gut in response to a 1-day 4 °C acclimation. Membrane fluidity for these two tissues was unaltered. In addition, the degree of lipid desaturation increased in the fat body, the silk glands, and the body wall, although these increases were moderate. This moth does not have pronounced cold hardiness even with acclimation, thus a moderate change in lipid composition might be expected for this species [40]. Although no genes were implicated in this study, insects such a *Drosophila* and many moths have multiple desaturase genes which could potentially be responsible for altering membrane fluidity [41], especially since de novo lipid synthesis from fat stores was not found in the arctiid study [40].

Exciting studies in cyanobacteria and yeast has recently revealed the role of membrane fluidity as the primary signal in cold reception. When the ambient temperature drops, decreasing membrane fluidity leads to membrane transport perturbations [19]. To counter this, cynaobacteria have developed a system by which the histidine kinases, Hik33 and Hik19, act in concert with the transcription regulator, Rer1, in response to decreasing fluidity [42,43]. The cell's response to this cascade features the induction of membrane desaturase genes (desA, desB, oleI) as well as other cold-acclimating genes [19,44–47]. Membrane desaturase genes increase the cell's membrane fluidity, restoring transport functions [19]. A GenBank BLAST search reveals that the *Anopheles* genome has two ESTs with weak similarity to the Hik33 and Hik19 genes in *Synechocystis* sp. (7e-11, 1e-10). *Drosophila* Hsp83 and Gp93 chaperones have a histidine kinase-like ATPase domain, thus further supporting the possibility that this pathway is involved in insect cold tolerance.

5. Established mechanisms of cold-hardiness

There are four known physiological mechanisms for insect cold hardiness. Any one of these mechanisms or any combination of these mechanisms may be utilized by an insect to survive suboptimal temperatures. Generally, the more mechanisms employed or the greater the induction is for a particular mechanism, the more cold hardy the insect becomes.

5.1. Polyols and other low-molecular weight substances

Polyhydric alcohols (polyols) and other low-molecular weight compounds are manufactured by many insects either in response to or in preparation for a low temperature insult. Seasonally, these compounds are manufactured in the fat body where they are released into the hemolymph to colligatively (0.2 mol/l or greater concentration) protect the entire body from low-temperature damage by either reducing the supercooling point or increasing the osmolarity of the cell [4,48]. Some insects upregulate low-molecular weight compounds to levels far below 0.2 mol/l and still increase cold-hardiness [48,49]. Noncolligative effects of polyols include stabilization of nascent proteins, increased repair of damaged protein by molecular chaperones [50], and membrane stabilization [51]. Low-molecular weight compounds known to protect insects from cold include glycerol, sorbitol, mannitol, trehalose, and proline [4,52,53].

Seasonally, many insects upregulate polyols and other low-molecular weight compounds in response to short daylength and low temperatures over a period of days or weeks [4,24]. Seasonal increases in these compounds may be attributed to freeze-tolerance [48], freeze-avoidance, or diapause [4]. Additionally, some insects can upregulate these compounds on a time scale from 20 min to 8 h in a process known as rapid cold hardening, although the level of polyol upregulation is lower than that seen for seasonal acclimation [49,54,55]. Rapid cold hardening may not be a strategy found in freeze-tolerant insects [56].

The mechanism of induction for glycerol involves the temperature-dependent activation of glycogen phosphorylase, which, upon its induction, frees glucose molecules to be cleaved into glycerol [52]. Glycerol synthesis may be further enhanced by the diversion of carbon flow to the pentose phosphate pathway [57,58]. In the rice stem borer, *Chilo suppressalis*, glycerol production results from the inhibition of fructose 1,6-bisphosphate and pyruvate kinase [59]. Glycogen phosphorylase, glyceraldehyde-3-phosphatase and polyol dehydrogenase are all activated in the stem borer during seasonal acclimation [58]. Inhibition of protein phosphatase-1 during glycerol synthesis is found in both freeze-tolerant and freeze-avoiding insects [60]. In the goldenrod moth, *Epiblema scudderiana*, hexokinase is strongly activated (300%) in the presence of glycerol-3-phosphate and low temperatures [61]. For the freeze-tolerant *Eurosta solidaginis*, glycerol is made utilizing the pentose phosphate pathway, but after temperatures drop below 5 °C, phosphofructo-kinase is strongly inhibited, diverting the insect's metabolism from glycerol to sorbitol synthesis in a one-step process [62,63].

Clearly, more research needs to be done to match the identity of the cryoprotective compound with cold-hardy insect species, measure rates of induction, and identify enzymes involved in these pathways. The information thus gleaned would serve to further define the relationship between these compounds and low-temperature survival, possibly highlighting common mechanisms that occur within or across insect lineages.

5.2. AFPs and INAs

Antifreeze proteins (AFPs) and ice-nucleating agents (INAs) are used by some insects to prevent injury from ice crystal formation. INAs are produced in freeze-tolerant insects to drive the crystallization temperature of the hemolymph upward, forcing ice crystals to form in the extracellular spaces at higher subzero temperatures. Ice crystals pull water out of solution extracellularly, driving the osmolarity of the cells higher and higher because water flows from the intracellular space to the extracellular space to compensate for water lost to ice [64]. In the end, the insect is quite well protected from intracellular ice formation. This attribute is well developed in Northern hemisphere insects that are known to be able to survive freezing to several tens of degrees below their supercooling points [1]. INAs have not been observed in freeze-avoiding insects.

Some insects, particularly beetles, produce AFPs in preparation for overwintering [65]. AFPs protect the insect by preventing the growth of ice crystals that have nucleated by adhering to the surface of the crystal, hindering the addition of new water molecules to the ice lattice. AFPs lower the freezing point of insect hemolymph up to 8.5 °C without affecting the melting point in a condition known as thermal hysteresis [66]. Fish have five different classes of AFPs, each with preferential binding to a specific surface of the growing ice crystal lattice [67]. Insect AFPs have not been subdivided into as many classes, but evidence shows insect AFPs bind to ice with comparable affinity and greater effectiveness than fish AFPs as measured by the degree of thermal hysteresis [68]. AFP activity is enhanced by protein enhancers [69], polyols, and organic anions [70].

5.3. Heat shock proteins

If cold tolerance is not sufficient to sustain an insect through a particularly strong low-temperature insult without injury, heat shock proteins (Hsps) must be manufactured to repair, contain, or remove damaged proteins. Thus far, investigations into Hsp expression after cold exposure in insects have been limited to *S. crassipalpis* [27–29], *Drosophila* (four species) [24,71], and the Colorado potato beetle (*Leptinotarsa decemlineata*) [29]. In all of these cases, Hsp transcripts are upregulated from 1 to 12 hours during recovery from cold shock.

The most commonly studied transcript is the inducible form of heat shock protein 70, *hsp70*. The protein (~70 kDa) product of this transcript is highly conserved (>50%) across all kingdoms of organisms and is expressed after cold shock in all six of the above insects. Hsp70 aids in stress survival by refolding damaged protein, redissolving insoluble protein [72], and tagging irreparable protein for degradation [73], although the specific function of insect Hsp70 for low-temperature survival has not been studied. However, induction of *S. crassipalpis* Hsps by heat shock and diapause has been correlated with increased survival to cold [7,27,74]. Stronger cold shocks induce stronger and longer induction of *hsp70* transcripts for *S. crassipalpis*, but the induction is delayed when compared to milder cold shocks [27]. Acclimation to lower developmental temperatures reduces the threshold of *hsp70* expression in *Drosophila triauraria*, but this has not been observed in the other two *Drosophila* species tested for *hsp70* expression thresholds [71].

The constitutive form of heat shock protein 70 (Hsc70) normally does not change its expression profile in response to stress, but *S. crassipalpis hsc70* transcripts are upregulated in response to cold shock [27]. The role of Hsc70 in stress signalling is important in that it is primarily responsible for the release of heat shock transcription factor (HSF) [22], although the purpose of Hsc70 upregulation after cold stress remains unclear.

Small heat shock proteins (sHsps) are a diverse family of proteins (12–40 kDa) that are identified by the presence of an alpha-crystalline domain. Their role in stress tolerance involves refolding local domains of damaged proteins, tagging aberrant protein in the early stages of denaturation for other chaperones to fold, and inhibition of proteolysis [22,75]. In addition, sHsps are effective in preserving the actin cytoskeleton in mammalian hypothermia, a feature that is particularly important for cold tolerance because cold is known to break down the cytoskeleton in vitro [76,77]. In *S. crassipalpis*, *hsp23* transcripts are upregulated in response to cold shock, heat shock, and during pupal diapause [26,29].

The 90-kDa family of heat shock proteins in flesh flies are also upregulated in response to cold shock [26], but not diapause [28]. Normally, *hsp90* transcripts are expressed at low constitutive levels but are induced quickly after cold shock (1 h), peak after 4 h, and remain expressed at high levels even after 12 h post-cold shock [28]. Hsp90 recognizes and repairs damaged proteins that are bound by Hsc70, sequesters HSF in the same manner as Hsc70, and targets protein for degradation in the ubiquitin-dependent proteosome pathway [78]. Hsp90 is also known to activate the ecdysone receptor–ultraspiracle complex. This may be the reason it is not expressed, like other Hsps, during diapause, a stage dependent on the absence of ecdysteroids [28,78].

Although HSPs have been correlated with cold survival, there is little direct evidence in the literature to confirm this. Fortunately, new RNA interference (RNAi) technology allows for the functional study of transcripts in a variety of ectothermic organisms, notably insects [23], and our laboratory's unpublished data indicates a loss of cold tolerance when Hsps are knocked down using RNAi.

6. Frontiers in cold-hardiness mechanisms

6.1. The role of the cytoskeleton

Studies of plant responses to cold have emphasized the increasing importance of the plant cytoskeleton in conferring tolerance to low temperatures. In addition, cold tolerance of the cytoskeleton has been documented in the Atlantic cod [79]. Cold tolerance may be acquired through two cytoskeletal methods: depolymerization of cytoskeletal elements trigger cellular responses to cold, and microtubules may be assembled in a cold-stable configuration in anticipation of low-temperature. In the former process, calcium channels are attached to the depolymerising actin cytoskeleton, and consequently the ability to prevent Ca^{2+} from entering the cell is lost at low temperature due to cytoskeletal breakdown [80]. The ensuing Ca^{2+} cascade leads to an undetermined signaling mechanism that results in cold-stable cells [81,82].

Post-translational modification of tubulin polymers [83], addition of cold-stabilizing proteins [76,84] such as Hsps [83,85], or tubulin amino acid substitutions [79,86] are added to the growing microtubules to increase the stability of the cytoskeleton. A cold-stable cytoskeleton presumably will maintain the structure, function, and organization of cells upon exposure to potentially damaging low temperatures.

The role of the cytoskeleton for low-temperature survival has not been investigated in insects, although it is known that sHsps associate with the cytoskeleton in *D. melanogaster* [87]. Preliminary results from cross-species microarrays (*S. crassipalpis* cDNA on *Drosophila* arrays) indicate changes in tubulin transcripts as a result of cold treatments, especially short-term acclimation (our unpublished data).

6.2. Insect genes upregulated by cold

A number of proteins and transcripts are upregulated as a result of low-temperature treatment in insects, although none of these genes have been the object of low-temperature studies at the functional level. Table 1 highlights many of the genes identified. Included in the table are transcripts found in other model systems (bacteria, mouse, rat) with similarities to known insect ESTs on GenBank.

6.3. Genome-wide studies in other organisms

Recent advances in functional genomics have provided valuable tools in the forms of cDNA macro- and microarrays. Through the use of this technology, thousands of genes can be screened for a particular treatment, even across species. Certainly, the field of insect cryobiology will benefit from the application of this technology to the various cold treatments and strategies, including recovery from cold shock, rapid cold hardening, seasonal acclimation, and freeze tolerance.

Table 1
Transcripts and proteins upregulated from cold treatments

Gene	Species	Observations	Reference
hsp70	*Drosophila* (4 species),	Upregulation during recovery from cold shock	[71]
	Sarcophaga crassipalpis,	Upregulation during diapause; recovery from	[27,30]
	Leptinotarsa decemlineata	cold shock.	
hsc70	*S. crassipalpis*	Upregulation during diapause; recovery from cold shock	[27]
hsp23	*S. crassipalpis*	Upregulation during diapause; recovery from cold shock	[22,29]
hsp90	*S. crassipalpis*	Recovery from cold shock	[22,28]
dca	*D. melanogaster*	Upregulation from 15 °C acclimation	[88]
Fst	*D. melanogaster*	Upregulation during recovery from a 0 °C cold shock	[89]
Hsr-omega	*Drosophila* (3 species)	Induction of the 93 kDa heat shock puff after cold shock	[90]
Svp	*Bombyx mori*	Transcription factor upregulated from chilling	[91]
sorbitol dehydro-genase	*B. mori*	Upregulation after chilling for 50 days	[91]
Samui	*B. mori*	Chill-inducible protein that transmits low temperature signals	[92,93]
c-fos-like	*Galleria mellonella*	Induction in brain during 3h chilling at 0 °C	[94]
Cp1, Cp2	*Spodoptera exigua*	Proteins induced after 2h treatments at 0 °C & 5 °C	[95]
hik19	*Synechocystis* sp. (cyanobacteria)	Cytoplasmic; induces desaturases upon membrane fluidity loss; similar gene in insects	[42,43]
hik33	*Synechocystis* sp. (cyanobacteria)	Membranal; induces desaturases upon membrane fluidity loss; similar gene in insects	[42,43]
cmr1	*Rattus rattus* (rat)	Responsible for cold signaling in neurons; similar gene in insects	[37]
CIRP	*Mus musculus* (mouse)	Upregulation during hypothermia; similar gene in insects	[96]

Microarray analyses of low-temperature treatment in other model systems have revealed a great variety of genes related to cold. *Arabidopsis thaliana* exposed to 24 h at 4 °C increases expression of 40 transcription factors, 11 osmoprotective genes, 24 cellular metabolic genes, 20 carbohydrate metabolic genes, 4 heat shock genes, and 6 detoxification enzymes [97]. Similar results were obtained from rice treated in the same manner, although the number of genes tested was fewer [98]. Of note in these studies was the upregulation of beta tubulin in *Arabidopsis* and actin in rice, indicating changes in the cytoskeleton during cold acclimation. Glutathione-*S*-transferase was upregulated in *Arabidopsis* during cold acclimation, which was also noted on microarrays of freeze-injured yeast [99]. The only low-temperature transcriptome study in animals, performed on macroarrays of the channel catfish, *Ictalarus punctatus*, revealed considerable changes in ribosomal protein constituents and an increase in *hsp70*, calmodulin-inhibitor, and beta actin due to a shift from 24 to 12 °C [100].

Our laboratory's unpublished work on *S. crassipalpis* relies on cross-species hybridization with *D. melanogaster* EST's. Genes that appear to be upregulated in the flesh fly as a result of cold treatments include 11 defensive genes (including glutathione-*S*-tranfersase), 16 metabolic genes, 21 cytoskeletal genes (including both α- and β-tubulin), 36 genes related to transcription and translation (especially spliceosomal elements), and 13 signal transduction molecules (especially calcium-binding and proteins related to G-protein signalling). Although few of these genes have been confirmed by Northern blot hybridization at present, it is clear that microarray studies such as this will enable the field to make a quantum leap forward by allowing the identification of major gene networks not previously known to be involved in low temperature responses.

Acknowledgements

This study was funded in part by NSF grant IBN-9728573.

References

[1] B.J. Sinclair, Climatic variability and the evolution of insect freezing tolerance, Biol. Rev. 78 (2003) 181–195.

[2] P. Vernon, G. Vannier, Evolution of freezing susceptibility and freezing tolerance in terrestrial arthropods, C. R., Biol. 325 (2002) 1185–1190.

[3] R.W. Salt, Principles of insect cold hardiness, Annu. Rev. Entomol. 6 (1961) 55–74.

[4] R.E. Lee, Principles of insect low temperature tolerance, in: R.E. Lee, D.L. Denlinger (Eds.), Insects at Low Temperature, Chapman and Hall, New York, 1991, pp. 17–46.

[5] J.S. Bale, Insects and low temperatures: from molecular biology to distributions and abundance, Philos. Trans. R. Soc. Lond., B 357 (2002) 849–862.

[6] J.S. Bale, Insect cold hardiness: a matter of life and death, Eur. J. Entomol. 93 (1996) 369–382.

[7] R.E. Lee, D.L. Denlinger, Cold tolerance in diapausing and non-diapausing stages of the flesh fly, *Sarcophaga crassipalpis*, Physiol. Entomol. 10 (1985) 309–315.

[8] D.L. Denlinger, et al., Cold shock and heat shock, in: R.E. Lee, D.L. Denlionger (Eds.), Insects at Low Temperature, Chapman and Hall, New York, 1991, pp. 131–147.

[9] S.X. Yi, R.E. Lee, Detecting freeze injury and seasonal cold-hardening of cells and tissues in the gall fly larvae, *Eurosta solidaginis* (Diptera: Tephritidae) using fluorescent vital dyes, J. Insect Physiol. 49 (2003) 999–1004.

[10] S.D. Collins, A.L. Allenspach, R.E. Lee, Ultrastructural effects of lethal freezing on brain, muscle, and Malpighian tubules from freeze-tolerant larvae of the gall fly, *Eurosta solidaginis*, J. Insect Physiol. 43 (1997) 39–45.

[11] C.P. Chen, D.L. Denlinger, Reduction of cold injury in flies using an intermittent pulse of high temperature, Cryobiology 29 (1992) 138–143.

[12] G.D. Yocum, et al., Alteration of the eclosion rhythm and eclosion behavior in the flesh fly, *Sarcophaga crassipalpis*, by low and high temperature stress, J. Insect Physiol. 40 (1994) 13–21.

[13] A.A. Tezze, E.N. Botto, Effect of cold storage on the quality of *Trichogramma nerudai* (Hymenoptera: Trichogrammatidae), Biol. Control 30 (2004) 11–16.

[14] S.L. Garcia, et al., Effect of sequential cold shocks on survival and molting incidence in *Panstrongylus megistus* (Burmeister) (Hemiptera, Reduviidae), Cryobiology 41 (2001) 74–77.

[15] S.L. Garcia, et al., Effect of sequential heat and cold shocks on nuclear phenotypes of the blood-sucking insect, *Panstrongylus megistus* (Burmeister) (Hemiptera, Reduviidae), Mem. Inst. Oswaldo Cruz 97 (2002) 1111–1116.

[16] J.D. Kelty, K.A. Killian, R.E. Lee, Cold shock and rapid cold hardening of pharate adult flesh flies (*Sarcophaga crassipalpis*): effects on behaviour and neuromuscular function following eclosion, Physiol. Entomol. 21 (1996) 283–288.

[17] J.P. Rinehart, G.D. Yocum, D.L. Denlinger, Thermotolerance and rapid cold hardening ameliorate the negative effects of brief exposures to high or low temperatures on fecundity in the flesh fly, *Sarcophaga crassipalpis*, Physiol. Entomol. 25 (2000) 330–336.

[18] S.C. Coulson, J.S. Bale, Effect of rapid cold hardening on reproduction and survival of offspring in the housefly *Musca domestica*, J. Insect Physiol. 38 (1992) 421–424.

[19] L. Vigh, B. Maresca, J.L. Harwood, Does the membrane's physical state control the expression of heat shock and other genes? Trends Biochem. Sci. 23 (1998) 369–374.

[20] D.J. Davis, R.E. Lee, Intracellular freezing, viability, and composition of fat body cells from freeze-intolerant larvae of *Sarcophaga crassipalpis*, Arch. Insect Biochem. Physiol. 48 (2001) 199–205.

[21] D.A. Parsell, S. Lindquist, The function of heat shock proteins in stress tolerance—degradation and reactivation of damaged proteins, Annu. Rev. Genet. 27 (1993) 437–496.

[22] D.L. Denlinger, J.P. Rinehart, G.D. Yocum, Stress proteins: a role in insect diapause? in: D.L. Denlinger, J.M. Giebultowicz, D.S. Saunders (Eds.), Insect Timing: Circadian Rhythmicity to Seasonality, Elsevier, Amsterdam, 2001, pp. 155–171.

[23] G. Marchler, C. Wu, Modulation of *Drosophila* heat shock transcription factor activity by the molecular chaperone DROJ1, EMBO J. 20 (2001) 499–509.

[24] A.A. Hoffmann, J.G. Sorensen, V. Loeschcke, Adaptation of *Drosophila* to temperature extremes: bringing together quantitative and molecular approaches, J. Therm. Biol. 28 (2003) 175–216.

[25] D.N. Lerman, M.E. Feder, Laboratory selection at different temperatures modifies heat shock transcription factor (HSF) activation in *Drosophila melanogaster*, J. Exp. Biol. 204 (2001) 315–323.

[26] K.H. Joplin, G.D. Yocum, D.L. Denlinger, Cold shock elicits expression of the heat shock proteins in the flesh fly *Sarcophaga crassipalpis*, J. Insect Physiol. 36 (1990) 825–834.

[27] J.P. Rinehart, G.D. Yocum, D.L. Denlinger, Developmental upregulation of inducible hsp70 transcripts, but not the cognate form, during pupal diapause in the flesh fly, *Sarcophaga crassipalpis*, Insect Biochem. Mol. Biol. 30 (2000) 518–521.

[28] J.P. Rinehart, D.L. Denlinger, Heat-shock protein 90 is down-regulated during pupal diapause in the flesh fly, *Sarcophaga crassipalpis*, but remains responsive to thermal stress, Insect Mol. Biol. 9 (2000) 641–645.

[29] G.D. Yocum, K.H. Joplin, D.L. Denlinger, Upregulation of a 23 kDa small heat shock protein transcript during pupal diapause in the flesh fly, *Sarcophaga crassipalpis*, Insect Biochem. Mol. Biol. 28 (1998) 677–682.

[30] G.D. Yocum, Differential expression of two HSP70 transcripts in response to cold shock, thermoperiod, and adult diapause in the Colorado potato beetle, J. Insect Physiol. 47 (2001) 1139–1145.

[31] R. Loftus, G. Corbiere-Tichane, Response of antennal cold receptors of the catopid beetles *Speophyes lucidulus* Delar. and *Choleva angustata* Far. to very slowly changing temperature, J. Comp. Physiol., A Sens. Neural Behav. Physiol. 161 (1987) 399–406.

[32] L. Liu, et al., Identification and function of thermosensory neurons in *Drosophila* larvae, Nat. Neurosci. 6 (2003) 267–273.

[33] H. Altner, R. Loftus, Ultrastructure and function of insect thermo- and hygroreceptors, Annu. Rev. Entomol. 30 (1985) 273–295.

[34] T. Zars, Hot and cold in *Drosophila* larvae, Trends Neurosci. 26 (2003) 575–577.

[35] W.D. Tracey, et al., *Painless*, a *Drosophila* gene essential for nociception, Cell 113 (2003) 261–273.

[36] M.J. Caterina, et al., The capsaicin receptor: a heat-activated ion channel in the pain pathway, Nature 389 (1997) 816–824.

[37] A.M. Peier, et al., A TRP channel that senses cold stimuli and menthol, Cell 108 (2002) 705–715.

[38] M. Holmstrup, K. Hedlund, H. Boriss, Drought acclimation and lipid composition in *Folsomia candida*: implications for cold shock, heat shock and acute desiccation stress, J. Insect Physiol. 48 (2002) 961–970.

[39] M. Hodkova, P. Berkova, H. Zahradnickova, Photoperiodic regulation of the phospholipid molecular species composition in thoracic muscles and fat body of *Pyrrhocoris apterus* (Heteroptera) via an endocrine gland, corpus allatum, J. Insect Physiol. 48 (2002) 1009–1019.

[40] V. Kostal, P. Simek, Changes in fatty acid composition of phospholipids and triacylglycerols after cold-acclimation of an aestivating insect prepupa, J. Comp. Physiol., B 168 (1998) 453–460.

[41] D.C. Knipple, et al., Evolution of the integral membrane desaturase gene family in moths and flies, Gen. Soc. Am. 162 (2002) 1737–1752.

[42] I. Suzuki, et al., The pathway for perception and transduction of low-temperature signals in *Synechocystis*, EMBO J. 19 (2000) 1327–1334.

[43] I. Suzuki, A. Los, N. Murata, Perception and transduction of low-temperature signals to induce desaturation of fatty acids, Biochem. Soc. Trans. 28 (2000) 628–630.

[44] L. Carratu, et al., Membrane lipid perturbation modifies the set point of the temperature of heat shock response in yeast, Proc. Natl. Acad. Sci. U. S. A. 93 (1996) 3870–3875.

[45] M. Inaba, et al., Gene-engineered rigidification of membrane lipids enhances the cold inducibility of gene expression in *Synechocystis*, J. Biol. Chem. 278 (2003) 12191–12198.

[46] K. Mikami, et al., The histidine kinase Hik33 perceives osmotic stress and cold stress in *Synechocystis* sp. PCC 6803, Mol. Microbiol. 46 (2002) 905–915.

[47] L. Vigh, et al., The primary signal in the biological perception of temperature: Pd-catalyzed hydrogenation of membrane lipids stimulated the expression of the desA gene in *Synechocystis* PCC6803, Proc. Natl. Acad. Sci. U. S. A. 90 (1993) 9090–9094.

[48] KB. Storey, Organic solutes in freezing tolerance, J. Comp. Physiol., B. Biochem. Syst. Environ. Physiol. 117A (3) (1997) 319–326.

[49] R.E. Lee, C.P. Chen, D.L. Denlinger, A rapid cold-hardening process in insects, Science 238 (1987) 1415–1417.

[50] F.G. Meng, Y.D. Park, H.M. Zhou, Role of proline, glycerol, and heparin as protein folding aids during refolding of rabbit muscle creatine kinase, Int. J. Biochem. Cell Biol. 33 (2001) 701–709.

[51] PJ. Quinn, A lipid-phase separation model of low-temperature damage to biological membranes, Cryobiology 22 (1985) 128–146.

[52] C.P. Chen, D.L. Denlinger, Activation of phosphorylase in response to cold and heat stress in the flesh fly, *Sarcophaga crassipalpis*, J. Insect Physiol. 36 (1990) 549–553.

[53] S.R. Misener, C.P. Chen, V.K. Walker, Cold tolerance and proline metabolic gene expression in *Drosophila melanogaster*, J. Insect Physiol. 47 (2001) 393–400.

[54] C.P. Chen, D.L. Denlinger, R.E. Lee, Cold-shock injury and rapid cold hardening in the flesh fly *Sarcophaga crassipalpis*, Physiol. Zool. 60 (1987) 297–304.

[55] R.E. Lee, et al., Ontogenetic patterns of cold-hardiness and glycerol production in *Sarcophaga crassipalpis*, J. Insect Physiol. 33 (1987) 587–592.

[56] B.J. Sinclair, S.L. Chown, Rapid responses to high temperature and desiccation but not to low temperature in the freeze tolerant sub-Antarctic caterpillar *Pringleophaga marioni* (Lepidoptera, Tineidae), J. Insect Physiol. 49 (2003) 45–52.

[57] T. Kageyama, Pathways of carbohydrate metabolism in the eggs of the silkworm moth, *Bombyx mori*, Insect Biochem. 6 (1976) 507–511.

[58] F.E. Wood Jr., J.H. Nordin, Activation of the hexose monophosphate shunt during cold-induced glycerol accumulation by *Protophormia terranovae*, Insect Biochem. 10 (1980) 87–93.

[59] Y.P. Li, L. Ding, M. Goto, Seasonal changes in glycerol content and enzyme activities in overwintering larvae of the Shonai ecotype of the rice stem borer, *Chilo suppressalis* Walker, Arch. Insect Biochem. Physiol. 50 (2002) 53–61.

[60] T.D. Pfister, K.B. Storey, Purification and characterization of protein phosphatase-1 from two cold-hardy goldenrod gall insects, Arch. Insect Biochem. Physiol. 49 (2002) 56–64.

[61] A.M. Muise, K.B. Storey, Regulation of hexokinase in a freeze avoiding insect: role in the winter production of glycerol, Arch. Insect Biochem. Physiol. 47 (2001) 29–34.

[62] K.B. Storey, Regulation of cryoprotectant metabolism in the overwintering gall fly larva, *Eurosta solidaginis*. Temperature control of sorbitol and glycerol levels, J. Comp. Physiol. 149 (1983) 495–502.

[63] H. Tsimuki, et al., The fate of [^{14}C]glucose during cold-hardening in *Eurosta soildiaginis* (Fitch), Insect Biochem. 17 (1987) 347–352.

[64] K.E. Zacchariassen, Physiology of cold tolerance in insects, Physiol. Rev. 65 (1985) 799–832.

[65] J.G. Duman, et al., Antifreeze proteins in Alaskan insects and spiders, J. Insect Physiol. 50 (2004) 259–266.

[66] J.G. Duman, A.S. Serianni, The role of endogenous antifreeze protein enhancers in the hemolymph thermal hysteresis activity of the beetle *Dendriodes canadensis*, J. Insect Physiol. 48 (2002) 103–111.

[67] C.C. Cheng, C.J. Brown, F.D. Sonnichsen, The structure of fish antifreeze proteins, in: K.V. Ewart, C.L. Hew (Eds.), Fish Antifreeze Proteins, World Scientific, London, 2002, pp. 109–138.

[68] C.B. Marshall, et al., Partitioning of fish and insect antifreeze proteins into ice suggests they bind with comparable affinity, Biochemistry 43 (2004) 148–154.

[69] J.G. Duman, The inhibition of ice nucleators by insect antifreeze proteins is enhanced by glycerol and citrate, J. Comp. Physiol., B 172 (2002) 163–168.

[70] N. Li, C.A. Andorfer, J.G. Duman, Enhancement of insect antifreeze protein activity by solutes of low molecular mass, J. Exp. Biol. 201 (1998) 2243–2251.

[71] S.G. Goto, M.T. Kimura, Heat- and cold-shock responses and temperature adaptations in subtropical and temperature species of *Drosophila*, J. Insect Physiol. 44 (12) (1998) 1233–1239.

[72] S. Lindquist, The heat shock response, Annu. Rev. Biochem. 55 (1986) 1151–1191.

[73] S.R. Terlecky, et al., Protein and peptide binding and simulation of in vitro lysomal proteolysis by the 73-KDa heat-shock protein, J. Biol. Chem. 267 (1992) 9202–9209.

[74] C.P. Chen, R.E. Lee, D.L. Denlinger, Cold shock and heat shock: a comparison of the protection generated by brief pretreatment at less severe temperatures, Physiol. Entomol. 16 (1991) 19–26.

[75] M.E. Feder, G.E. Hofmann, Heat-shock proteins, molecular chaperones, and the stress response: evolutionary and ecological physiology, Annu. Rev. Physiol. 61 (1999) 243–282.

[76] D. Job, et al., Recycling of cold-stable microtubules: evidence that cold stability is due to substoichiometric polymer blocks, Biochemistry 21 (1982) 509–515.

[77] G. Russotti, et al., Studies of heat and PGA$_1$-induced cold tolerance show that HSP27 may help preserve actin morphology during hypothermia, Tissue Eng. 3 (1997) 135–147.

[78] J.C. Young, Moarefi, F.U. Hard, Hsp90: a specialized but essential protein-folding tool, J. Cell Biol. 154 (2001) 267–273.

[79] H.W. Detrich, et al., Cold adaptation of microtubule assembly and dynamics. Structural interpretation of primary sequence changes present in the α- and β-tubulin of Antarctic fishes, J. Biol. Chem. 275 (2000) 37038–37047.

[80] H. Knight, A.J. Trehavas, M.R. Knight, Cold calcium signaling in *Arabidopsis* involves two cellular pools and a change in calcium signature after acclimation, Plant Cell 8 (1996) 489–503.

[81] B.L. Orvar, et al., Early steps in cold sensing by plant cells: the role of actin cytoskeleton and membrane fluidity, Plant J. 23 (2000) 78–794.

[82] O.A. Timofeeva, et al., Microtubules regulate activity of cell wall lectins in cells of *Triticum aestivum* L. plants during cold hardening, Cell Biol. Int. 27 (2003) 281–282.

[83] P. Liang, T.H. MacRae, Molecular chaperones and the cytoskeleton, J. Cell. Sci. 110 (1997) 1431–1440.

[84] C. Barroso, et al., Two kinesin-related proteins associated with the cold-stable cytoskeleton of carrot cells: characterization of a novel kinesin, DcKRP120-2, Plant J. 24 (2000) 859–868.

[85] W.F. Bluhm, et al., Specific heat shock proteins protect microtubules during simulated ischemia in cardiac myocytes, Am. J. Physiol. 275 (1998) H2243–H2249.

[86] A.Y. Nyporko, O.N. Demchuk, Y.A. Blume, Cold adaptation of plant microtubules: structural interpretation of primary sequence changes in a highly conserved region of α-tubulin, Cell Biol. Int. 27 (2003) 241–243.

[87] B.G. Leicht, et al., Small heat shock proteins of *Drosophila* associate with the cytoskeleton, Proc. Natl. Acad. Sci. U. S. A. 83 (1986) 90–94.

[88] S.G. Goto, Expression of *Drosophila* homologue of senescence marker protein-30 during cold acclimation, J. Insect Physiol. 46 (1998) 1111–1120.

[89] S.G. Goto, A novel gene that is up-regulated during recovery from cold shock in *Drosophila melanogaster*, Gene 270 (2001) 259–264.

[90] A.K. Singh, S.C. Lakhotia, Lack of effects of microtubule poisons on the 93D and the 93D like heat shock puffs in *Drosophila*, Indian J. Exp. Biol. 20 (1984) 569–576.

[91] H. Katoh, et al., Enhanced expression of *Bombyx* seven-up, an insect homolog of chicken ovalbumin upstream promoter-transcription factor, in diapause eggs exposed to 5 °C, J. Insect Biotechnol. Sericology 71 (2002) 17–24.

[92] Y. Moribe, et al., *Samui*, a novel cold-inducible gene, encoding a protein with a BAG domain similar to silencer of death domains (SODD/BAG4), isolated from *Bombyx* diapause eggs, Eur. J. Biochem. 268 (2001) 3432–3442.

[93] Y. Moribe, et al., Differential expression of the two cold-inducible genes, Samui and sorbitol dehydrogenase, in *Bombyx* diapause eggs exposed to low temperature, J. Insect Biotechnol. Sericology 71 (2002) 167–171.

[94] B. Cymborowski, Expression of C-fos-like protein in the brain and prothoracic glands of *Galleria mellonella* larvae during chilling stress, J. Insect Physiol. 42 (1996) 367–371.

[95] Y. Kim, N. Kim, Cold hardiness in *Spodoptera exigua* (Lepidoptera: Noctuidae), Environ. Entomol. 26 (1997) 1117–1123.

[96] J. Fujita, Cold shock response in mammalian cells, J. Mol. Microbiol. Biotechnol. 1 (1999) 243–255.

[97] M. Seki, et al., Monitoring the expression profiles of 7000 *Arabidopsis* genes under drought, cold and high-salinity stresses using a full-length cDNA microarray, Plant J. 31 (2002) 279–292.

[98] M.A. Rabbani, et al., Monitoring expression profiles of rice genes under cold, drought, and high-salinity stresses and abscisic acid application using cDNA microarray and RNA gel-blot analyses, Plant Physiol. 133 (2003) 1755–1767.

[99] O. Odani, et al., Screening of genes that respond to cryopreservation stress using yeast DNA microarray, Cryobiology 47 (2003) 155–164.

[100] A. Ju, R.A. Dunham, Z. Liu, Differential gene expression in the brain of channel catfish (*Ictalurus punctatus*) in response to cold acclimation, MGG, Mol. Gen. Genomics 268 (2002) 87–95.

International Congress Series 1275 (2004) 47–54

ELSEVIER

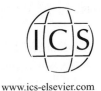

www.ics-elsevier.com

Molecular mechanisms of anoxia tolerance

Kenneth B. Storey*

Institute of Biochemistry, Carleton University, 1125 Colonel By Drive, Ottawa, Canada K1S 5B6

Abstract. Facultative anaerobiosis occurs widely across phylogeny and comparative studies with multiple animal models are identifying conserved molecular mechanisms that support anoxia tolerance. Our studies of freshwater turtles have analyzed metabolic, signal transduction and gene expression responses to anoxia. A key mechanism is reversible protein phosphorylation, which provides coordinate suppression of the rates of ATP-producing versus ATP-utilizing cellular processes to achieve strong metabolic rate depression (MRD). Anoxia tolerance is also supported by selective gene expression as revealed by cDNA library and cDNA array screening. Prominent groups of genes that are up-regulated under anoxia in turtle organs include mitochondrially encoded subunits of electron transport chain proteins and several serine protease inhibitors. © 2004 Elsevier B.V. All rights reserved.

Keywords: Gene expression; Anaerobiosis; Metabolic rate depression; cDNA array; Turtle

1. Introduction

Oxygen deprivation is rapidly lethal for humans and many other organisms but the realities of environment or lifestyle have lead to the evolution of facultative anaerobiosis in diverse group of animals. Among vertebrates, the premier facultative anaerobes are freshwater turtles of the *Trachemys* and *Chrysemys* genera. These endure apnoic dives of many hours and can survive for 3–4 months submerged in cold deoxygenated water, a capacity that serves winter hibernation in ice-locked ponds and lakes that can become severely hypoxic or anoxic [1]. Known molecular mechanisms of anoxia tolerance include: (a) large organ reserves of fermentable fuels, chiefly glycogen, (b) strategies for buffering or excreting end products, (c) alternative routes of anaerobic carbohydrate catabolism with higher ATP yields than are achieved from glycolysis ending in lactate, (d) well-developed antioxidant defenses to minimize oxidative stress when oxygen is

* Tel.: +1 613 520 3678; fax: +1 613 520 2569.
E-mail address: kenneth_storey@carleton.ca.

0531-5131/ © 2004 Elsevier B.V. All rights reserved.
doi:10.1016/j.ics.2004.08.072

reintroduced, (e) strong metabolic rate depression (MRD), and (f) up-regulation of selected genes whose protein products aid anoxia survival [1–3].

Of these, the most important factor overall is MRD. Maintenance of cellular energetics is the most pressing concern for anaerobic survival because fermentative pathways yield just a fraction of the ATP per mole of substrate catabolized as is available from oxygen-based catabolism; e.g. net ATP output is just 2 mol ATP/mol glucose converted to lactate versus 36 ATP/mol for conversion to CO_2 and H_2O. Hence, by strongly suppressing metabolic rate in anoxia, animals lower ATP demand and greatly extend the time that endogenous carbohydrate reserves can support survival. For example, freshwater turtles typically suppress metabolic rate to just 10–20% of the aerobic rate at the same body temperatures [1]. MRD involves coordinated controls on the rates of both ATP-producing and ATP-utilizing cell reactions so that two outcomes are achieved: (a) net ATP turnover is strongly reduced, and (b) the priorities for ATP expenditure are reorganized. Indeed, these outcomes have been well-documented in studies with isolated turtle hepatocytes [4]. Incubation under anoxia decreased ATP turnover by 94% and dramatically changed the proportion of ATP turnover devoted to five main ATP-consuming processes: ion motive ATPases, protein synthesis, protein degradation, gluconeogenesis and urea synthesis. As a result the Na^+K^+ATPase pump became the dominant energy sink in anoxic hepatocytes, consuming 62% of total ATP turnover compared with 28% in normoxia. Protein synthesis and degradation were largely shut down in anoxia (by >90%) and urea synthesis was halted.

2. Metabolic regulation via reversible protein phosphorylation

Studies by my laboratory and others have shown that the primary mechanism controlling MRD is reversible protein phosphorylation [2]. The mechanism controls ATP production via glycolysis under anoxia in both vertebrates (turtles, goldfish) and invertebrates including regulation of glycogen phosphorylase, phosphofructokinase and pyruvate kinase [2,5]. Recent work has also shown reversible phosphorylation control of various ATP-consuming reactions. Key targets of phosphorylation-mediated suppression include ion motive ATPases such Na^+K^+ATPase of the plasma membrane and Ca^{2+}-ATPase of the sarco(endo)plasmic reticulum [2]. Regulation of ion pumps as well as ion channels and membrane receptors contribute to the control of neuronal activity in brain of anoxic turtles [3,6]. Ion pumps (that move ions against concentration gradients) and ion channels (that facilitate movement down gradients) need coordinated regulation to maintain transmembrane potential difference despite a much lower ATP turnover under anoxia. Several mechanisms of ion channel arrest have been identified with reversible phosphorylation of voltage-gated channels (Na^+, Ca^{2+}, K^+) and receptor subunits (e.g. N-methyl-D-aspartate-type glutamate receptor) playing a substantive role [6].

The rate of gene transcription is also suppressed in hypometabolic states although this is done with little change in global mRNA transcript levels. For example, total RNA levels were unaffected in turtle organs and mRNA content was constant in four out of five organs over 16 h of submergence anoxia [7]. In addition, mRNA remains largely intact during hypometabolism, creating an effective life-extension of transcripts so that these are immediately available when aerobic conditions return. However, instances of specific transcriptional repression are known; for example, mRNA transcripts of voltage-dependent potassium channels in turtle brain were reduced to 18.5% of normoxic levels after 4 h of anoxia but rebounded after reoxygenation [8]. Mechanisms of transcriptional control can be global (e.g. inhibition of RNA polymerase) or specific to families of genes sharing a common response element. Both mechanisms can involve reversible phosphorylation; for example, the former can arise from the phosphorylation of core subunits of RNA polymerase II [9,10] and the latter from suppression of signal transduction pathways involving mitogen-activated protein kinases (MAPKs) and transcription factors, most of which are regulated by reversible protein phosphorylation [11]. Still unstudied in comparative systems, mechanisms of global transcriptional repression are obviously a key area that needs future study in facultative anaerobes and other systems of MRD. A little more is known about gene-specific repression. For example, extracellular signal regulated kinases (ERKs) showed no response to anoxia in turtles or freezing in freeze tolerant frogs and turtles [11–13] suggesting that the genes that they control are not up-regulated under these stresses. This is not surprising since the ERK module primarily transduces signals that stimulate growth and proliferation, cellular activities that would be curtailed under anoxic conditions. However, the c-Jun N-terminal kinases (JNKs) appear to play a role in the response to anoxia. JNK activity rose during survivable anoxia exposure in tissues of both adult and hatchling turtles; in both cases, JNK activity peaked after 5 h of anoxic submergence but fell with longer exposure [11–13]. This suggests a role for JNK activation in the hypoxia transition period during the early hours of submergence with JNK suppressed again when metabolic arrest is fully developed in support of long-term anoxia survival.

Protein synthesis is major energy expense in cells and is strongly suppressed during anaerobiosis [4,14,15] and in other hypometabolic states (e.g. mammalian hibernation) [2]. Two mechanisms that contribute to protein synthesis arrest have been studied: (1) reversible phosphorylation control of the translational machinery, and (2) the state of ribosome assembly. Both have been seen during MRD in multiple systems, e.g. anoxia exposure in *Artemia* and the marine snail *Littorina littorea* and mammalian hibernation [2]. Reversible phosphorylation control is directed at key ribosomal regulatory proteins, such as the alpha subunit of the eukaryotic initiation factor 2 (eIF-2α) and the eukaryotic elongation factor-2 (eEF-2) [2,16,17]. Translation is also suppressed by the stress-induced dissociation of polysomes (that conduct active translation) into monosomes (translationally silent) with the movement of a high proportion of total mRNA into the monosome fraction [2]. Both mechanisms aid global suppression of protein synthesis but leave open ways to achieve selective expression of specific anoxia-responsive genes. For example, under stress conditions (including hypoxia, ischemia, starvation, etc.) message selection for translation changes to favour only those messages that contain an internal ribosome entry site (IRES) [16] whereas the vast majority of cellular mRNAs (m^{7}G-capped mRNAs) cannot bind to the small ribosomal subunit due to stress-induced fragmentation of eIF4G [17]. Of note for studies of anoxia-responsive protein translation is the fact that an IRES is present in the mRNA of the hypoxia-inducible factor-1α (HIF-1α) [18] and this provides a way to elevate HIF-1α protein which, in turn, mediates a variety of gene expression responses to hypoxia. Interestingly, the mRNA of vascular endothelial growth factor (VEGF), one of the targets of HIF-1 action, also has an IRES [19]. It will be interesting to explore anoxia-responsive genes in facultative anaerobes to determine if they also possess an IRES (the IRES is typically found within a long and GC-rich 5′ -

untranslated region) that permits their translation under the ATP-restricted conditions of the anoxic state.

3. Anoxia-induced gene expression in freshwater turtles

Although anoxia survival is aided by global suppression of transcription and translation, recent studies have documented several instances of anoxia-responsive up-regulation of selected protein types. For example, selected heat shock proteins are up-regulated in an organ-specific manner under anoxia in turtles [20–22]; their chaperone actions may aid long-term stability of other proteins over extended periods of hypometabolism. Recent work in my laboratory has explored anoxia-induced gene expression in the red-eared slider turtle, *Trachemys scripta elegans*. Initial studies used differential screening of cDNA libraries and, interestingly, revealed multiple examples of the up-regulation of genes encoded on the mitochondrial genome under anoxia. Screening of a heart library made from adult turtles submerged for 20 h in N_2-bubbled water at 7 °C showed anoxia-responsive up-regulation of *Cox1* that encodes cytochrome *c* oxidase subunit 1 (COX1), *Nad5* that encodes subunit 5 of NADH-ubiquinone oxidoreductase (ND5), and the mitochondrial WANCY (tryptophan, alanine, asparagine, cysteine, tyrosine) tRNA gene cluster [23,24]. Transcripts of all three rose within 1 h of anoxia exposure to levels that were 4.5-, 3- and 3.5-fold higher than controls for *Cox1*, *Nad5* and WANCY, respectively. Levels remained high after 20 h of anoxia and then declined during aerobic recovery. *Cox1* and *Nad5* also responded to anoxia in red muscle, brain and kidney [23]. Other mitochondrially encoded genes were anoxia responsive in liver: transcripts of *Cytb*, encoding cytochrome *b*, and *Nad4*, encoding subunit 4 of ND, rose by 5- and 13-fold, respectively, within 1 h of anoxia exposure [25].

The reason for mitochondrial gene up-regulation in anoxia is not yet known but we have also seen the phenomenon in other animals under low oxygen. For example, *Cox2* transcripts rose 6–7-fold in *L. littorea* under an N_2 atmosphere (K. Larade, unpublished) and freezing (which causes ischemia) triggered the up-regulation of mitochondrially encoded genes in freeze tolerant turtles (*Chrysemys picta*) and frogs (*Rana sylvatica*). *Cox1* and *Nad5* were freeze-responsive in turtle liver [23] as was *Nad4* in frog liver and subunits 6 and 8 of F_0F_1 ATPase in frog brain (S. Wu and K.B. Storey, unpublished). Furthermore, four genes on the mitochondrial genome (*Nad2*, *Cox1*, ATPase subunits 6 and 8) were also up-regulated during mammalian hibernation [2] which suggests that the phenomenon is a general principle of hypometabolism. The proteins encoded by these mitochondrial genes all belong to large complexes on the mitochondrial inner membrane that are made up of multiple subunits coded on both the nuclear and mitochondrial genomes (e.g. 3 of the 13 subunits of COX and 6 of the 41 subunits of ND are on the mitochondrial genome) [26,27]. However, we have found no case to date where a nuclear-encoded subunit of these proteins was up-regulated in a hypometabolic state (anoxia, freezing, hibernation). Mitochondrial DNA has only one promoter on each of the L and H strands and genes are transcribed as one RNA precursor from the same initiation site (except for rRNA genes) [28]. Long polycistronic messages are then cleaved to give individual RNA species. This mode of transcription explains the parallel increases in *Cox1*, *Nad5* and WANCY transcripts in anoxic turtle heart but not the tissue-specific differences in gene up-regulation. For example, transcripts of

Cox1 and *Nad5* rose in anoxic turtle heart but not in liver whereas *Cytb* transcripts rose in liver but not in heart [23,25]. Further study of the responses to anoxia by the mitochondrial genome in tissues of a single anoxia-tolerant species may resolve the question.

4. cDNA array screening

One of the hottest new technologies in biology is cDNA array screening. Microarrays spotted with thousands of unique cDNAs on a single glass slide provide researchers with the opportunity to screen for changes in the expression genes representing hundreds of different cell functions. We have made extensive use of human 19,000 gene cDNA arrays produced by the Ontario Cancer Institute (University of Toronto) to provide a comprehensive overview of gene responses to environmental stress in multiple animal systems including hibernating mammals, freeze tolerant frogs, and anoxia tolerant turtles and snails (Refs. [2,29,30] and unpublished). Cross-reaction is never 100% with heterologous probing and therefore cannot give a full picture of all gene changes under stress, but the method still allows thousands of genes to be screened and many putatively up-regulated genes to be highlighted. Moreover, cDNA array screening provides the key advantage of allowing the researcher to look for coordinated responses by groups of genes, e.g. genes representing families of proteins, pathways, signal transduction cascades, etc.

Indeed, one outstanding result from our screening of turtle liver, heart, skeletal muscle and brain was the repeated identification of members of one such family as putatively up-regulated in anoxia. These are the serine protease inhibitors (serpins). Several serpins, as well as tissue factor pathway inhibitor (TFPI), were putatively up-regulated (by 2-fold or more) in organs from anoxic turtles, compared with aerobic controls (Table 1). Array screening indicated that four proteinase inhibitors were up-regulated in liver, a main site of synthesis of these proteins, three in heart, two in muscle and one in brain.

Serpins are a superfamily of proteins with 16 clades. All show a common core domain of three β-sheets and 8-9 α-helices and most are glycoproteins of 40–60 kDa [31]. The majority of serpins are extracellular (except those in clade B) and most exhibit serine or cysteine proteinase inhibition although some have evolved to take on other tasks such as hormone transport (e.g. corticosteroid and thyroxin binding globulins) or blood pressure regulation (angiotensinogen). Serpins are irreversible covalent inhibitors of proteases that cleave specific proteins. Many are specific inhibitors of proteases that act as critical checkpoints in self-perpetuating proteolytic cascades such as the proteases involved in blood coagulation (e.g. thrombin, factor Xa and XIa), fibrinolysis (e.g. plasmin, tissue

Table 1
Proteinase inhibitors identified from cDNA array screening as putatively up-regulated during anoxia in turtle organs: aerobic control versus 4 h of anoxic submergence in nitrogen-bubbled water

Inhibitor	Full name	Organ	Function
SERPINA1	α_1-antitrypsin	Brain, muscle	inhibits elastase, trypsin, chymotrypsin, thrombin, plasmin, kallikrein, collagenase
SERPINC1	antithrombin	Liver, heart	inhibits thrombin, factor Xa, IXa
SERPIND1	heparin cofactor II	Liver, muscle	inhibits thrombin
SERPINF1	pigment epithelium derived factor (PEDF)	Liver, heart	noninhibitory towards proteinases; acts as an anti-angiogenic factor
TFPI	tissue factor pathway inhibitor	Liver, heart	TF–FVIIa complex inhibitor

plasminogen activator, urokinase plasminogen activator), inflammation (e.g. elastase, cathepsin G), and complement activation [31].

Up-regulation of selected serpins under anoxia could be important for inhibiting proteolytic reactions and cascades that could otherwise cause cumulative damage to tissues over the long term in an energy-restricted state. This suggests that another key aspect of MRD is the suppression of proteolytic cascades. SERPIN1A (α_1-proteinase inhibitor or α_1-antitrypsin), the most abundant of the circulating serpins, has a primary physiological role in protecting the lower respiratory tract from proteolytic destruction by neutrophil elastase which hydrolyzes structural proteins as part of its attack on bacterial infections [32]. Low circulating SERPIN1A is associated with chronic obstructive pulmonary emphysema caused by excessive elastase attack on lung tissue. Anoxia-responsive up-regulation of SERPINA1 may act to suppress the action of these circulating proteases involved in inflammation during periods of breath-hold (apnea) when the intake of air-borne pathogens is interrupted. This would help to avoid nonspecific damage to tissues over what could be days or weeks of anoxia exposure, a time when cellular repair mechanisms that require de novo protein synthesis to replace damaged proteins would be suppressed as part of MRD.

Other serpins target proteinases associated with the clotting cascade. SERPINC1 (antithrombin) inhibits thrombin and, thereby, also blocks feedback activation of the cascade by thrombin. SERPIND1 (heparin cofactor II) also inhibits thrombin. Both are activated by binding to heparin or other glycosaminoglycans by one of two main ways: (1) the glycosaminoglycan can simultaneously bind both serpin and proteinase to bring them together, or (2) glycosaminoglycan binding to a serpin can alter its conformation to one that is more reactive towards the proteinase [31]. Clotting capacity could be reduced during anaerobiosis to minimize the risk of thrombosis in the microvasculature under the low blood flow conditions caused by bradycardia during hypometabolism. Indeed, reduced clotting capacity is a component of another form of hypometabolism that is also associated with profound bradycardia—mammalian hibernation. Using array screening, we have similarly noted putative up-regulation of SERPINC1 (and SERPINA1) in liver of hibernating ground squirrels [33] and other mechanisms for clotting inhibition during hibernation have been previously reported including up-regulation in liver and export of α_2-macroglobulin (a non-serpin general inhibitor of clotting cascade proteases) [34] and reduced circulating levels of platelets and several clotting factors [35].

Inhibition of clotting under low blood flow conditions during hypometabolism can also be aided by up-regulation of TFPI, another protein targeted by our array screening. Tissue factor (TF) is an initiator of coagulation. Injury to blood vessel walls exposes TF to circulating Factor VII and TF forms a complex with the active (a) form of FVII (TF–FVIIa) that induces a conformational change in the protease domain of Factor VIIa to activate it [36]. This allows the protease to activate Factors IX and X which then go on to stimulate the conversion of prothrombin to thrombin. TFPI is an inhibitor of the TF–FVIIa complex and the main regulator of the tissue factor pathway [36]. Hence, TFPI has an important anticoagulant action and its up-regulation under anoxia in turtles may further suppress spontaneous clot formation during hypometabolism.

SERPINF1, also known as pigment epithelium-derived factor (PEDF), is a serpin that does not inhibit a proteinase. Instead, PEDF has potent anti-angiogenic and neurotrophic actions and counterbalances the angiogenic effects of VEGF [37,38]. PEDF was first described as a factor that inhibited aberrant blood vessel growth in models of ischemia-induced retinopathy; PEDF acts by inducing apoptosis in actively dividing endothelial cells [39]. New work has shown that PEDF also inhibits vascular growth and tissue mass in prostate and pancreas [40]. Circulating levels of PEDF in humans are high enough to be physiologically relevant indicating that systemic delivery of PEDF could affect angiogenesis throughout the body [38]. Although no research has yet been done, the putative up-regulation of PEDF in anoxia-tolerant turtles is highly intriguing. Low oxygen typically activates HIF-1 that, in turn, up-regulates a variety of genes whose protein products address two main goals: (1) improvement of oxygen delivery to tissues (e.g. up-regulation of VEGF and erythropoietin), and (2) improvement of glycolytic ATP output (e.g. up-regulation of glycolytic enzymes and glucose transporters). For facultative anaerobes, enhanced capillary growth during natural hypoxia/anoxia excursions is counterintuitive as it is energy-expensive at a time when energy savings are crucial and unproductive since low tissue oxygen levels cannot be improved by enhanced oxygen delivery under apnoic conditions. Hence, up-regulation of PEDF could serve to counteract an angiogenic response to low oxygen under conditions (e.g. breath-hold diving, submerged hibernation) that cannot be aided by enhanced capillary growth.

In conclusion, much is already known about intermediary energy metabolism and the mechanisms of metabolic arrest under anoxia but new explorations of anoxia-induced gene expression are producing many new leads into areas of metabolic function that that have never before been considered as contributing to facultative anaerobiosis. For the comparative biochemist, the opportunities for significant new discoveries are exciting.

Acknowledgements

Thanks to J.M. Storey for editorial review of the manuscript. K.B.S. holds the Canada Research Chair in Molecular Physiology and research is supported by a Discovery grant from the Natural Sciences and Engineering Research Council of Canada. To learn more about vertebrate anoxia tolerance, visit www.carleton.ca.

References

[1] D.C. Jackson, in: K.B. Storey (Ed.), Molecular Mechanisms of Metabolic Arrest, BIOS Scientific Publishers, Oxford, 2001, pp. 103–114.
[2] K.B. Storey, J.M. Storey, Biol. Rev. Camb. Philos. Soc. 79 (2004) 207–233.
[3] P.W. Hochachka, P.L. Lutz, Comp. Biochem. Physiol., B 130 (2001) 435–459.
[4] P.W. Hochachka, et al., Proc. Natl. Acad. Sci. U. S. A. 93 (1996) 9493–9498.
[5] K.B. Storey, Comp. Biochem. Physiol., B 113 (1996) 23–35.
[6] P.E. Bickler, P.H. Donohoe, L.T. Buck, in: K.B. Storey (Ed.), Molecular Mechanisms of Metabolic Arrest, BIOS Scientific Publishers, Oxford, 2001, pp. 77–102.
[7] D.N. Douglas, et al., J. Comp. Physiol., B 164 (1994) 405–414.
[8] H.M. Prentice, et al., Comp. Biochem. Physiol. 285 (2003) R1317–R1321.
[9] K. Gaston, P.S. Jayaraman, Cell. Mol. Life Sci. 60 (2003) 721–741.
[10] A. Shilatifard, Biochim. Biophys. Acta 1677 (2004) 79–86.
[11] K.J. Cowan, K.B. Storey, J. Exp. Biol. 206 (2003) 1107–1115.
[12] S.C. Greenway, K.B. Storey, J. Exp. Zool. 287 (2000) 477–484.
[13] S.C. Greenway, K.B. Storey, J. Comp. Physiol. 169 (1999) 521–527.
[14] K. Larade, K.B. Storey, Mol. Cell. Biochem. 232 (2002) 121–127.

[15] K.P. Fraser, et al., J. Exp. Biol. 204 (2001) 4353–4360.
[16] A.C. Gingras, B. Raught, N. Sonenbert, Ann. Rev. Biochem. 68 (1999) 913–963.
[17] D.J. DeGracia, et al., J. Cereb. Blood Flow Metab. 22 (2002) 127–141.
[18] K.J.D. Lang, A. Kappel, G.J. Goodall, Mol. Biol. Cell 13 (2002) 1792–1801.
[19] D.L. Miller, et al., FEBS Lett. 434 (1998) 417–420.
[20] H.M. Prentice, et al., J. Cereb. Blood Flow Metab. 24 (2004) 826–828.
[21] M.A. Scott, M. Locke, L.T. Buck, J. Exp. Biol. 206 (2003) 303–311.
[22] J. Chang, A.A. Knowlton, J.S. Wasser, Am. J. Physiol. 278 (2000) R209–R214.
[23] Q. Cai, K.B. Storey, Eur. J. Biochem. 241 (1996) 83–92.
[24] Q. Cai, K.B. Storey, Genome 40 (1997) 534–543.
[25] W.G. Willmore, T.E. English, K.B. Storey, Copeia 2001 (2001) 628–637.
[26] A. Azzi, M. Muller, N. Labonia, in: J.M. Tager, A. Azzi, S. Papa, F. Guerrieri (Eds.), Organelles in Eukaryotic Cells, Plenum Press, New York, 1989, pp. 2–8.
[27] T. Ohnishi, J. Bioenerg. Biomembranes 25 (1993) 325–329.
[28] N.W. Gilham, Organelle genes and genomes, Oxford University Press, Oxford, 1994.
[29] K.B. Storey, Adv. Exp. Med. Biol. 543 (2003) 21–38.
[30] K.B. Storey, Cryobiology 48 (2004) 134–145.
[31] P.G.W. Gettins, Chem. Rev. 102 (2002) 4751–4803.
[32] N. Kalsheker, S. Morley, K. Morgan, Biochem. Soc. Trans. 30 (2002) 93–98.
[33] K.B. Storey, J. Investig. Med. 52 (2004) (in press).
[34] H.K. Srere, et al., Am. J. Physiol. 268 (1995) R1507–R1512.
[35] R.M. McCarron, et al., in: K.B. Storey (Ed.), Molecular Mechanisms of Metabolic Arrest, BIOS Scientific Publishers, Oxford, 2001, pp. 23–42.
[36] G.C. Price, S.A. Thompson, P.C.A. Kam, Anaesthesia 59 (2004) 483–492.
[37] E.J. Duh, et al., Investig. Ophthalmol. Vis. Sci. 43 (2002) 821–829.
[38] S.V. Petersen, Z. Valnickova, J.J. Enghild, Biochem. J. 374 (2003) 199–206.
[39] V. Stellmach, et al., Proc. Natl. Acad. Sci. U. S. A. 98 (2001) 2593–2597.
[40] J.A. Doll, et al., Nat. Med. 9 (2003) 774–780.

International Congress Series 1275 (2004) 55–62

ELSEVIER

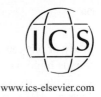

www.ics-elsevier.com

Daphnia and *Drosophila*: two invertebrate models for O_2 responsive and HIF-mediated regulation of genes and genomes

Thomas A. Gorr*

*Division of Hematology, Department of Medicine, Brigham and Women's Hospital, Harvard Medical School,
221 Longwood Avenue, Boston, MA 02115, USA*

Abstract. A brief comparison of hypoxia-tolerant versus hypoxia-sensitive strategies to cope with periods of oxygen deprivation (hypoxia, anoxia) is presented with a particular focus on oxygen sensing via hypoxia-inducible factors (HIF) in two hypoxia-tolerant invertebrate models: *Daphnia magna* and *Drosophila melanogaster*. In *Daphnia*, HIF controls the hypoxic induction of multiple globin genes, which, not only causes a visible development of color, but also greatly facilitates O_2 delivery to hypoxic tissues as do HIF-driven erythropoiesis and angiogenesis in mammals. In contrast, expression of the single-copy drosophilid globin gene is HIF-dependently suppressed in hypoxic SL2 cells from late fly embryos. Invertebrate globin genes, therefore, demonstrate HIF's ability to confer trans-activation and trans-inactivation onto target genes. Strategies to acquire hypoxia-tolerance center around a regulated and reversible metabolic depression throughout which cellular ATP supply and demand functions are coordinatedly reduced. Our microarray-based elucidation of *Drosophila*'s genome-wide response to graded hypoxia revealed indeed numerous transcriptional inductions or suppressions that suggested an overall down-regulation of major ATP consuming processes (e.g. protein synthesis, cell cycle progression) in severely oxygen depleted SL2 cells. HIF control was implicated in some of these regulations and thus, might play an essential role to conserve energy during periods of limited O_2 supply in hypoxia-tolerant animals. © 2004 Elsevier B.V. All rights reserved.

Keywords: Daphnia; Drosophila; Hypoxia; HIF; Hypometabolism

1. Introduction

This review presents new information on the freshwater crustacean *Daphnia magna* and the fruitfly *Drosophila melanogaster*, two hypoxia-tolerant invertebrate models for the

---
* Corresponding author. Tel.: +1 617 732 7951; fax: +1 617 739 0748.
  E-mail address: tgorr@rics.bwh.harvard.edu.

0531-5131/ © 2004 Elsevier B.V. All rights reserved.
doi:10.1016/j.ics.2004.08.068

study of oxygen-responsive genes and genomes. It begins by comparing hypoxia-sensitive versus hypoxia–tolerant strategies with a particular focus on the transcriptional adaptation to falling oxygen tensions (hypoxia) as mediated by hypoxia-inducible transcription factors (HIF) in both systems. When appropriate, the review will incorporate recent insights and discussions from my own work on the hypoxic and HIF-mediated regulation of *Daphnia* and *Drosophila* globin genes, and will include some results from our microarray-centered elucidation of *Drosophila*'s 'hypoxia genome', to suggest that HIF function also is critical for developing and maintaining hypoxia-tolerance in this insect model. In the interest of space however, this review will not recapitulate recent advances on structural, functional and regulatory aspects of HIF proteins and oxygen-sensing. The reader is referred to Refs. [1,4], and papers cited therein, for details.

2. Biochemical concepts in hypoxia-tolerant versus hypoxia-sensitive models

Hypoxia tolerance, the ability to survive and recover from hours to weeks or even months of exposure to little (hypoxia) or no (anoxia) oxygen present in the environment, is a widespread adaptation amongst invertebrates and can provide researchers with an unrivaled diversity of model organisms to study oxygen-responsive adaptations at the DNA level that might underlie or contribute to the organism's resilience to lack of oxygen. For example, *D. magna* (Crustacea, Cladocera) or *D. melanogaster* (Insecta, Diptera) are particularly suited to further our understanding of oxy-genes and -genomes. They both express HIF, the key regulator protein in the transcriptional response to hypoxia (*Daphnia*: [1]; *Drosophila*: flies [2], cell culture [3,4]) and therefore make use of a phylogenetically conserved signaling pathway (i.e., oxygen sensing) to relay environmental cues such as declining oxygen tensions through the hypoxia-specific stabilization of the HIFα subunit protein, followed by heterodimerization with its partner protein ARNT, into the nucleus. In contrast, under normoxic conditions, the HIFα subunit is oxidatively modified and subsequently degraded by proteolysis, thus abrogating HIF function. The unique aspect about *Daphnia* and *Drosophila* HIF (and that of many more invertebrates, e.g. the nematode *C. elegans*) is that the oxygen sensing pathway and the transcriptional regulation of oxy-genes/-genomes works within the framework of a hypoxia-tolerant organism. Only here can we begin to understand HIF's relevance in establishing biochemical alterations that might lead to the phenotypic tolerance toward lack of oxygen in these lower metazoans and compare these insights with HIF's role in the hypoxic response in sensitive models (e.g. mammals+birds (aka endotherms), primary and transformed mammalian cell lines), where it primarily limits cell death through enhanced delivery of oxygen (induced erythropoiesis and angiogenesis) and minimized ATP-losses (induced high-flux glycolysis, aka Pasteur-effect) during periods of oxygen deprivation. To better appreciate the physiological distinction between hypoxia-tolerant (e.g. *Drosophila*, *Daphnia*, *C. elegans*) and -sensitive animals (e.g. endotherms), however, a few more comparative details seem necessary.

Adult daphnids and fruitflies are able to withstand, without signs of mortality, up to 4 hours (*Drosophila* [5]) or even 24 h (*Daphnia* [6]) of anoxia (N_2 atmosphere) which they survive by virtue of (a) immediate development of anoxic stupor which ranges from loss of coordination to complete immobility (*Drosophila*: [5,7,8]), (b) strongly depressed metabolism as revealed through decreases in O_2-consumption to ~20–30% of normoxic controls (*Drosophila*: [5,9]) or through slowed heart beat and hemolymph perfusion rates (*Daphnia* [6]), and (c) anaerobiosis with, typical for arthropods [10], lactate as prime end product and substantial glycogen stores for sustenance (*Daphnia* [6]). Thus, *Daphnia* and *Drosophila* cope with acute scarcity of O_2 through key adaptations characteristic of hypoxia-tolerance [11]: regulated and reversible metabolic depression along with transition to glycogen-based fermentative glucose consumption in order to balance reduced ATP synthesis with reduced ATP demand [12,13]. Such a metabolic framework for investigating HIF function is very different from the commonly used "mammalian", i.e. human plus rodent, in vivo or in vitro models which are quickly and irreversibly debilitated by lack of oxygen [14,15]. HIF regulation in organisms that are actually adapted to face hypoxia as a physiological, rather than pathological, signal, therefore, might lead to novel insights on oxygen sensing, gene function and metabolic control, and might also bring us closer in understanding HIF's archetypal function(s).

Metabolic control in hypoxia-sensitive models of mammalian brain or liver entails a strong up-regulation of the glycolytic glucose consumption once oxygen partial pressure (pO_2) falls below a critical level [16]. This inverse relationship between glycolytic flux and oxygen availability is known as Pasteur effect and marks the switch from aerobic (mitochondrial) to anaerobic (glycolytic) metabolism and energy production. In mammalian cells, this switch is regulated by HIF [17]. Out of a total of 12 functionally distinct glycolytic reactions, 8–10 are coordinately induced through HIF-dependent enhanced transcription of the enzyme-encoding gene when mammalian cells are exposed to 0–2% O_2 [18–24]. This prominent stimulation of glycolytic flux by low pO_2 is a short-term attempt of hypoxia-sensitive cells, where ATP turnover is not reprogrammed to a reduced steady-state [11–13], to compensate for continuing ATP utilization demands [25]. Due to the ~10-fold lower efficiency of glycolytic (2–3 mol ATP/mole glucosyl unit) versus oxidative ATP production (36 mol ATP/mole glucose), however, high-flux glycolysis soon amasses toxic levels of end products while it, in the absence of energy expenditure reductions, still fails to meet ATP maintenance demands of ionic and osmotic equilibrium, thus producing an ultimately fatal ATP imbalance in the cell [12–16,25,26].

The ability to reversibly enter a state of a *regulated* metabolic depression, characterized by a greatly (sometimes >90%) reduced, yet balanced ATP supply=ATP demand steady-state [11–13] prevents lethal falls in cellular ATP levels and is the single most protective and unifying feature of hypoxia-tolerant organisms [13]. Since ~80% of mitochondrial O_2-consumption is coupled to ATP synthesis [27], metabolic depressions are frequently reported by declining measures of oxygen consumption rates during periods of hypoxia/anoxia (see above). As a stress-coping mechanism, regulated metabolic depression (or hypometabolism) 'buys time' (i.e., enables long-term survival (hours–months) in anoxia) and relies not on energy *compensation* but rather on energy *conservation*. This involves the coordinated suppression of every major ATP-utilizing function in the cell (i.e., predominantly: (a) protein synthesis (~30%), (b) protein degradation (~20%) and (c) ion-motive ATPases, notably Na^+-K^+-ATPase (~25%) (with fractional proportion in % of total normoxic ATP turnover given in parentheses [11,12,27–29] to match the synchronously declining ATP production in an O_2-depleted cell. A depressed metabolism, therefore, does not require hypoxia/anoxia-induced high-flux glycolysis, and it should come as no surprise that numerous hypoxia-tolerant organisms only display a weak or transient, if any, Pasteur

Table 1
Metabolic strategies employed by hypoxia-sensitive and hypoxia-tolerant model organisms during O_2 deprivation

Features/strategy	Hypoxia-sensitive	Hypoxia-tolerant
Representatives	most endotherms (mammals, birds)	many invertebrates; few reptiles, frogs+fish (e.g. bivalve mollusks); (e.g. freshwater turtles)
Metabolic capacity	strongly aerobic	facultative anaerobic
Metabolic depression	absent	present
ATP turnover	non-steady-state (declining)	steady-state at reduced level
ATP-costly functions	maintained	suppressed
Pasteur effect	standard	weak or reversed
Fermentation yields	lactate	lactate, succinate, acetate, propionate

effect [25,30], or even develop a glycolytic rate inhibition (i.e., reverse Pasteur effect) and formation of little lactate during anoxia as seen in insect brains [31].

Rather than increasing glycolytic flux, strongly tolerant intertidal bivalve mollusks and annelids often supplement the glycolytic lactate production (3) with more ATP-efficient mitochondrial fermentations that yield succinate (5), acetate (5) or propionate (7) (moles ATP/mole glycogen-derived glucosyl unit given in parentheses) [10–12,32]. As a final note on the importance of a reduced energy status, the extent of an animal's metabolic depression is known to be inversely related to the period of anoxic tolerance of it, i.e., animals with a lower ATP turnover during anoxia survive for longer [33,34]. Table 1 above is adopted from various seminal reports by the late Dr. P. Hochachka [35,36] in order to summarize this general comparison between selected strategies employed by hypoxia-tolerant versus hypoxia-sensitive models when facing prolonged periods of O_2 lacks.

3. HIF stimulates or inhibits gene expression in *Daphnia* and *Drosophila*

As pointed out above, gene silencing of ATP-costly cell functions is an essential aspect of hypoxia tolerance. One important discovery with relevance for a possible HIF contribution to confer hypoxic tolerance, is that HIF, once bound to DNA, can act either as transactivator ($\rightarrow$ gene induction) or -inactivator ($\rightarrow$ gene silencing). This functional duality of HIF was found to apply to the hypoxic expression of daphnid versus drosophilid globin genes [1,4]. Despite *Daphnia*'s tolerance toward *acute* anoxic stresses and strong anaerobic capacity (see above and [6]), a *gradual* decline in pO_2 over days rather than minutes–hours, will be met through the HIF-mediated induced transcription of several of its globin genes (notably hb2, see Fig. 1 below) once the active HIF α/β heterodimer has bound to multiple specific binding sites called HREs (hypoxia response elements) within the promoter of these genes [1]. *Daphnia* hemoglobin is a ~500 kDa 16-subunit extracellular oxygen carrier, with each these subunits containing not one, but two hemes [37]. Remarkably, oxygen acquisition in hypoxic daphnids improves because of increases not only in hemoglobin concentration but also in oxygen affinity (see Ref. [1] and references cited therein). On a systemic level, these adaptations benefit hemoglobin-rich animals with improved stress-tolerance by extending the pO_2 range of their aerobic and regulated metabolism down to critical oxygen tensions (pC) of ~1.3% oxygen, whereas pale animals begin to transition into anaerobiosis at pC's around 4.8% oxygen [38,39]. Consequentially, red animals show improved survival and reproduction rates, as well as enhanced O_2 consumption along with ameliorated acidosis compared to pale individuals [39]. *Daphnia*'s hemoglobin-supported extension of oxidative metabolism during low pO_2

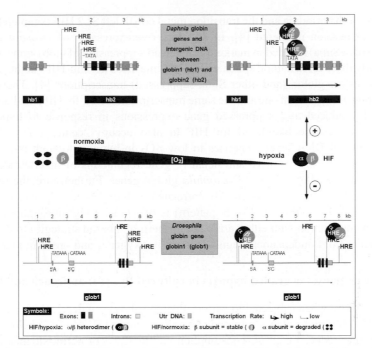

Fig. 1. HIF's dual function. The HIF complex is depicted as functional α/β heterodimer under hypoxic pO₂ where it either stimulates (*Daphnia* globin genes, top) or inhibits (*Drosophila* globin gene, bottom) the oxygen dependent expression of target genes through binding to specific cis elements (hypoxia response elements, HREs). Functional HIF-binding HREs are illustrated as determined in [1] for *Daphnia* globin 2 gene (hb2), but are hypothetical for *Drosophila* globin at this point. At normoxic tensions, the HIFα, but not the β, subunit is oxidatively modified, and subsequently degraded by the proteasome, thereby restricting any HIF action to low pO_2. Transcription of *Drosophila* globin (glob1) yields, in fly embryos, two mRNAs (A or C), initiated from two distinct promoters adjacent to respective 5′ utr exons (5′A or 5′C). See box at bottom for symbol explanation.

poses intriguing parallels to hypoxia-stimulated erythropoiesis and angiogenesis in mammals, which also serve to enhance O_2 delivery in times of need.

The recently discovered single-copy globin gene (glob1) of *Drosophila* encodes for a intracellular high O_2-affinity (P_{50}~0.1–0.2 Torr) hemoglobin in association with the tracheal system and the fat body of fly embryos, larvae and adults [40,41]. The gene is flanked by multiple HRE's (Fig. 1), yet steady-state levels of glob1 transcripts were found, in hypoxic cultures of SL2 cells from late fly embryos, not to be up-, but down-regulated [4]. Moreover, this silencing of glob1 expression correlated with differential stimulation of SL2 HIF activity by either hypoxia or various chemicals, which, in insect but not mammalian cells, result in the following distinctive levels of HIFα subunit stabilization [3,4]: hypoxia (H) > iron chelation (desferrioxamine, DFO) ≫ cobalt (Co)~normoxia (N) (stimuli are ranked from strong (H) to ineffective (Co, N)). In other words: glob1 expression was most severely suppressed when SL2 HIF was maximally active (H=1% oxygen), as judged by in vitro HRE binding assays. DFO treatment yielded moderate HIF activity and moderate inhibition of glob1, while both normoxia and the transition metal cobalt left SL2 HIF completely inactive and glob1 expression unaltered [4]. In addition, overexpression of *Drosophila*'s HIFα homologue (aka Sima) resulted in markedly enhanced suppression of glob1 transcript levels, while a newly discovered natural splice variant of Sima acted as 'anti-HIF' in that it was able to partially restore globin (and other Sima-suppressed) transcriptions [4]. These findings provide strong evidence that one and the same transcription factor, fly HIF, mediates, at least in SL2 cells, induced *and* suppressed gene expressions in response to hypoxia, and, therefore, increases the likelihood for HIF to also occupy 'center stage' during the reprogramming of DNA level responses to low pO_2 in hypoxia-tolerant models. Fig. 1 below summarizes these positive and negative gene regulations of invertebrate HIFs, as exemplified through *Daphnia* and *Drosophila* globin genes. Furthermore, the finding that differential SL2 HIF activity was directly correlated with expression changes of candidate target genes (i.e. H > DFO ≫ Co, N pattern) is of use as a high-throughput screening technique in conjunction with either array or Northern blot based strategies to discriminate HIF-dependent from -independent regulations of fly oxygenes and -genomes (see below).

4. Genomic responses to graded hypoxia in cultured fly cells: approach and highlights

Adult fruitflies, when subjected to various degrees of oxygen deprivation, start between pO_2's of 1.6–3.0% to develop a symptomatic anoxic stupor [7]. At pO_2's below this value (~1–1.5%), flies reduced their O_2-consumption rate to ~20% of normoxic measures [5,9]. Therefore, the 1.6–3.0% oxygen range corresponds, in good agreement with respiratory switches in other insect species [42–46], to the critical oxygen tension (pC) of adult D. melanogaster flies, below which the animals' aerobic metabolism ceases to be regulated and transition into anaerobiosis and metabolic depression occurs [5,7–9,47,48] (see above). In order to probe the genetic/genomic alterations behind this biochemical transition, we exposed cultured cells *Drosophila* from embryos (SL2) for 16 h to 4% (assumed oxyregulation sampling with $pO_2 > pC$), 1% (assumed aerobe/anaerobe transition sampling with $pO_2 \sim pC$), and 0.2% oxygen (assumed metabolic depression sampling, with $pO_2 < pC$). Normoxic SL2 (16 h/21% oxygen) were used as controls. RNA-derived cDNAs were synthesized in the presence of cyanine 5 (cy5—all three hypoxia categories) or cyanine 3 (cy3-normoxia) fluorophores. Three combinations of cDNA mixes (a: 4%/cy5+21%/cy3; b: 1%/cy5+21%/cy3; c: 0.2%/cy5+21%/cy3) were then used to each hybridize five replicates of *Drosophila* DNA arrays (manufactured at Harvard Medical School, Biopolymers Laboratory). Normalized and averaged ($n=5$) cy5/cy3 fluorescence ratios were calculated and used to detect either hypoxically induced (i.e. more mRNA/cDNA with cy 5 label, corresponding to: cy5 signal > cy3 signal) or -suppressed genes (i.e. more mRNA/cDNA with cy 3 label, corresponding to cy5 signal < cy3 signal). In addition, complete or partial cDNAs of 50 marker genes, predicted by the obtained cy5/cy3 ratio charts to either be strongly induced or suppressed by hypoxia, were cloned via reverse transcription-PCR in order to (a) validate their expression changes at 4, 1 and 0.2% oxygen, relative to normoxia, by an independent method (Northern blot), and (b) generate array (log2[cy5/cy3] ratios) versus Northern (log2[hypoxia/normoxia transcript level ratios]) regressions which allowed us to calculate the cy5/cy3-ratios in each hypoxia category that corresponded to at least a Northern-detected 2-fold change in expression (up-

or down-regulated). Since a complete presentation of our methodology and findings will be published elsewehere, I would now like to conclude this report by highlighting two results of relevance to the aforementioned discussion of metabolic strategies employed by hypoxia-tolerant organisms during periods of O_2 deprivation.

4.1. Glycolysis

The number (#) of hypoxically induced ($\geq$2-fold) glycolytic genes changed as follows as a function of pO_2: 4% O_2: #=1 gene (Lactate dehydrogenase, Ldh); 1% O_2: #=2 genes, (Ldh and Phosphofructokinase, Pfk); 0.2% O_2: #=6 genes (Ldh, Pfk, Glucose transporter homolog, Hexokinase A, Triosephosphate isomerase, Phosphoglucomutase). In accord with weak or even reverse Pasteur effects in insects (see above), fewer reactions are hypoxia-responsive in fly glycolysis (2–6) than they are in mammalian glycolysis (8–10). As judged by H > DFO ≫ Co, N patterns, HIF control was implicated in Ldh and Pfk transcription.

4.2. Protein synthesis and cell cycle progression

Evidence for the down-regulation at 1% and 0.2% (but not 4%) O_2 of both these ATP-costly cell functions was seen in HIF-mediated (H > DFO ≫ Co, N patterns) induction of translation repressor proteins as well as in the suppression of cell cycle maintenance factors.

HIF, therefore, appears to be critically important for conserving energy during periods of low pO_2 in hypoxia-tolerant models.

References

[1] T.A. Gorr, et al., J. Biol. Chem. 279 (2004) 36038–36047.
[2] S. Lavista-Llanos, et al., Mol. Cell. Biol. 22 (2002) 6842–6853.
[3] M. Nagao, et al., FEBS Lett. 387 (1996) 161–166.
[4] T.A. Gorr, et al., J. Biol. Chem. 279 (2004) 36048–36058.
[5] S.N. Krishnan, et al., J. Insect Physiol. 43 (1997) 203–210.
[6] R.J. Paul, et al., Comp. Biochem. Physiol., A 120 (1998) 519–530.
[7] L. Csik, Z. Vgl. Physiol. 27 (1939) 304–310.
[8] G.G. Haddad, J. Appl. Physiol. 88 (2000) 1481–1487.
[9] E. Ma, T. Xu, G.G. Haddad, Mol. Brain Res. 63 (1999) 217–224.
[10] M.K. Grieshaber, et al., Rev. Physiol., Biochem. Pharmacol. 125 (1994) 43–147.
[11] P.W. Hochachka, G.N. Somero, Oxford University Press, New York, 2002.
[12] P.W. Hochachka, et al., Proc. Natl. Acad. Sci. U. S. A. 93 (1996) 9493–9498.
[13] R.G. Boutilier, J. Exp. Biol. 204 (2001) 3171–3181.
[14] T.E. Duffy, S.R. Nelson, O.H. Lowry, J. Neurochem. 19 (1972) 959–977.
[15] L.T. Buck, S.C. Land, P.W. Hochachka, Am. J. Physiol. 265 (1993) R49–R56.
[16] R.K. Suarez, et al., Am. J. Physiol. 257 (1989) R1083–R1088.
[17] T.N. Seagroves, et al., Mol. Cell. Biol. 21 (2001) 3436–3444.
[18] G.L. Semenza, et al., J. Biol. Chem. 269 (1994) 23757–23763.
[19] G.L. Semenza, et al., J. Biol. Chem. 271 (1996) 32529–32537.
[20] B.L. Ebert, et al., Biochem. J. 313 (1996) 809–814.
[21] N.V. Iyer, et al., Genes Dev. 12 (1998) 149–162.
[22] G.L. Semenza, Curr. Opin. Genet. Dev. 8 (1998) 588–594.
[23] B.L. Ebert, H.F. Bunn, Blood 94 (1999) 1864–1877.
[24] K.A. Webster, J. Exp. Biol. 206 (2003) 2911–2922.
[25] K.B. Storey, Mol. Physiol. 8 (1985) 439–461.

[26] G. Krumschnabel, et al., J. Exp. Biol. 203 (2000) 951–959.
[27] D.F.S. Rolfe, G.C. Brown, Physiol. Rev. 77 (1997) 731–758.
[28] S.C. Land, L.T. Buck, P.W. Hochachka, Am. J. Physiol. 265 (1993) R41–R48.
[29] S.C. Land, P.W. Hochachka, Am. J. Physiol. 266 (1994) C1028–C1036.
[30] H. Schmidt, G. Kamp, Experientia 52 (1996) 440–448.
[31] G. Wegener, in: P.W. Hochachka, P.L. Lutz, T. Sick, M. Rosenthal, G. van den Thillart (Eds.), Surviving Hypoxia: Mechanisms of Control and Adaptation, CRC Press, Boca Raton, 1993, pp. 417–434.
[32] G. Wegener, in: H. Acker (Ed.), Oxygen Sensing in Tissues, Springer, Berlin, 1988, pp. 13–35.
[33] A. De Zwaan, V. Putzer, Symp. Soc. Exp. Biol. 39 (1985) 33–62.
[34] M. Guppy, P. Withers, Biol. Rev. 74 (1999) 1–40.
[35] P.W. Hochachka, Science 231 (1986) 234–241.
[36] P.W. Hochachka, Intensive Care Med. 12 (1986) 127–133.
[37] E. Ilan, E. Weisselberg, E. Daniel, J. Biochem. 207 (1982) 297–303.
[38] M. Kobayashi, T. Hoshi, Comp. Biochem. Physiol., A 72 (1982) 247–249.
[39] R. Pirow, C. Bäumer, R.J. Paul, J. Exp. Biol. 204 (2001) 3425–3441.
[40] T. Burmester, T. Hankeln, Mol. Biol. Evol. 16 (1999) 1809–1811.
[41] T. Hankeln, et al., J. Biol. Chem. 277 (2002) 29012–29017.
[42] R. Galun, Nature 185 (1960) 391–392.
[43] M. Keister, J. Buck, in: M. Rockstein (Ed.), The Physiology of Insecta, vol. 6, Academic Press, New York, 1974, pp. 469–509.
[44] S.M. Tenney, Respir. Physiol. 60 (1985) 121–134.
[45] C. Loudon, J. Insect Physiol. 34 (1988) 97–103.
[46] R. Arieli, C. Lehrer, J. Insect Physiol. 34 (1988) 325–328.
[47] L.E. Chadwick, D. Gilmour, Physiol. Zool. 13 (1940) 398–410.
[48] C. Loudon, J. Exp. Biol. 147 (1989) 217–235.

International Congress Series 1275 (2004) 63–70

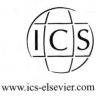

www.ics-elsevier.com

Adaptive mechanisms in mice constitutively overexpressing erythropoietin

Johannes Vogel*, Max Gassmann

Institute of Veterinary Physiology, Vetsuisse Faculty, University of Zürich, Switzerland

Abstract. Oxygen supply of mammalian tissues requires a sufficient number of red blood cells that is regulated by erythropoietin (Epo). Although extreme hematocrit values may result in threatening cardiovascular complications, some high altitude dwellers cope well with extreme hematocrit values. To investigate adaptive mechanisms to excessive erythrocytosis, we generated transgenic (tg6) mice that, due to constitutive expression of human Epo, reach hematocrit values around 0.85. Tg6 mice had signs of chronic heart failure (cardiac dilatation, increased central venous pressure) but normal blood pressure, heart rate and cardiac output. Plasma volume was unchanged, whereas blood volume was as much as 25% of the body weight in tg6 mice compared to 8% in wildtype (wt) siblings. While plasma viscosity did not differ between tg6 and wt, tg6 whole-blood viscosity increased to a lower degree (fourfold) than expected from correspondingly hemoconcentrated wt blood (eightfold) due to an up to threefold higher flexibility of tg6 erythrocytes. The fact that our tg6 mice show nitric oxide-mediated vasodilatation, too, implies different adaptive mechanisms acting in parallel to limit the strain on the heart in excessive erythrocytosis. However, these mechanisms appear to be exhausted already under normal conditions since tg6 mice are not able to compensate properly for exercise and have a reduced life expectancy. © 2004 Elsevier B.V. All rights reserved.

Keywords: Erythrocytosis; Polyglobulia; Nitric oxide; Blood viscosity; Erythrocyte flexibility

1. Introduction

In erythrocytosis (such as polycythemia vera, or paraneoplasic syndroms), chronic mountain sickness, as well as in lowlanders at high altitude and after Epo-abuse hematocrit

* Corresponding author. Tel.: +41 1 6358814; fax: +41 1 6358932.
E-mail address: jvogel@vetphys.unzh.ch (J. Vogel).

0531-5131/ © 2004 Elsevier B.V. All rights reserved.
doi:10.1016/j.ics.2004.08.091

is markedly elevated resulting in severe clinical complications such as hypertension and thromboembolism often leading to death [1]. However, some individuals can cope well with excessive erythrocytosis. For example, some Peruvian miners living and working at high altitude and being exposed to cobalt (known to induce erythropoietin (Epo) expression) have hematocrit levels of 0.75–0.91 [2,3] without major life threatening complications. Excessive erythrocytosis is also found in sports medicine: An endurance athlete with an autosomal dominant erythrocytosis resulting in hematocrit levels up to 0.68 has won several Olympic gold medals in the past [4]. Due to the lack of a suitable model, however, there is little data available on adaptive mechanisms to excessive erythrocytosis in vivo. Thus, we generated a transgenic (tg) mouse line that, due to oxygen independent overexpression of human erythropoietin, reaches hematocrit values up to 0.9 during the first 8–9 postnatal weeks [5,6].

Here, we report the adaptive mechanisms in our transgenic mice that have been discovered so far.

2. Basic characteristics of the transgenic Epo-overexpressing mouse

The transgenic mouse line was generated by pronuclear microinjection of the full-length human Epo cDNA driven by the human platelet-derived growth factor (PDGF) B-chain promotor as described [5]. The resulting transgenic mouse line TgN(PDGFBE-PO)321ZbZ (termed tg6) was bred by mating hemizygous males to wildtype (wt) C57Bl/6 females since transgenic females are infertile.

Table 1 summarizes the blood parameters and cardiovascular parameters measured in transgenic mice and wildtype siblings. Plasma Epo levels were about 12 times higher in tg6 mice compared to wt siblings. This resulted in almost doubling of the hematocrit values, hemoglobin concentration and reticulocyte counts. In transgenic mice the mean corpuscular volume (MCV) was significantly higher and the mean corpuscular hemoglobin concentration (MCHC) in tendency lower (not significant). Unexpectedly,

Table 1
Blood parameters and physiological values in wildtype and transgenic mice (mean±S.D., *$p<0.05$, **$p<0.01$, Student's *t*-test for independent samples) [5,7]

	Wildtype mice	Transgenic mice
Plasma Epo (U/L)	22.1±5.2	259±79**
Hematocrit (%)	43.1±3	87.8±2**
Red blood cell count (10^{12}/L)	6.2±0.5	13.8±1**
Hemoglobin (g/dL)	14±1	26±1**
Mean corpuscular volume (fL)	44.8±1.8	57.4±5.1*
Mean corpuscular hemoglobin concentration (g/dL)	33±2	29.9±3
Reticulocyte count (%)	1.7±0.6	3.4±1.6**
Mean arterial blood pressure (mm Hg)	99±12	100±7
Heart rate (min^{-1})	548±44	573±31
Cardiac output (ml/min)	17.2±3.2	14.5±6.9
Central venous pressure (mm Hg)	3.9±0.8	6.6±0.9**
Blood volume (ml)	1.99±0.45	5.6±0.31**
Plasma volume (ml)	1.2±0.2	1.1±0.3

blood pressure and heart rate was not elevated. Cardiac output has been measured with three different methods, using an ultrasonic flow probe placed around the ascendant aorta after median sternotomy [5], non-invasively by echocardiography [6] and with an indicator dilution method [7]. All three methods revealed no significant differences between tg6 and wt mice. The lowest average values were measured with the first method, the open chest preparation [5], most probably due to the operation stress itself. Both other methods revealed similar mean values. The indicator dilution method however revealed a much higher scatter of the measurements in transgenic mice, since in those mice with the most extreme hematocrit values cardiac output was lowest. The elevation of the central venous pressure, also measured by two independent researchers [6,7], indicates a congestive heart failure in line with an about 50% larger systolic diameter and a 25% reduced fractional shortening of the left ventricle [6]. Blood volume was nearly doubled in the transgenic mice, basically due to the increased red blood cell mass since the plasma volume was not altered by Epo-overexpression [6,7].

3. NO-mediated chronic vasodilatation

The most significant problem for the tg6 mice is the fact that the increased hematocrit results in an increased total peripheral resistance (TPR), which is mainly determined by the radius of the vessels and the blood viscosity. TPR also depends on the length of the vasculature which is anatomically fixed and cannot be regulated like blood vessel radius or blood viscosity. Based on this knowledge, we investigated the impact of NO and blood viscosity as possible adaptive mechanisms.

In situ hybridisation and immunohistochemical analysis showed about three- to sixfold increased endothelial nitric oxide synthase (eNOS) expression exclusively confined to the endothelium of large transgenic arterial vessels such as the aorta and pulmonary artery. Keeping in mind that an increased expression of eNOS not necessarily means an increased NO production, since eNOS can be regulated post-translational [8–10] and possesses an autoinhibitory NO-dependent negative feedback mechanism [11], we also assessed the NO production of the vessel walls. Circulating nitrate (stable end product of endogenous NO oxidation) levels as well as nitrate levels in the aorta and pulmonary artery were markedly increased in tg6 mice [5]. Of note, the increased plasma NO levels could be measured despite the high levels of hemoglobin which might scavenge NO in vivo [12,13]. These results demonstrate a higher bioavailability of NO in the tg6 mice.

Functional relevance of the enhanced NO production was proven by two additional experiments, measurement of the NO-mediated endothelium dependent relaxation of aortic rings and by adding of the NOS inhibitor N^G-nitro-L-arginine methyl ester (L-NAME) to the drinking water (Fig. 1).

NO-mediated endothelium-dependent relaxation was markedly increased in transgenic mice as depicted in Fig. 1 (left panel). These findings indicate a chronic NO-dependent general vasodilatation in tg6 mice and an increased vascular NO bioavailability. Alterations in the response of the smooth muscle cells could be excluded since endothelium-independent vasodilatation using an exogenous NO donor (sodium nitroprusside) was not different between wt and tg6 mice.

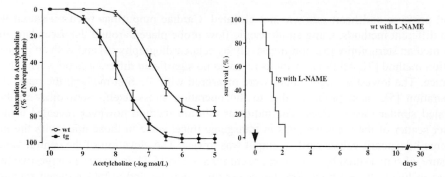

Fig. 1. Enhanced NO-dependent relaxation of aortic rings in tg6 mice (left panel) and its biological effect as adaptive mechanism (right panel). Left panel: Acetylcholine-mediated relaxation of aortic rings previously contracted with norepinephrine (precontraction did not differ between tg6 and wt mice) is increased in tg6 mice. Half-maximal response to acetylcholine (expressed as negative logarithm): 8.36 ± 0.1 vs. 7.43 ± 0.1, $p<0.0001$; area under the curve: 153 ± 10 vs. 283 ± 18, $p<0.0001$; maximal relaxation: -97.5 ± 3.3 vs. -76.8 ± 3.4, $p<0.001$ (mean$\pm$SEM, tg6 vs. wt). Right panel: Toxic effect of L-NAME added to the drinking water (arrow) in tg6 mice. All tg6 mice died within 52 h, whereas wt mice do not increase mortality.

To further prove the importance of the increased bioavailability of NO in vivo, L-NAME was added to the drinking water. Wt mice showed an increase of the systolic blood pressure from 118 ± 3 to 170 ± 3 mm Hg but appeared otherwise healthy. In contrast, all tg6 died within 52 h after adding L-NAME to their drinking water (Fig. 1, right panel). In analogy to wt mice, tg6 mice also increased initially systolic blood pressure after L-NAME administration but then blood pressure rapidly dropped followed by a circulatory breakdown most probably due to a congestive left ventricular failure.

Of note, the expression of endothelin-1 (ET-1), a potent vasoconstrictor, was two- to fivefold increased in larger vessels of tg6 mice. However, aortic rings of tg6 mice exhibited a markedly reduced reactivity to ET-1 compared to wt littermates, an effect that was abrogated by pre-treatment with L-NAME or de-endothelialization. In line with these findings, the survival time of tg6 mice after adding L-NAME to their drinking water could be doubled using the ET_A receptor antagonist darusentan [14]. This study demonstrated for the first time that in excessive erythrocytosis the tissue endothelin system is activated despite enhanced bioavailability of NO.

4. Blood viscosity is regulated in tg6 mice

Next to the chronic NO-mediated vasodilatation of the tg6 mice, we hypothesized that regulation of blood viscosity could be an additional adaptive mechanism in tg6 mice.

The results of the blood and plasma viscosity measurements are shown in Fig. 2. As expected, the viscosity of tg6 blood was much higher compared to wt blood. However, compared to wt blood concentrated to the same hematocrit found in tg6 mice, the viscosity of tg6 blood was only half (Fig. 2, left panel). Since plasma viscosity (Fig. 2, upper right panel) and plasma protein composition (Fig. 2, lower right panel) did not differ between

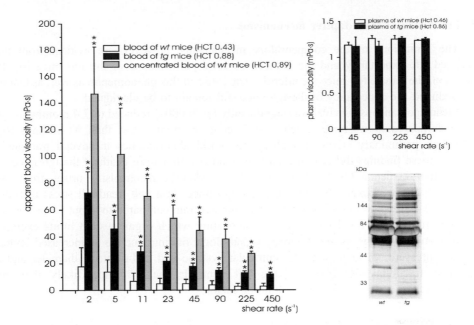

Fig. 2. Blood and plasma viscosity of tg6 and wt mice. Left panel: Tg6 blood was four times as viscous as normal wt blood but only half as viscous as hemoconcentrated wt blood reaching the same hct as tg6 blood. Plasma viscosity (upper right panel) and plasma protein pattern (lower right panel, SDS–PAGE) was the same in tg6 and wt mice. **$p < 0.01$.

both mouse lines, it appeared likely that the lower than expected viscosity of tg6 blood is associated with the tg6 erythrocytes. Indeed, we found an up to threefold higher flexibility of the tg6 erythrocytes compared to wt red blood cells (Fig. 3) which is most probably due to the increased MCV and a higher percentage of juvenile erythrocytes in tg6 mice. Both an increased MCV and a higher percentage of juvenile erythrocytes (proven by an increased reticulocyte count, cf. Table 1) are known to increase erythrocyte flexibility [15,16].

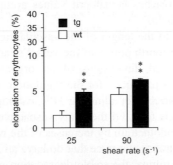

Fig. 3. Ektacytometry of tg6 and wt erythrocytes at physiological shear rates. Tg6 erythrocytes were up to three times more elongable at shear rates similar to those found in the vasculature in vivo (11.5–115 s^{-1} [17]). Moreover, enhanced elongation of tg6 erythrocytes was also observed at the maximal experimental shear rate (2500 s^{-1}, not shown) that can be applied without damaging the red blood cells. **$p < 0.01$.

5. Limitation of the adaptive mechanisms

The limitations of the compensatory mechanisms, however, are evident from the reduced life expectancy and the reduced exercise performance of the tg6 mice [6]. In addition, the female tg6 mice are infertile. The cause of this phenomenon as well as that of the reduced life expectancy of the tg6 mice still remain to be elucidated.

Mean spontaneous survival was significantly ($p < 0.0001$) reduced to 7.4 months in tg6 mice compared to wt mice which is in average 6 months less than wt siblings [6]. Although preliminary studies revealed histological abnormalities in several transgenic organs, these findings did not univocally explain the premature death of the tg6 mice.

Another evidence for the limitation of the adaptive mechanisms arises from the drastically reduced exercise performance in tg6 mice. In a belt treadmill stress test, the time until exhaustion in tg6 mice was only about 10 min compared to about 75 min in wt siblings [6]. We do not have direct data indicating which organ system limits exercise performance in the tg6 mice but numerous pathologic findings such as an increased central venous pressure, an increased left ventricular systolic and end-diastolic diameter and a reduced fractional shortening of the left ventricle make it very likely that the cardiovascular system is one major limiting factor.

6. Discussion

Red blood cells are essential for the oxygen transport to the tissues and more red blood cells, at the first glance, appear to improve oxygen delivery and thus efficiency of peripheral tissues—an idea that resulted in Epo-doping in human athletes. However, blood viscosity increases exponentially with the number of red blood cells leading to massive strain on the heart, blood cell aggregation and subsequently reduced tissue perfusion. As a consequence, oxygen supply of the tissues might be threateningly lowered or even collapsed. However, in situations where the organism is faced with reduced availability of oxygen, e.g., during high altitude habitation or in lung disease, there is no other possibility than increasing the number of red blood cells to maintain the oxygen supply of peripheral tissues. Additional adaptive mechanisms might therefore be mandatory to control the raise of the TPR as a side effect of the increased blood viscosity. Our erythropoietin overexpressing mouse that reaches hematocrit values around 0.85 is an ideal model to study such adaptive mechanisms.

The TPR is proportional to the length of the vasculature and the blood viscosity and inversely proportional to the fourth power of the vessel's radius (Hagen–Poiseuille law). Due to the anatomically fixed dimensions of an organism, the total length of the vasculature is static and not a parameter for the regulation of the TPR. The radius of the vessels, the most effective variable for adjusting TPR, can rapidly be changed by variation of the vascular smooth muscle tone. Of the many vasoactive factors, nitric oxide (NO) is released from the vascular endothelium by increases of the wall shear stress that increases with blood viscosity. In our transgenic mice that do have an increased blood viscosity, the plasma levels of nitrite and nitrate, the stable degradation products of NO are markedly elevated indicating a chronically increased NO production. This is in line with the higher tissue levels of endothelial NO synthase in transgenic arteries, the increased NO-mediated endothelium-dependent relaxation of aortic rings and the fact that the NO synthase inhibitor L-NAME, when added to the drinking water, is toxic to tg6 mice. These results clearly demonstrate that one adaptive mechanism to extreme erythrocytosis is NO-mediated chronic vasodilatation.

As an additional adaptive mechanism, a lower than expected blood viscosity could be detected; tg6 blood was four times as viscous as wt blood but only half as viscous as wt blood hemoconcentrated to hematocrit values similar to those found in tg6 mice. Since plasma viscosity and plasma protein composition was the same in tg6 and wt mice the unexpected low blood viscosity appeared to be connected somehow to the red blood cells. Indeed, at physiological shear rates erythrocytes from tg6 mice were up to three times more flexible than wt red blood cells. To elucidate the reason for this higher flexibility of tg6 erythrocytes, we had a look at reticulocyte counts, MCV and MCHC. All these parameters determine the flexibility of the red blood cells. An increased number of reticulocytes, as we have measured in our tg6 mice, is indicative for a higher percentage of juvenile erythrocytes which are known to be more deformable [16]. A higher MCV, also measured in our tg6 mice, is as well associated with a higher red blood cell flexibility [18]. The internal viscosity of erythrocytes is mainly determined by the MCHC, e.g., a lower MCHC is associated with a higher flexibility of the erythrocytes. In our tg6 mice the MCHC tended to be reduced although this observation did not reach statistical significance. To summarize, all these erythrocyte parameters were changed in the way to explain the increased erythrocyte flexibility.

Our transgenic mice overexpressing human Epo gain hematocrit values as high as 0.85 during the first 3 months of life. They are an excellent model to study adaptive mechanisms to excessive erythrocytosis that occurs in humans, e.g., in severe respiratory disease or in high altitude dwellers. At least two adaptive mechanisms might act in parallel in our tg6 mice to limit the strain on the heart resulting from the increased TPR as a consequence of the increased blood viscosity. First, rise in TPR is restricted by a chronic vasodilatation due to continuous overproduction of NO. Withdrawal of this mechanism by adding L-NAME to the drinking water is lethal for the transgenic mice. Second, increase in blood viscosity as a result of the excessive hematocrit is only fourfold and not eightfold as expected from measurements in wt blood concentrated to hematocrit values similar to those of tg6 mice. This unexpected low increase of blood viscosity is most probably due to an increased flexibility of the tg6 erythrocytes which might be caused by an increased population of juvenile erythrocytes and a slightly increased MCV. Whether or not these adaptations to excessive erythrocytosis found in tg6 mice are general physiological mechanisms and if they can be utilized for therapeutic interventions remains to be elucidated by future research.

Acknowledgements

This work was supported by grants from the Roche Foundation, the Käthe Zingg-Schwichtenberg Fonds, the Stiftung für wissenschaftliche Forschung an der Universität Zürich, the EMDO-Stiftung, the Swiss National Science Foundation, the Forschungs-förderungsprogramm of the University of Heidelberg and the Deutsche Forschungs-gemeinschaft.

References

[1] G. Bertinieri, et al., Hemodilution reduces clinic and ambulatory blood pressure in polycythemic patients, Hypertension 3 (31) (1998) 848–853.

[2] R.B. Santolaya, et al., Respiratory adaptation in the highest inhabitants and highest Sherpa mountaineers, Respir. Physiol. 2 (77) (1989) 253–262.

[3] J.A. Jefferson, et al., Excessive erythrocytosis, chronic mountain sickness, and serum cobalt levels, Lancet 9304 (359) (2002) 407–408.

[4] E. Juvonen, et al., Autosomal dominant erythrocytosis caused by increased sensitivity to erythropoietin, Blood 11 (78) (1991) 3066–3069.

[5] F.T. Ruschitzka, et al., Nitric oxide prevents cardiovascular disease and determines survival in polyglobulic mice overexpressing erythropoietin, Proc. Natl. Acad. Sci. U. S. A. 21 (97) (2000) 11609–11613.

[6] K.F. Wagner, et al., Chronic inborn erythrocytosis leads to cardiac dysfunction and premature death in mice overexpressing erythropoietin, Blood 2 (97) (2001) 536–542.

[7] J. Vogel, et al., Transgenic mice overexpressing erythropoietin adapt to excessive erythrocytosis by regulating blood viscosity, Blood 6 (102) (2003) 2278–2284.

[8] T. Michel, O. Feron, Nitric oxide synthases: which, where, how, and why? J. Clin. Invest. 9 (100) (1997) 2146–2152.

[9] M.A. Corson, et al., Phosphorylation of endothelial nitric oxide synthase in response to fluid shear stress, Circ. Res. 5 (79) (1996) 984–991.

[10] G. Garcia-Cardena, et al., Dynamic activation of endothelial nitric oxide synthase by Hsp90, Nature 6678 (392) (1998) 821–824.

[11] H.M. Abu-Soud, et al., Neuronal nitric oxide synthase self-inactivates by forming a ferrous-nitrosyl complex during aerobic catalysis, J. Biol. Chem. 39 (270) (1995) 22997–23006.

[12] A.J. Gow, et al., The oxyhemoglobin reaction of nitric oxide, Proc. Natl. Acad. Sci. U. S. A. 16 (96) (1999) 9027–9032.

[13] A.J. Gow, J.S. Stamler, Reactions between nitric oxide and haemoglobin under physiological conditions, Nature 6663 (391) (1998) 169–173.

[14] T. Quaschning, et al., Erythropoietin-induced excessive erythrocytosis activates the tissue endothelin system in mice, FASEB J. 2 (17) (2003) 259–261.

[15] N.S. Hill, G.L. Sardella, L.C. Ou, Reticulocytosis, increased mean red cell volume, and greater blood viscosity in altitude susceptible compared to altitude resistant rats, Respir. Physiol. 2 (70) (1987) 229–240.

[16] W. Tillmann, et al., Rheological properties of young and aged human erythrocytes, Klin. Wochenschr. 11 (58) (1980) 569–574.

[17] A.J. Erslev, J. Caro, A. Besarab, Why the kidney? Nephron 3 (41) (1985) 213–216.

[18] T. Shiga, N. Maeda, K. Kon, Erythrocyte rheology, Crit. Rev. Oncol. Hematol. 1 (10) (1990) 9–48.

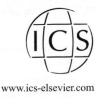

www.ics-elsevier.com

Hypoxic stabilization and proteolytic degradation of erythroid-specific 5-aminolevulinate synthase

Mohamed Abu-Farha, William G. Willmore*

Institute of Biochemistry, Carleton University, Ottawa, Ontario, Canada

Abstract. Eukaryotes have acquired a broad range of post-translational modifications to place controls and checks on metabolic pathways. Included among these is hydroxylation. Hydroxylases catalyze the oxygen-, iron (II)-, ascorbate- and 2-oxoglutarate-dependent hydroxylation of protein substrates. Until recently, few studies examined hydroxylation as a post-translational modification, focusing primarily on hydroxylation of structural proteins such as collagen and elastin. With the discovery of hydroxylase-dependent destabilization of transcription factors, the role of hydroxylation in gene expression has renewed the interest in these enzymes. The paramount example of this is the hydroxylation of the transcription factor involved in hypoxic-inducible gene expression, Hypoxia-Inducible Factor-1 (HIF-1). The possibility exists that other proteins are hydroxylated in a manner similar to HIF-1 and are degraded and/or have altered enzymatic activities. These proteins may be involved in pathways that maintain oxygen homeostasis. A database search of potential targets of HIF-1 prolyl hydroxylases has revealed erythroid-specific 5-aminolevulinate synthase (ALAS2). Here we provide evidence that ALAS2 is broken down under normoxic conditions by the proteosome and that the prolyl-4-hydroxylase/E3 ubiquitin ligase pathway may be involved. The implications to oxygen sensing are discussed. © 2004 Published by Elsevier B.V.

Keywords: Hypoxia; Hydroxylation; Hydroxylases; E3 ubiquitin ligases; Erythroid-specific 5-aminolevulinate synthase; von Hippel-Lindau protein; Proteosomal degradation; Protein–protein interactions

1. Introduction

Organisms encounter low oxygen conditions (hypoxia) under a variety of physiological and pathological conditions. These include environmental conditions such as high altitude,

* Corresponding author. Tel.: +1 613 520 2600x1211; fax: +1 613 520 3539.
E-mail address: Bill_Willmore@carleton.ca (W.G. Willmore).

0531-5131/ © 2004 Published by Elsevier B.V.
doi:10.1016/j.ics.2004.08.073

diving, hibernation and intensive exercise as well as ischemic clinical conditions such as cardiac arrest, stroke, and chronic lung disease. Managing oxygen demand in relation to oxygen supply remains the fundamental challenge to surviving hypoxia. Oxygen-dependent organisms have therefore evolved a wide range of cellular responses to adapt to changes in oxygen availability.

The cellular response to hypoxia is characterized by changes in gene expression and protein function. These changes may be in response to either acute (intermittent) or chronic (sustained) exposure to hypoxia. A key regulator of hypoxia-inducible gene expression is Hypoxia-Inducible Factor-1 (HIF-1). HIF-1 is a heterodimeric tran-scription factor that binds to a Hypoxia Response Element, an 8-bp consensus sequence (5'-TACGTGCT-3') found in the promoters or enhancers of hypoxia-inducible genes (for recent reviews, see Refs. [1–7]). HIF-1 is composed of an α and a β subunit. The level of functional HIF-1 heterodimer in the cell is directly controlled by the amount of ambient oxygen present. The β subunit of the heterodimer is constitutively stable and is present in the cell under both normoxic and hypoxic conditions. The α subunit, however, is rapidly ubiquitinated and degraded by the proteosome in normoxia.

The oxygen sensitivity of HIF-1 α was a subject of intensive study in recent years. It was found that HIF-1 α contains two oxygen regulatory sequences (LXXLAP, where L is leucine, A is alanine, P is proline, and X is any amino acid) which, when deleted, renders the protein stable under normoxic conditions [8–12]. Hydroxylation of the prolines in these regulatory motifs promotes recognition of HIF-1 α by the von Hippel-Lindau (vHL) tumor suppressor protein [13]. vHL forms the substrate recognition subunit of a much larger complex that functions as an E3 ubiquitin ligase [14,15]. The binding of vHL to hydroxylated HIF-1 α results in its rapid ubiquitination by the E3 ubiquitin ligase and degradation by the proteosome. vHL neither recognizes nor binds to non-hydroxylated HIF-1α, allowing HIF-1α to travel to the nucleus, dimerize with HIF-1β and activate transcription. The regulation of HIF-1 by oxygen tension provides an elegant means of regulating hypoxic gene expression.

With the discovery of the mechanisms by which HIF-1 is regulated by oxygen, renewed interest in hydroxylation as a post-translational modification has occurred. Previous studies focused (a) on the hydroxylation of structural proteins, such as collagen, (b) the synthesis of catecholamines and neurotransmitters and (c) the metabolism of Vitamin D and steroid hormones by hydroxylases. With the new role of hydroxylases in transcrip-tional regulation, identification of other targets of hydroxylases will become the focus of future studies.

Protein targets of hydroxylases may be involved in hypoxia-inducible, but HIF-1-independent, metabolic pathways. As with HIF-1 α, hydroxylation may result in ubiquitination and proteolytic degradation of the modified protein, or it may result in more subtle alterations, such as changes in enzyme kinetics. The lack of hydroxylation under hypoxic conditions may convert inactive proteins to their active state. As a post-translational modification, hydroxylation may be as important as phosphorylation/dephosphorylation control of protein function under hypoxic conditions.

A database search for the LXXLAP sequence within proteins has revealed a number of potential candidates that could be recognized by the vHL E3 ubiquitin ligase in various eukaryotes. The present study describes one such protein, erythroid-specific 5-amino-levulinate synthase (ALAS2), which may be hydroxylated and degraded under normoxic conditions. ALAS1 is ubiquitous to all cells and catalyzes the rate-limiting step of heme synthesis for cytochromes and heme containing enzymes. ALAS2 catalyzes the first step of heme synthesis specifically for hemoglobin. Playing a key role in oxygen delivery to tissues, ALAS2 may be regulated in an oxygen-dependent manner in erythroid cells.

2. Materials and methods

2.1. Database search for LXXLAP

SWISS-PROT and TrEMBL databases were searched for proteins containing the LXXLAP subsequence and the results were sorted using a PERL-based algorithm. Proteins were grouped according to identity, number of species the protein appeared in and possible involvement in oxygen-sensing pathways.

2.2. Chemicals and cell culture

All chemicals were purchased from Sigma (St. Louis, MO) with the exception of the kits listed below. Human chronic myelogenous leukemia cells (K562) were purchased from the American Type Culture Collection (Manassas, VA) and maintained in Iscove's Modified Dulbecco's Medium supplemented with 10% fetal calf serum, 100 Units/ml penicillin, 100 µg/ml streptomycin and 0.25 mg/ml amphotercin B. Cultures were maintained at 1×10^6 cells/ml at 37 °C and 5% CO_2 in humidified tissue culture incubator (Thermo Forma, Marietta, OH). Erythroid differentiation of K562 cells was induced with sodium butyrate (NaBu; 1.5 mM) for 24 h. Cells were treated with hypoxia (1% O_2) using a triple-gas incubator (Thermo Forma) and anoxia using an anaerobic chamber (10 L) with AnaeroGEN anaerobic generation systems and BR55 oxygen indicator (Oxoid, Nepean, Ontario).

2.3. Reverse transcriptase-polymerase chain reaction (RT-PCR), cloning and site-directed mutagenesis

Total RNA was extracted from K562 cells using RNeasy kit (Qiagen, Missisauga, Ontario). RT-PCR was performed using 1 µg of total RNA and the Access RT-PCR System (Promega, Madison, Wisconsin). Oligonucleotides used for RT-PCR are mature ALAS2 forward with FLAG and BamHI site: 5′-TGTGGATCCATGGACTACAAGGACGAC-GATGACAAACATATGCAAATCCACCTTAAGGCAAC-3′ and ALAS2 reverse with EcoRI: 5′-TTAGGCTGAATTCAGCTAGAGGCACACAA-3′.

PCR products were TOPO-cloned into pCR2.1, and digested with BamHI/EcoRI. The insert was ligated into pCR3.1 using T4 DNA ligase. After transformation and isolation of plasmids, constructs were screened for FLAG using Hpy99I digestion and sequenced for proper insert orientation and full length. Proline 520 of the premature form of ALAS2 was mutated to alanine using the QuikChange Site-Directed Mutagenesis Kit from Stratagene (La Jolla, CA) according to the manufacturer's protocol.

2.4. ALAS2 enzyme assay

The enzymatic activity of ALAS2 was measured in K562 cells using Cary 100 spectrophotometers (Varian, Victoria, Australia) at 30 °C over a period of 5 min. The assay measures the reduction of NAD^+ to NADH at 340 nm. The reaction mixture contained 20 mM HEPES, pH 7.2, 1 mM α-ketoglutarate, 1 mM NAD^+, 3 mM $MgCl_2$, 0.25 mM thiamine pyrophosphate, 100 mM glycine, 20 μM succinyl-CoA, 0.25 Units α-ketoglutarate dehydrogenase. Cells were homogenized in 20 mM HEPES, pH 7.2. PMSF was added to inhibit protease activity. The reaction was initiated with the addition of cell lysate. Protein concentration was determined according to the method described by Bradford [16] using bovine serum albumin as a standard. One unit of enzyme activity is defined as the activity to convert 1 nmol of substrate to product per hour at 30 °C.

2.5. Protein synthesis inhibition

K562 cells were treated with a wide range of cyclohexamide (CHX) (0.01–20 μg/ml of media) to test the toxicity of CHX on the K562 cells. The CHX solutions are made in DMSO. Viability was determined using a tetrazolium dye assay.

2.6. Transient transfection

The transfection of K562 cells was done using Lipofectamine 2000 (Invitrogen, Burlington, Ontario). The transfection was done in a 24-well plate over 48 h. The optimal concentration of DNA was found to be 1.2 μg of DNA/0.5 ml of K562 cells suspended at 1.2×10^6 cells/ ml.

2.7. Western blot analysis

After transfection, K562 cells were harvested by centrifugation and then washed twice with cold PBS (20 mM phosphate-buffered saline, pH 7.4) and lysed using cell lysis buffer (PBS containing 1% NP40, 0.5% sodium deoxycholate, 0.1% SDS, and 0.01% protease inhibitor cocktail). Five micrograms of crude protein from the different treatments was boiled in Laemmli sample buffer, subjected to electrophoresis in a 10% polyacrylamide gel, and the proteins were transferred to a nitrocellulose membrane. Western blot analysis for ALAS2 was performed with monoclonal HRP-labeled mouse anti-FLAG M2 antibodies (1:2000 dilution) and for β-tubulin was performed with a monoclonal antibody against β-tubulin (1:2000 dilution) and an HRP-labeled anti-mouse IgG antibody (1:5000 dilution) (Fig. 1).

```
                                        LXXLAP
Human ALAS2           509 VPRGEELLRLAPSPHHSP 526
Rat ALAS2             509 VPRGEELLRLAPSPHHSP 526
Mouse ALAS2          509 VPRGEELLRLAPSPHHSP 526
Beluga Whale ALAS2   504 VPRGEELLRLAPSPHHSP 521
Zebrafish ALAS2      504 VPRGEELLRLAPSPFHNP 521

Human ALAS1          563 VPRGEELLRIAPTPHHTP 580
Rat ALAS1            565 VPRGEELLRIAPTPHHTP 582
Mouse ALAS1          564 VPRGEELLRIAPTPHHTP 581
Beluga Whale ALAS1   563 VRRGEELLRIAPTPHHTP 580
Zebrafish ALAS1      536 VARGEELLRIAPTPHHTP 553

Drosophila ALAS      459 VARGQEKLRLAPTPFHTF 576
```

Fig. 1. Multiple alignment of ALAS2 and ALAS1 amino acid sequences from multiple organisms showing conservation of the LXXLAP sequence in ALAS2 but not ALAS1.

3. Results

3.1. Down regulation of ALAS1 activity in undifferentiated K562 cells

Differentiation of the K562 cells with NaBu induces the expression of the erythroid specific form of ALAS2. The activity of ALAS was measured before and after chemical induction of differentiation by NaBu. Hypoxic treatment of K562 cells for 24 h diminished the enzyme activity ALAS1. ALAS1 activity was also measured in K562 treated with 10 μM of proteosome inhibitor also reduced the activity of ALAS1 to about 60% compared to normoxia (Fig. 2A).

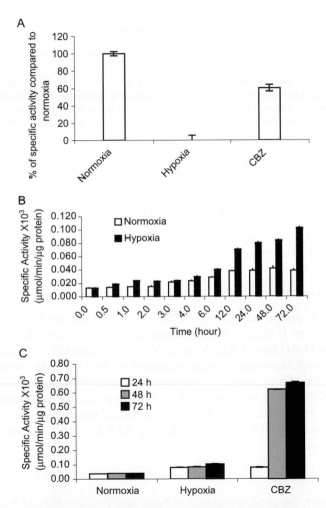

Fig. 2. Enzyme activity of ALAS under different treatments. (A) Activity of ALAS1 in undifferentiated K562 cells treated for 24 h with normoxia, hypoxia and proteosome inhibitor (CBZ). (B) ALAS2 activity in K562 cells under normoxia and hypoxia over 72-h time course treatment after induction of differentiation with 1.5 mM NaBu. (C) ALAS2 activity from K562 cells after 24-, 48- and 72-h treatment with normoxia, hypoxia and CBZ after induction of differentiation with 1.5 mM NaBu.

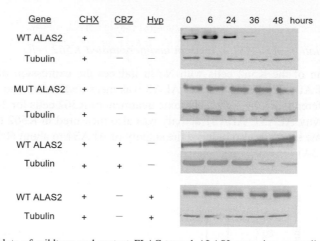

Fig. 3. Western blots of wildtype and mutant FLAG-tagged ALAS2 over time normalized to tubulin gene expression. K562 cells were transiently transfected with mammalian expression vectors containing wildtype or mutant ALAS2 constructs and treated with normoxia (21% oxygen), hypoxia (Hyp) (1% oxygen) or proteosome inhibitor (CBZ) (10 μM). Protein synthesis was inhibited using cyclohexamide (CHX) (0.05 mg/ml).

3.2. Increase of enzyme activity of ALAS2 in differentiated K562 cells under hypoxia

It is assumed that the enzyme activity after differentiation is caused by the increased expression of the erythroid specific form of ALAS2. In general, ALAS2 showed an increase in activity after differentiation with NaBu (Fig. 2B). The enzyme activity under hypoxia increased about two-fold over the 72-h treatment of hypoxia compared to normoxia (Fig. 2B). The biggest change occurred during proteosome inhibition where the activity increased from 2- to 25-fold compared to normoxia (Fig. 2C).

3.3. ALAS2 protein profile

ALAS2 protein profile was studied by transiently transfection FLAG-tagged mature ALAS2, mature form is missing the mitochondria localizing sequence. Fig. 3 shows the Western blots of FLAG tagged ALAS2 under different treatments after inhibiting protein synthesis using cyclohexamide. Protein expression of ALAS2 under normoxia starts to decrease after 24 h of treatment with cyclohexamide and diminishes after 48 h of CHX treatment. ALAS2 protein was stabilized by both hypoxia and proteosome inhibition. Mutation of the proline site in the LXXLAP sequence also caused the stabilization of ALAS2 under normoxia after treatment with CHX. ALAS2 expression was normalized to β tubulin expression.

4. Discussion

ALAS catalyzes the rate-limiting step of heme synthesis in cells. ALAS exists in two forms, the housekeeping enzyme ALAS1 present in all tissues and the erythroid-specific ALAS2 responsible for heme synthesis for hemoglobin. Interest in the ALAS2 gene is driven by the fact that deficiency of ALAS2 leads various types of X-linked sideroblastic anemias.

Differentiation switches the major cellular form of ALAS from ALAS1 to ALAS2 in K562. Differentiation was confirmed in K562 by measuring heme content of cells [data not shown]. Prior to differentiation, hypoxia decreased ALAS1 activity. The specific activity of ALAS2 was greatly increased by both hypoxia and proteosome inhibition, especially after 48 h of both treatments.

The increase in hypoxia may be due partially to the increase in ALAS2 gene expression. Previous studies found the ALAS2 gene to be induced by hypoxia in a HIF-1-independent manner [17]. Our transient transfection studies utilized CHX to inhibit translation, removing the influences of increased ALAS2 gene expression during hypoxia. Over-expression of wildtype recombinant FLAG-tagged ALAS2 in K562 resulted in protein turnover after 36 h. Hypoxia and proteosome inhibition resulted in stabilization of recombinant ALAS2 beyond 36 h. Mutation of the key proline in the LXXLAP subsequence of ALAS2 also stabilized the protein under normoxia. This evidence suggests that ALAS2 is hydroxylated under normoxic conditions and is subsequently ubiquitinated by vHL E3 ubiquitin ligase.

Hydroxylation may play a broad role in HIF-1-independent responses to hypoxia. Hydroxylation, under normoxic conditions, may alter the activities of enzymes, transcription factors, receptors, etc. involved in pathways that maintain oxygen homeostasis. In organisms adapted to survive chronic hypoxic exposure, this may also include pathways involved in metabolic arrest. A general strategy utilized by hypoxia-tolerant organisms is to have a general suppression of protein synthesis in the face of decreased ATP turnover [18]. Control would therefore have to target the basal transcription/translation machinery. A recent study [19] has shown that the hyperphosphorylated form of the major subunit of RNA polymerase II, RPB1, is hydroxylated by the HIF-1 α prolyl hydroxylase and is ubiquitinated by the vHL E3 ubiquitin ligase. RPB1 contains the HIF-1 α LXXLAP motif. Hyperphosphorylated RPB1 disappears rapidly from hypoxic cells and the role of phosphorylation in RPB1 hydroxylation remains to be elucidated. Further studies may reveal other proteins regulated in a similar fashion that are involved in maintaining oxygen homeostasis.

Acknowledgments

This research is supported by Discovery Operating and Equipment grants from Natural Sciences and Engineering Research Council (NSERC) of Canada, New Opportunities grants from the Canadian Foundation for Innovation (CFI) and the Ontario Innovation Trust (OIT), and an Institutional Development grant from the Canadian Institutes of Health Research (CIHR).

References

[1] G. Semenza, Signal transduction to hypoxia-inducible factor 1, Biochem. Pharmacol. 64 (2002) 993–998.

[2] R.H. Wenger, Cellular adaptation to hypoxia: O_2-sensing protein hydroxylases, hypoxia-inducible transcription factors, and O_2-regulated gene expression, FASEB J. 16 (2002) 1151–1162.

[3] R.K. Bruick, Oxygen sensing in the hypoxic response pathway: regulation of the hypoxia-inducible transcription factor, Genes Dev. 17 (2003) 2614–2623.

[4] N. Masson, P.J. Ratcliffe, HIF prolyl and asparaginyl hydroxylases in the biological response to intracellular O_2 levels, J. Cell. Sci. 116 (2003) 3041–3049.

[5] M. Safran, W.G. Kaelin Jr., HIF hydroxylation and the mammalian oxygen-sensing pathway, J. Clin. Invest. 111 (2003) 779–783.

[6] E. Metzen, P.J. Ratcliffe, HIF hydroxylation and cellular oxygen sensing, Biol. Chem. 385 (2004) 223–230.

[7] P.H. Maxwell, HIF-1's relationship to oxygen: simple yet sophisticated, Cell Cycle 3 (2004) 156–159.

[8] P. Jaakkola, et al., Targeting of HIF-1 α to the von Hippel Lindau ubiquitylation complex by O_2-regulated prolyl hydroxylation, Science 292 (2001) 468–472.

[9] M. Ivan, et al., HIFα targeted for vHL-mediated destruction by proline hydroxylation: implications for O_2 sensing, Science 292 (2001) 464–468.

[10] N. Masson, et al., Independent function of two destruction domains in hypoxia-inducible factor-α chains activated by prolyl hydroxylation, EMBO J. 20 (2001) 5197–5206.

[11] E. Yu, et al., HIF-1α binding to vHL is regulated by stimulus-sensitive proline hydroxylation, Proc. Natl. Acad Sci. U. S. A. 98 (2001) 9630–9635.

[12] R.K. Bruick, S.L. McKnight, A conserved family of prolyl-4-hydroxylases that modify HIF, Science 294 (2001) 1337–1340.

[13] P.H. Maxwell, et al., The tumour suppressor protein vHL targets hypoxia-inducible factors for oxygen-dependent proteolysis, Nature 399 (1999) 271–275.

[14] K. Iwai, et al., Identification of the von Hippel-Lindau tumor-suppressor protein as part of an active E3 ubiquitin ligase complex, Proc. Natl. Acad Sci. U. S. A. 96 (1999) 12436–12441.

[15] J. Lisztwan, et al., The von Hippel-Lindau tumor suppressor protein is a component of an E3 ubiquitin–protein ligase activity, Genes Dev. 13 (1999) 1822–1833.

[16] M.M. Bradford, A rapid and sensitive method for the quantitation of microgram quantities of protein utilizing the principle of protein-dye binding, Anal. Biochem. 72 (1976) 248–254.

[17] T. Hofer, et al., Hypoxic up-regulation of erythroid 5-aminolevulinate synthase, Blood 101 (2003) 348–350.

[18] K.B. Storey, Mammalian hibernation. Transcriptional and translational controls, Adv. Exp. Med. Biol. 543 (2003) 21–38.

[19] A.V. Kuznetsova, et al., von Hippel-Lindau protein binds hyperphosphorylated large subunit of RNA polymerase II through a proline hydroxylation motif and targets it for ubiquitination, Proc. Natl. Acad Sci. U. S. A. 100 (2003) 2706–2711.

ELSEVIER

www.ics-elsevier.com

HIF and anapyrexia; a case for crabs

Steve Morris[*]

Morlab, School of Biological Sciences, University of Bristol, Bristol BS8 1UG, UK

Abstract. Hypometabolism is an effective hypoxia defence. Anapyrexia–hypoxia induced lowering of preferred temperature can bring immediate improvements in survival of ectothermic animals able to seek out lower ambient temperatures. At the same time, the regulation of gene expression by hypoxia-inducible factors (HIF) is appearing to be ubiquitous in animals and affords a different strategy for responding to hypoxia. Anapyrexia in ectotherms appears to be initiated at O_2 levels above those allowing the HIF response, allowing for a tiered response to hypoxia in ectothermic species. There are few data for invertebrate species, including crustaceans, yet both anapyrexia and HIF responses would seem to offer advantages. This review examines the physiological phenomena in context of ectotherm ecophysiology and crustaceans particularly. © 2004 Elsevier B.V. All rights reserved.

Keywords: Hypoxia; HIF; Anapyrexia; Hypometabolism; Behaviour; Crustaceans

1. Introduction

Hypometabolism is the most effective of available hypoxia defence mechanisms [1]. The benefits of suppressed metabolism have been appreciated for some time [2] and details of the regulative processes are being elucidated at the molecular level [3]. The relatively recent description of regulators of hypoxia-inducible factors (HIF) [4,5], which regulate gene expressions, has revealed a sophisticated O_2-sensing and signalling mechanism [6,7]. HIF-mediated regulation may thus usefully alter metabolism in response to hypoxia. There is a graded response of HIF to hypoxia such that it becomes apparent only at relatively low O_2 levels [8]. The vast majority of this new information is derived from mammalian models, especially human. Environmental hypoxia can also induce anapyrexia in animals—that is a lowering of preferred body temperature (T_b) due to a

---

* Tel.: +44 117 928 9181; fax: +44 117 928 8520.
  E-mail address: Steve.Morris@bristol.ac.uk.

0531-5131/ © 2004 Elsevier B.V. All rights reserved.
doi:10.1016/j.ics.2004.08.056

lowering of the thermoregulatory set-point [9]. Reduced temperature lowers metabolic rate and thus O_2 demand. In homeothermic animals, anapyrexia mostly requires adjustments in physiological processes. Anapyrexia seems to occur at O_2 levels above those normally required to allow HIF accumulation. Behavioural components to anapyrexia have been apparent in mammals selecting lower environmental temperature [10]. In this regard, ectothermic animals present an interesting experimental tool since they are largely limited to behavioural responses only. A variety of ectothemic species respond to hypoxia by selecting lower ambient and thereby T_b. A question thus arises as to the relative importance and utility of ubiquitous HIF-mediated responses to hypoxia compared to anapyrexia which seeks to remove or at least minimise the effects of environmental hypoxia on metabolism—perhaps obviating the HIF response. This question seems particularly germane to both vertebrate and invertebrate ectotherms.

2. Hypoxia induced changes in gene expression

In animals, a reduced supply of oxygen (environmental hypoxia) eventually elicits an internal hypoxia and a suite of physiological responses which are supported by changes in gene expression. In mammalian systems, many genes inducible by hypoxia are regulated by a DNA-binding protein, hypoxia-inducible factor 1 (HIF-1) [11,12]. This HIF-1 is a heterodimeric transcription factor, composed of an α and a β subunit (schematic in Fig. 1). The α subunit is unstable and rapidly degraded under normoxia [13]. HIF(s) are widely, probably universally, expressed in the cells of animals [14]. Heterodimers composed of HIF-1α and HIF-1β subunits bind to small hypoxic response elements [HRE] (5' - RCGTG-3') in conserved regions associated with genes encoding the proteins regulated in response to hypoxia. The β subunit is abundantly expressed independently of oxygen tension. In contrast, HIF-1α is only detected when cells are challenged by hypoxia, although its transcription and thus mRNA levels are essentially invariant [15]. Above a critical intracellular O_2 tension, HIF-1α is subject to post-translational modification and rapidly degraded in proteasomes after its ubiquitination (ubiquitin molecules are added to facilitate degradation) (Fig. 1). HIF-1α contains an oxygen-dependent degradation domain with a highly conserved region: a binding site for the tumour suppressor pVHL (von Hippel–Lindau protein). The pVHL organizes the assembly of a complex that activates the ubiquitin E3 ligase, targeting HIF-1α for degradation.

2.1. The pivotal role of prolyl and asparaginyl hydroxylases (FIH)

The cellular O_2 sensing mechanism that determines the HIF-1α/pVHL interaction includes an O_2-dependent enzymatic hydroxylation of highly conserved proline residues [7,6,16]. In human HIF-1α, hydroxylation of proline564 and proline402 promotes degradation (Fig. 1). Human HIF hydroxylases (PH) have been cloned [17–19] and belong to the family of O_2-, iron-, and 2-oxoglutarate-dependent dioxygenases (O_2, 2-OG) (review Refs. [24–26]; Fig. 1). Hydroxylation of the proline is required for pVHL binding to HIF-1α. In addition, O_2-dependent hydroxylation of the conserved asparagine803 residue within the C-terminal transactivation domain (CTAD) of HIF-1α has been identified as a regulator of its transactivating capacity and ability to interact with transcriptional coactivator proteins, such as CBP/p300 [20–22]. Modification of the

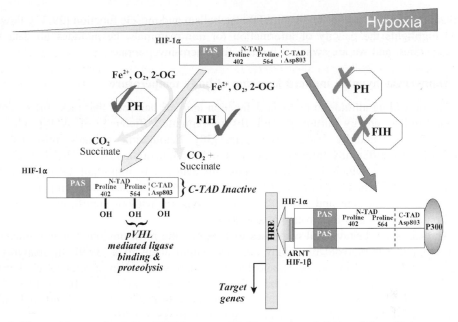

Fig. 1. The persistence and activity of HIF-1α are regulated by two separate hydroxylations. Under normoxia, proline hydoxylase (PH) acts on proline402 and proline564 which allows the binding of pVHL and associated ligase complex (polyubiquitination) and proteolysis in the proteasomes. Oxygen also allows the hydroxylation of asparagine803 by FIH (identical to asparagine hydroxylase) which inactivates the C-terminal transactivation domain (CTAD). Under sufficiently hypoxic conditions, PH and FIH are inactivated which allows the dimerisation of HIF-1α and HIF-1α, and the recruitment of p300/CBP co-factor. This complex then promotes target gene transcription through binding to HRE [PAS—Per/ARNT/Sim: protein interaction domains involved in dimerisation]. 2-OG=2-oxoglutarate-dependent dioxygenases. Based on mammalian HIF functioning and adapted from Metzen and Ratcliffe [25], and Bracken et al. [26].

asparagine is inhibited by hypoxia, facilitating recruitment of CBP/p300. Inhibition of this asparagyl hydroxylation in hypoxia allows the full transactivation of target genes. Under normoxic conditions, this interaction is blocked by hydroxylation of an asparagine residue within the CTAD [20]. A factor that interacts with the CTAD, FIH-1 [21], has been found to possess CTAD asparagine-hydroxylase activity [20,22,23]. Similarly to the proline hydroxylases, FIH-1 is an O_2, 2-OG enzyme [23] and it has also been reported to mediate suppression of CTAD function, via interaction with pVHL [21].

Thus, experimental inhibition of prolyl and/or asparagyl hydroxylation may be a powerful approach for studying oxygen-independent activation of HIF. A variety of PH inhibitors have been shown to inhibit the HIF-1α/pVHL interaction, stabilize HIF-1α, and induce HIF target genes in vivo [27,28].

The many significant biomedical implications [27,29] have stimulated a plethora of studies in mammalian models [30] and although HIF-1 is apparently ubiquitous in animals [31] there are few other data on oxygen-dependent gene expression. HIF-1 regulation occurs in fish [32], nematodes [17] and was recently reported in crustaceans [33,34]. Over 120 genes are hypoxia regulated in one fish species [35] and the HIF in fish is 61% similar to mammalian [36]. In mammals, up-regulated genes include those involved in glucose utilization, amino acid, metabolism, ATP metabolism and muscle function [29,37]. Powell [31] highlights the paucity of information for non-mammals, he includes no data for invertebrates, and we are aware of no data for macro-invertebrates.

3. Anapyrexia–hypoxia induced lowering of body temperature

The prevailing attitude to hypoxia defence in animals has been that they: (a) severely down-regulate energy turnover; and (b) up-regulate efficiency of ATP-producing pathways, regulated by O_2-sensitive genes [38]. Ectothermic animals must manage metabolic rate differently from homeotherms and the functioning of the HIF-1 system in an ectotherm, in which body temperature fluctuates, has important bearing on the evolution of both homeothermy and hypoxia tolerance. Increased body temperature can increase metabolic rate and induce an internal hypoxia without significant changes in environmental O_2, and the inverse is also true.

Animals show behavioural responses to hypoxia, the most obvious being avoidance. When hypoxia is unavoidable, many animals exhibit anapyrexia [39,9]. In anapyrexia, hypoxia induces a decrease in T_b and has been demonstrated in species ranging from protozoa to mammals but the number of species studied remains insufficient [9,39,41]. Furthermore, there have been few attempts to integrate the biochemical and molecular concepts with the physiological phenomenon of anapyrexia [9,39].

Non-homeothermic animals have almost no mechanisms to physiologically alter T_b and tend to be in equilibrium with ambient temperature (T_a). Behavioural adaptations provide a measure of control of T_b. Most ectotherms display a preferred T_b which is influenced by a number of factors, e.g. behavioural fever in lizards [42], amphibians and fish [43]. In ectotherms, anapyrexia manifests as a behaviourally induced hypothermia (hypoxia induced behavioural hypothermia—HIBH) whereby the animal selects a lower T_a to reduce T_b; that is, the response to hypoxia is behavioural. Predicted by Wood [44], it was promptly confirmed in lizards [45] which showed HIBH at a threshold of ~10% ambient oxygen. HIBH has now been demonstrated in reptiles, amphibians and fish [45,46,48]. There are some significant implications for the evolution of homeothermy, since it seems that facultative physiological lowering of T_b has probably been inherited from a system eliciting a behavioural response in a putative ectothermic ancestor. Hyperventilation is a normal response to hypoxia but is an extra energetic cost. Clearly under circumstances where oxygen supply becomes limiting moderate hypothermia (anapyrexia) can be beneficial in (a) reducing O_2 demand and matching it to reduced supply, (b) reducing the need for hyperventilation, (c) increasing the oxygen affinity of the respiratory pigment, and (d) avoiding increased cardiac and ventilatory activity. A decrease in T_b in response to hypoxia increases survival [9,46]. However, despite the importance of HIBH in ectotherms, this phenomenon remains to be properly explained.

4. Hypoxia induced behavioural hypothermia in crustacean

Prior to 1997, there had been only one report of HIBH in an invertebrate, encouraging researchers to dismiss this as an important phenomenon. However, crayfish clearly selected a lower T_a under hypoxic conditions [47]. This observation has now been substantiated in the shore crab, *Carcinus maenas* [48], confirming the existence of this response and requiring detailed further investigation. HIBH maybe of over-riding importance in aquatic invertebrates, such as crustaceans, presented with frequent environmental hypoxia in a heterothermic environment [49–52] but so far remains almost completely un-assessed. Aquatic habitats often offer a variety of thermal environments that could be exploited by species using HIBH and thus there exist realistic benefits of HIBH to some species.

4.1. The basis of HIBH

The threshold for HIBH of 10% ambient O_2 appears to relate to the functioning of the respiratory pigment but exactly how blood-gas conditions are translated to behavioural hypothermia is unclear [46]. The relationship between decreasing blood O_2 and the initiation of hypothermia also remains largely obscure. However, on this basis, it seems possible that HIBH is initiated before HIF-1α degradation is appreciably slowed [8]. The degree of HIF activation thus depends on the extent and rate at which environmental hypoxia is translated into an internal cellular hypoxia in a large metazoan animal.

The respiratory pigment of crustaceans is copper-based haemocyanin. The oxygen dissociation curve of haemocyanin, like haemoglobin, is sigmoidal and O_2-binding co-operative. As inspired air (normally ~21% oxygen) is reduced in oxygen (mild hypoxia), the arterial oxygen saturation is initially maintained on the flat part of the curve and the pigment well saturated ($PaO_2(1) \rightarrow PaO_2(2)$ in Fig. 2). Reduction to 10% ambient O_2 elicits a marked deoxygenation ($PaO_2(3)$) compromising oxygen delivery. The progressive hypoxia would normally elicit increased ventilation and often blood perfusion to sustain O_2 uptake. Decreasing T_b not only reduces O_2 uptake but also promotes a left shift of the curve (i.e. increased O_2 affinity), both preserving a higher arterial O_2 (Fig. 2).

4.2. Mediation of behavioural hypothermia

The explicit assumption with regards to HIBH mediation appears to have long been that a blood borne message, the concentration of which is sensitive to systemic O_2, directly permeates some part of the CNS. This message then 'resets the thermostat' to lower body temperature and that physiological consequences are largely passive effects of

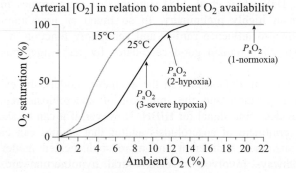

Fig. 2. Model O_2 equilibrium curves showing the benefit of lowered temperature during hypoxia. (1) Curve under normoxia, (2) hypoxia and (3) sever hypoxia. PaO_2=accompanying partial pressure of O_2 in the arterial blood supply.

lowered temperature on existing processes [9]. The result has been two decades of searching for the mediating circulating message. For example, ethanol as a product of anaerobiosis in goldfish induces fish to select T_b ~8 °C lower [53]. L-Lactate from anaerobiosis promoted behavioural hypothermia in *Bufo* [54]. These data led to suggestions that critically reduced blood O_2 may be transduced to HIBH via the initiation of anaerobiosis. Attempts to establish direct links between blood oxygenation and hypothermia in *Bufo* remain inconclusive [46]. Also in clear contrast, it has been suggested that HIBH in frogs has the primary function of delaying the onset of plasma acidosis [55], which would be a clear benefit. Infusion of L-lactate into *Bufo* promoted an increase in metabolic rate which could be inhibited, however, by inhibition of either the Lac^-H^+ or Na^+/H^+ transporters [56].

There has been an increase in the interest and perceived importance of HIBH in crustaceans and in identifying some of the possible transduction messages [48]. Injection of isosmotic Na-lactate into *C. maenas* induced behavioural hypothermia [48]. However, such L-lactate levels are usually associated with pronounced hypoxia and significant acidosis. Extreme and/or persistent hypoxia normally occurs only at O_2 levels well below those stimulating HIBH. In addition, the accompanying acidosis elicits a marked reduction in blood oxygen affinity, an effect opposite to that promoted by lowered temperature. If lactate is an important signal in HIBH, then the re-oxidation of lactate to pyruvate is an important process, and would be slowed by lowered T_b [57], perpetuating the O_2 debt and the duration of HIBH. The importance of hypoxia induced transcription of genes such as LDH [58] which have an HRE is hitherto unconsidered.

It seems physiologically inappropriate that L-lactate should be the signal to initiate HIBH for the purposes of avoiding a systemic hypoxia since in simple terms it is too late! The suggestion of Tatersall and Boutilier [55] that HIBH slows lactic acid release seems more likely. Petersen et al. [40] suggest that adenosine stimulates HIBH in lizards at levels of blood oxygenation above that promoting lactate production. Clearly the nature of the HIBH stimulus, the transduction and messenger systems, and the ecophysiological benefits remain to be resolved.

Additional putative mediators of HIBH include arginine, vasopressin, histamine and adenosine [9,40]. DeWachter et al. [48] suggest that neuroamines might be involved but the data remain highly preliminary. In so much as monoamine hormones and adenosine are known to influence cardiac and ventilatory function in crustaceans under hypoxic conditions, they remain good candidates for messenger/transducer molecules [59,60].

Despite some apparent deficiencies in the available models, the evidence is that the balance between respiration and the initiation of anaerobiosis represents a crucial condition and provides some signal for HIBH. However, if it can be shown that HIBH is initiated before recruitment of anaerobiosis and/or that amines can elicit HIBH in the absence of L-lactate, then a different and more sophisticated model will result. The physiological pathways involved in behavioural hypothermia are, however, quite speculative [9]. Factors that appear to elicit an anapyrexia also influence haemoglobin-oxygen saturation, blood flow, and oxygen content of the blood. Thus, it is not surprising that numerous potential triggers have been suggested to induce anapyrexia [40].

Clearly investigation of respiratory, blood gas, blood pigment physiology and thermal biology should be carried out at this time. Pre-exposure, acclimation and adaptation must be addressed if the import of HIBH is to be revealed.

In endotherms, hypoxia has long been understood to induce hypothermia by reducing heat production (hypometabolism) [1,2,61]. General consensus is the HIBH is a consequence of resetting of the thermostatic set-point or preferred temperature. This must result in systemic down-regulation of metabolism including key aspects of energy metabolism [2] and especially the enzymes whose genes are apparently regulated in hypoxia by HIF-1[3]. It seems impossible that regulation of gene expression by HIF-1 and anapyrexia/HIBH can operate independently.

HIBH might slow metabolic demand simply through lowered T_b and the Q_{10} effect on metabolism but having done so would surely change the O_2 threshold at which HIF-1α increased—this represents a modulation of HIF regulated changes in gene expression. Yet ectotherms that exhibit HIBH apparently utilize HIF-1α, and at least one fish and one crustacean have the hypoxic-responsive element (HRE) in key genes, that for lactate dehydrogenase [33,58]. Conversely, anapyrexia/HIBH may itself depend, in part, on HIF-1α regulated gene expression but the time course argues for some mediation by existing signal systems. Thus, hypoxic acclimation, in which HIF-1α becomes chronically elevated, must lower the threshold for HIBH. Similarly, in ectothermic animals, thermal acclimation can reduce the Q_{10}. Thus warm acclimation would be expected to raise the threshold for both HIBH and HIF-1α elevation.

The apparent contradictions in the mediating mechanism in HIBH might be explainable if HIBH was in fact part of the suite of consequences of HIF induction of gene expression. Indeed, the observations of Pinz and Pörtner [56] support different potential signalling effects for lactate depending on whether membrane channels were modified as part of the hypoxic response. It seems unlikely that animals when faced with hypoxia elect *between* anapyrexia or a HIF-mediated change in gene expression. HIF-1α responds nearly instantaneously and has a half-life <5 min [29] and thus the rate limiting step would be only in the transcription and translation of the message from the genes activated/ deactivated by HIF. It is physiologically much more elegant for HIBH to be part of the HIF-mediated response. Another possibility is that HIBH and inhibition of HIF-1α degradation have different threshold O_2 sensitivities—in which case HIBH (or anapyrexia) may serve to maintain O_2 levels and thereby delay the accumulation of HIF-1α and consequent large-scale change in gene expression.

The interrelation of temperature and the prevailing systemic PO_2 is considerably more interesting (and useful) in ectotherms compared to homeotherms (anapyrexia notwithstanding). Generally, metabolic rate increases with higher temperature and thus O_2 supply will fall short of demand more quickly if animals are held at warmer temperatures. Thus, it would be expected that HIF-1α degradation would slow and/or HR genes would change expression, at a higher ambient PO_2 when the animals were held at warmer temperatures. The converse applies at lower temperature when the ambient PO_2 might be much lower to activate HIF—which is the basis of the contention that HIBH should delay expression changes in HR genes.

To our knowledge, these obvious linkages between HIF-1α regulated transcription and anapyrexia (in this case as HIBH) have not even been discussed in the literature and are yet to be investigated in any fashion. Clearly, anapyrexia and hypometabolism represent transitory solutions to some problems of hypoxia and longer-term changes in gene expression profile may follow.

References

[1] P.W. Hochachka, P.L. Lutz, Mechanism, origin, and evolution of anoxia tolerance in animals, Comp. Biochem. Physiol., A 130 (2001) 435–459.

[2] K.B. Storey, J.M. Storey, Metabolic-rate depression and biochemical adaptation in anaerobiois, hibernation and estivation, Q. Rev. Biol. 65 (2) (1990) 145–174.

[3] K.B. Storey, J.M. Storey, Metabolic rate depression in animals: transcriptional and translational controls, Biol. Rev. 79 (1) (2004) 207–233.

[4] G.L. Wang, G.L. Semenza, Purification and characterization of hypoxia-inducible factor 1, J. Biol. Chem. 270 (1995) 1230–1237.

[5] G.L. Wang, et al., Hypoxia-inducible factor 1 is a basic-helix-loop-helix-PAS heterodimer regulated by cellular O2 tension, Proc. Natl. Acad. Sci. U. S. A. 92 (1995) 5510–5514.

[6] M. Ivan, et al., HIF targeted for VHL-mediated destruction by proline hydroxylation: implications for O_2 sensing, Science 292 (2001) 464–468.

[7] P. Jaakkola, et al., Targeting of HIF-alpha to the von Hippel–Lindau ubiquitylation complex by O-2-regulated prolyl hydroxylation, Science 292 (2001) 468–472.

[8] B.-H. Jiang, et al., Hypoxia-inducible factor 1 levels vary exponentially over a physiologically relevant range of O_2 tension, Am. J. Physiol. 271 (1996) C1172–C1180.

[9] A.A. Steiner, L.G.S. Branco, Hypoxia-induced anapyrexia: implications and putative mediators, Annu. Rev. Physiol. 64 (2002) 263–288.

[10] C.J. Gordon, L. Fogelson, Comparative effects of hypoxia on behavioural thermoregulation in rats, hamsters, and mice, Am. J. Physiol. 260 (1991) R120–R125.

[11] G. Wang, G.L. Semenza, General involvement of hypoxia-inducible factor in transcriptional response to hypoxia, Proc. Natl. Acad. Sci. U. S. A. 90 (9) (1993) 4304–4308.

[12] H.F. Bunn, R.O. Poyton, Oxygen sensing and molecular adaptation to hypoxia, Physiol. Rev. 76 (1996) 839–885.

[13] S. Salceda, J. Caro, Hypoxia-inducible factor 1 (HIF-1α) protein is rapidly degraded by the ubiquitin–proteasome system under normoxic conditions. Its stabilization by hypoxia depends on redox-induced changes, J. Biol. Chem. 271 (1997) 22642–22647.

[14] H. Zhu, H.F. Bunn, How do cells sense oxygen? Science 292 (2001) 449–451.

[15] C.W. Pugh, et al., Activation of hypoxia-inducible factor-1; definition of regulatory domains within the α Subunit, J. Biol. Chem. 272 (1997) 11205–11214.

[16] N. Masson, et al., Independent function of two destruction domains in hypoxia-inducible factor-α chains activated by prolyl hydroxylation, EMBO J. 20 (2001) 5197–5206.

[17] A.C. Epstein, et al., C. elegans EGL-9 and mammalian homologs define a family of dioxygenases that regulate HIF by prolyl hydroxylation, Cell 107 (2001) 43–54.

[18] R.K. Bruick, S.L McKnight, A conserved family of prolyl-4-hydroxylases that modify HIF, Science 294 (2001) 1337–1340.

[19] F. Oehme, et al., Overexpression of PH-4, a novel putative proline 4-hydroxylase, modulates activity of hypoxia-inducible transcription factors, Biochem. Biophys. Res. Commun. 296 (2002) 343–349.

[20] D. Lando, et al., Asparagine hydroxylation in the HIF transactivation domain a hypoxic switch, Science 295 (2002) 858–861.

[21] P.C. Mahon, K. Hirota, G. Semenza, LFI H-1: a novel protein that interacts with HIF-1alpha and VHL to mediate repression of HIF-1 transcriptional activity, Genes Dev. 15 (2001) 2675–2686.

[22] D. Lando, et al., FIH-1 is an asparaginyl hydroxylase enzyme that regulates the transcriptional activity of hypoxia-inducible factor, Genes Dev. 16 (2002) 1466–1471.

[23] K.S. Hewitson, et al., Hypoxia-inducible factor (HIF) asparagine hydroxylase is identical to factor inhibiting HIF (FIH) and is related to the cupin structural family, J. Biol. Chem. 277 (2002) 26351–26355.

[24] K.I. Kivirikko, T. Pihlajaniemi, Collagen hydroxylases and the protein disulfide isomerase subunit of prolyl 4-hydroxylases, Adv. Enzymol. Relat. Areas Mol. Biol. 72 (1998) 325–398.

[25] E. Metzen, P.J. Ratcliffe, HIF hydroxylation and cellular oxygen sensing, Biol. Chem. 385 (2004) 223–230.

[26] C.P. Bracken, M.L. Whitelaw, D.J. Peet, The hypoxia-inducible factors: key transcriptional regulators of hypoxic responses, Cell. Mol. Life Sci. 60 (2003) 1376–1393.

[27] C. Warnecke, et al., Activation of the hypoxia-inducible factor pathway and stimulation of angiogenesis by application of prolyl hydroxylase inhibitors, FASEB J. 17 (2003) 1186–1188.

[28] N.J. Mabjeesh, et al., Dibenzoylmethane, a natural dietary compound, induces HIF-1α and increases expression of VEGF, Biochem. Biophys. Res. Comm. 303 (2003) 279–286.

[29] L.E. Huang, H.F. Bunn, Hypoxia-inducible factor and its biomedical relevance, J. Biol. Chem. 278 (2002) 19575–19578.

[30] G.L. Semenza, HIF-1: mediator of physiological and pathophysiological responses to hypoxia, J. Appl. Physiol. 88 (2000) 1474–1480.

[31] F.L. Powell, Functional genomics and the comparative physiology of hypoxia, Annu. Rev. Physiol. 68 (2003) 203–230.

[32] M. Nikinmaa, Oxygen-dependent cellular functions—why fishes and their aquatic environment are a prime choice of study, Comp. Biochem. Physiol. 133A (2002) 1–16.

[33] T.A. Gorr, et al., Hypoxia induced synthesis of hemoglobin in the crustacean *Daphnia magna* is HIF dependent. J. Biol. Chem. 279 (2004) 36038–36047.

[34] J.M. Head, N.B. Terwilliger, The role of HIF-1α in crustacean responses to hypoxia, Integr. Comp. Biol. 42 (6) (2002) 1242.

[35] A.Y. Gracey, J.V. Troll, G.N. Somero, Hypoxia-induced gene expression profiling in the euryoxic fish *Gillichthys mirabilis*, Proc. Natl. Acad. Sci. 98 (2001) 1993–1998.

[36] A.J. Soitamo, et al., Characterization of a hypoxia-inducible factor (HIF-1α) from rainbow trout, J. Biol. Chem. 23 (2001) 19699–19705.

[37] R.S.S. Wu, Hypoxia: from molecular responses to ecosystem responses, Mar. Pollut. Bull. 45 (2002) 35–45.

[38] P.W. Hochachka, G.N. Somero, Biochemical Adaptation—Mechanism and Process in Physiological Evolution, Oxford University Press, New York, 2002, pp. 101–157.

[39] S.C. Wood, Interactions between hypoxia and hypothermia, Annu. Rev. Physiol. 53 (1991) 71–85.

[40] A.M. Petersen, T.T. Gleeson, D.A. Scholnick, The effect of oxygen and adenosine on lizard thermoregulation, Physiol. Biochem. Zool. 76 (3) (2003) 339–347.

[41] S.C. Wood, Oxygen as a modulator of body temperature, Braz. J. Med. Biol. Res. 28 (11–12) (1995) 1249–1256.

[42] M.J. Kluger, Fever: role of pyrogens and cryogens, Physiol. Rev. 71 (1) (1991) 93–127.

[43] W.W. Reynolds, M.E. Casterlin, in: A.S. Milton (Ed.), Pyretics and Antipyretics, Springer-Verlag, Berlin, 1982, pp. 649–688.

[44] S.C. Wood, Cardiovascular shunts and oxygen-transport in lower vertebrates, Am. J. Physiol. 247 (1984) R3–R14.

[45] J.W. Hicks, S.C. Wood, Temperature regulation in lizards: effects of hypoxia, Am. J. Physiol. 248 (1985) R595–R600.

[46] C. Reidel, S.C. Wood, Effects of hypercapnia and hypoxia on temperature selection of the toad, *Bufo marinus*, Fed. Proc. 2 (1988) 500A.

[47] R.K. Dupré, S.C. Wood, Behavioral temperature regulation by aquatic ectotherms during hypoxia, Can. J. Zool. 66 (1988) 2649–2652.

[48] B. DeWachter, F.-J. Sartoris, H.-O. Pörtner, The anaerobic endproduct lactate has a behavioural signaling function in the shore crab *Carcinus maenas*, J. Exp. Biol. 200 (1997) 1015–1024.

[49] S. Morris, A.C. Taylor, Diurnal and seasonal variation in physico-chemical conditions within intertidal rock pools, Estuar. Coast. Shelf Sci. 17 (1983) 151–167.

[50] S. Morris, A.C. Taylor, Heart rate response of the intertidal prawn *Palaemon elegans* to simulated and in situ environmental changes, Mar. Ecol., Prog. Ser. 20 (1984) 127–136.

[51] S. Morris, A.C. Taylor, The respiratory response of the intertidal prawn *Palaemon elegans* (Rathke) to hypoxia and hyperoxia, Comp. Biochem. Physiol. 81A (1985) 633–639.

[52] S. Morris, A.C. Taylor, The response to temperature change of oxygen consumption by *Palaemon elegans* (Rathke): a determinant of distribution, Exp. Biol. 44 (1985) 255–268.

[53] L.I. Crawshaw, L.P. Woolmuth, C.S. O'Connor, Intracranial ethanol and ambient anoxia elicit selection of cooler water by goldfish, Am. J. Physiol. 256 (1989) R133–R137.

[54] H.-O. Pörtner, L.G.S. Branco, G.M. Malvin, S.C. Wood, A new function for lactate in the toad *Bufo marinus*, J. Appl. Physiol. 76 (1994) 2405–2410.

[55] G.J. Tattersall, R.G. Boutilier, Balancing hypoxia and hypothermia in cold-submerged frogs, J. Exp. Biol. 200 (1997) 1031–1038.

[56] P. Pinz, H.-O. Pörtner, Metabolic costs induced by lactate in the toad *Bufo marinus*: new mechanism behind oxygen debt? J. Appl. Physiol. 94 (2003) 1177–1185.

[57] T.T. Gleeson, Post-exercise lactate metabolism: a comparative review of sites, pathways, and regulation, Annu. Rev. Physiol. 58 (1996) 565–581.

[58] B.B. Rees, J.A.L. Bowman, B.B. Rees, Structure and sequence conservation of a putative hypoxia response element in the lactate dehydrogenase-B gene of *Fundulus*, Biol. Bull. 200 (2001) 1247–1251.

[59] J.L. Wilkens, Possible mechanisms of control of vascular resistance in the lobster *Homarus americanus*, J. Exp. Biol. 198 (1997) 2547–2550.

[60] E. Stegen, M.K. Grieshaber, Adenosine increases ventilation rate, cardiac performance and haemolymph velocity in the American lobster *Homarus americanus*, J. Exp. Biol. 204 (2001) 947–957.

[61] E. Gellhorn, Oxygen deficiency, carbon dioxide and temperature regulation, Am. J. Physiol. 120 (1937) 190–194.

www.ics-elsevier.com

Some considerations on calcium homeostasis in semi-terrestrial crabs

F.P. Zanotto[a,*], F. Pinheiro[a], L.A. Brito[a], M.G. Wheatly[b]

[a]University of São Paulo, Department of Physiology, São Paulo, SP, Brazil
[b]Wright State University, Biological Sciences Department, Dayton, OH, USA

Abstract. Calcium (Ca), deposited as $CaCO_3$ after molting events take place, indicates that Ca levels in semi-terrestrial crabs should be regulated at the dietary level as well as through whole animal net Ca flux. Two semi-terrestrial crabs found in salt marsh environments (*Sesarma rectum* and *Chasmagnathus granulata*) were fed purified diets with variable Ca concentrations (0%, 2.22% and 6.66% Ca). Both animals displayed similar feeding strategies through consumption of higher amounts of the diet containing more Ca (6.66% Ca). *Sesarma*, a predominantly herbivore crab, ate more quantities of all the diets offered when compared to *Chasmagnathus*, a more carnivorous crab. Whole animal net fluxes of Ca over 5 days in *Sesarma* show that fluxes vary from 2.5 to 1.5 mmol kg^{-1} h^{-1}, similar to values found earlier for a crayfish, *Procambarus clarkii*. However, the fluxes over 5 days did not decrease significantly compared to fluxes for the first day postmolt. Overall, semi-terrestrial crabs seem to maximize Ca influx through the gills and through dietary intake, a mineral that is known to have great importance for biomineralization in crustaceans. © 2004 Elsevier B.V. All rights reserved.

Keywords: Calcium net flux; Dietary calcium; Calcium balance; Semi-terrestrial crabs

1. Introduction

Calcium (Ca) is of primordial importance for crustaceans because calcium carbonate crystals ($CaCO_3$) must be deposited in the new exoskeleton to harden it after the old exoskeleton has been shed. Critical periods for mineral intake occur during molting

* Corresponding author. Present address: Universidade Presbiteriana Mackenzie, FCBEE, Rua da Consolação 930, 01302-907, São Paulo, SP, Brazil. Tel.: +55 11 3236 8145; fax: +55 11 3758 9803.
E-mail address: fzanotto@usp.br (F.P. Zanotto).

0531-5131/ © 2004 Elsevier B.V. All rights reserved.
doi:10.1016/j.ics.2004.09.018

related events, when crabs shed their old exoskeleton and calcify the new one during postmolt. Whole body Ca uptake in freshwater crayfish, for example, occurs mainly through the gills and changes from intermolt (zero net flux) to premolt (net efflux) and postmolt (net influx at the rate of 2 mmol kg^{-1} h^{-1}) [1,2]. Terrestrial crabs, on the other hand, should have evolved mechanisms for calcium regulation through the gills but additionally through dietary intake, and these regulatory mechanisms should be evident during the whole life cycle of these animals. Therefore, dietary intake of calcium should be especially important for terrestrial crabs, and it is already known that they display different strategies to conserve ions such as storage in the hemolymph and in the digestive system [3].

Specific work in the literature on crustacean nutrition using purified diets has been focused mainly on shrimp, due to their commercial economic importance as human food [4–8] (see Ref. [9]). Work on nutritional requirements of brachyuran crabs has been neglected because of their slow growth rate, cannibalism and low meat/ exoskeleton ratio, characteristics which do not encourage their economic exploitation. A few crabs from commercially important families such as Portunidae, Xanthidae and Cancridae have been studied at semi-intensive conditions, fed, however, with natural diets.

The focus of this study is to present an integrative view of calcium homeostasis in two semi-terrestrial crabs, *Sesarma rectum* and *Chasmagnathus granulata*, by measuring whole animal Ca net flux during postmolt as well as through the study of the effects of dietary Ca changes in purified diets offered to the animals.

2. Methods and results

2.1. Whole animal Ca flux during postmolt

To study the net influx of Ca^{2+} after ecdysis took place, Ca^{2+} net flux was measured in *S. rectum*, a mangrove crab from Brazil, for 5 days after ecdysis. The animals were unfed during the whole period. The net flux (Jca) was measured in μmol kg^{-1} h^{-1}, using the following equation:

$$Jca = \frac{initial\ Ca^{2+}concentration(\mu mol.L^{-1}) - final\ Ca^{2+}concentration(\mu mol.L^{-1}).volume\ of\ solution(L)}{mass\ (Kg).elapsed\ time(h)}$$

The artificial brackish water where the crabs were exposed contained the following salts (in g L^{-1}): NaCl 10.7; NaHCO$_3$ 0.1; NaBr (anhydrous) 0.03; Na$_2$SO$_4$ (anhydrous) 1.8; KCl 0.34; MgCl$_2 \cdot$6H$_2$O 4.84 and CaCl$_2$ (anhydrous) 0.51. Total Ca concentration in the water was around 5 mM.

Ca^{2+} net flux in *S. rectum*, a Brazilian crab, was quantitatively very similar to flux found in the crayfish *Procambarus clarkii*, a freshwater crustacean, at values around 2000 μmol kg^{-1} h^{-1} [1] (Fig. 1). The flux, however, did not decrease significantly over 5 days after ecdysis (Repeated-measures ANOVA, $P<0.05$). This fact raises the question as to what extent the uptake of Ca through the gills of semi-terrestrial crabs is an important variable for Ca balance in these animals. Semi-terrestrial crabs usually undergo ecdysis in burrows, where ground water is available. Therefore, these animals still need to have contact with water sources during the postmolt period. Another point to consider is that the

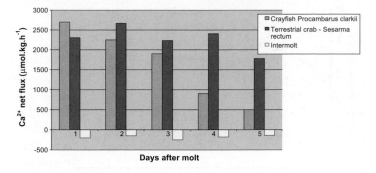

Fig. 1. Ca $^{2+}$ net flux (μmol kg h^{-1}) in *P. clarkii* and *S. rectum* for 5 days after ecdysis. Bars represent mean values. The lower bars represent values of Ca^{2+} flux for intermolt animals.

uptake of Ca in these crabs was qualitatively different from crayfish, showing a smaller decrease as time after ecdysis went on. Perhaps these animals, unable to feed during the experimental period, were relying on Ca uptake mainly through the gills. Moreover, semi-terrestrial crabs are heavily calcified compared to their aquatic counterparts and could partially explain why total Ca uptake over 5 days was apparently higher for the semi-terrestrial crab studied here.

Table 1
Diet composition offered to the crabs for 11 days

Ingredients	Diet A	Diet B	Diet C
Casein	20.5 g	20.5 g	20.5 g
Peptone	5 g	5 g	5 g
Sucrose	5 g	5 g	5 g
Starch	11 g	11 g	11 g
Salt mixture[a]	3 g	3 g	3 g
Vitamins[b]	0.1 g	0.1 g	0.1 g
Vitamin C	0.2 g	0.2 g	0.2 g
Betain	0.8 g	0.8 g	0.8 g
Corn oil	0.0019 L	0.0019 L	0.0019 L
Cod oil	0.0019 L	0.0019 L	0.0019 L
Cholesterol	0.5 g	0.5 g	0.5 g
CaCl$_2$	0 g	1.11 g	3.33 g
Total	49.9 g	51.01 g	54.34 g

Diets A, B and C differed only in relation to Ca content. Diet A contained 0% Ca, Diet B 2.22% Ca and Diet C 6.66% Ca.

[a] Calcium free salt mixture (ICN): KPO$_4$: 52.81%; NaPO$_4$: 10.31%; MgSO$_4 \cdot$ 7H$_2$0: 8.19%; NaCl: 23.13%; iron citrate: 4.5%; KI: 0.13%; MgSO$_4 \cdot$ 1H$_2$0: 0.74%; ZnCl: 0.08%; CuSO$_4 \cdot$ 5H$_2$0: 0.05%; sodium selenite: 0.001% and chromium potassium sulfate: 0.06%.

[b] AIN Vitamin Mixture 76 (ICN)—kg of mixture. Thiamine hydrochloride: 600 mg; riboflavin: 600 mg; pyridoxine hydochloride: 700 mg; nicotinic acid: 3 g; D-calcium pantothenate: 1.6 g; folic acid: 200 mg; D-biotin: 20 mg; vitamin B12: 1 mg; vitamin A: 1.6 g (250,000 UI/g); LD-tocopherol acetate: 20 g (250 UI/g); vitamin D3: 250 mg (400,000 UI/g); vitamin K$_2$: 5 mg and sucrose 972.9 g.

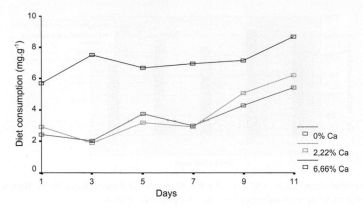

Fig. 2. Mean diet consumption (mg g^{-1}) for *S. rectum* for every 2 days (total of 11 days), fed purified diets which contained three different Ca concentrations (0%, 2.22% and 6.66% Ca). There was a higher consumption for diets containing 6.66% Ca compared to the other diets (Repeated-measures ANOVA, $P<0.01$; $N=10$).

2.2. Dietary effects of Ca during intermolt

Both *Sesarma* and *Chasmagnathus* were held without food for 48 h prior to experimentation. Then, the diets were offered to the animals for the next 4 days, every other day, before experiments started, to allow the animals to get used to the new purified food. After the pre-treatment, diets were offered for 1 h in the dry part of the box (considered day 1). The diets were removed and the animals were allowed to choose the dry or wet part of the box. The wet part of the box contained artificial seawater [10] (Table 1). The diets were offered for the next 11 days, on days 1, 3, 5, 7, 9 and 11, again for 1 h, and removed. The uneaten diets were dried for 48 h at 35 °C and weighed to calculate amounts eaten.

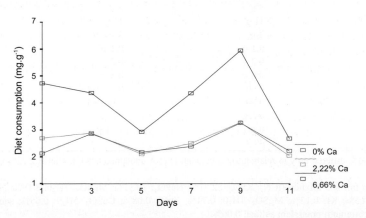

Fig. 3. Mean diet consumption (mg g^{-1}) for *C. granulata* for every 2 days (total of 11 days), fed purified diets which contained three different Ca concentrations (0%, 2.22% and 6.66% Ca). There was a higher consumption for diets containing 6.66% Ca compared to the other diets (Repeated-measures ANOVA, $P<0.01$; $N=5$ for diet with 0% Ca and $N=6$ for the other diets).

Table 2
Total Ca consumption (mg) over 11 days for *S. rectum* and *C. granulata* fed three different diets (mean±S.E.; $N=10$ for *Sesarma* and $N=6$ for *Chasmagnathus*)

Diet	*S. rectum* Ca consumption (mg)	*Chas. granulata* Ca consumption (mg)
0% Ca	0	0
2.22% Ca	11.39±2.15	12.78±6.28
6.66% Ca	48.29±5.52	28.29±1.19

S. rectum consumed more of the diet containing Ca at 6.66% compared to the other diets (Fig. 2; Repeated-measures ANOVA, $P<0.01$). The overall consumption was around 6 mg g^{-1} for the latter diet and around 3–4 mg g^{-1} for the other diets containing Ca at 0% and 2.22%. There was an effect of day (Repeated-measures ANOVA, $P<0.01$) showing that the overall consumption of diet varied over 11 days for all diets.

Chasmagnathus fed the three diets showed the same pattern of consumption as seen in *Sesarma* (Fig. 3). *Chasmagnathus* ate more of the diet containing Ca at 6.66% Ca, at values around 3–6 mg g^{-1} (Repeated-measures ANOVA, $P<0.01$). There was also a strong effect of days, the consumption over the days showing a large variation for all diets (Repeated-measures ANOVA, $P<0.001$). Again, the consumption for diets containing Ca at 2.22 and 0% was lower and around 2–2.5 mg g^{-1} (Fig. 3). Ca consumption was higher for diets containing 6.66% Ca, values around 4× higher compared to *Sesarma* fed diets containing 2.22% Ca (Table 2) and 2.2× higher Ca ingestion was seen for *Chasmagnathus* compared to animals fed 2.22% of Ca (Table 2).

3. General discussion

Earlier work has shown that terrestrial crabs display behavioral regulation during food intake [11,12]. Two species of herbivorous land crabs, *Gecarcoidea natalis* and *Cardisoma hirtipes* displayed different feeding strategies when offered leaves found in their natural environment [12] and as a result *G. natalis* had a higher intake of Ca in the field when compared to *Cardisoma*, achieved through selection of yellow leaves in their environment that already contained more Ca.

We found here that two phylogenetically related crabs with different feeding habits and different degrees of terrestriality show similar patterns of regulation of ingested Ca. *Sesarma* feeds on a mixed diet but the diet is composed mainly of mangrove leaves (around 75% of the diet, see Ref. [13]) and *Chasmagnathus* feeds on a diet composed of fewer plant matter, showing an opportunist behavior in relation to foods encountered [14]. The results showed that both crabs had the same behavioral response to food ingestion when offered different levels of Ca in the diet, i.e., through more consumption of the high Ca diet. The total consumption, however, was higher for *Sesarma* compared to *Chasmagnathus*.

Work on a salt marsh crab, *Armases cinereum*, revealed that salt added as NaCl to the diets stimulated feeding by *Armases*, in concentrations even higher than those found in their natural environment [15]. Overall, it seems that salts in general, as well as Ca, are upregulated for crabs living in salt marsh environments. This has been suggested before for terrestrial crabs that live in swamps far from the sea and where the water available is of reduced salinity [16–18].

Presently, we cannot discriminate how our crabs detected and consumed more of the high Ca diet. Interestingly, it has been found that hermit crab is able to behaviorally choose shells in the environment [19] and detect calcium through chemoreceptors in the dactyls which are sensitive to calcium [20]. This suggested "ion sensitivity" has also been noted in terrestrial isopod antennae which showed sensitivity to calcium solutions in the range of 10–100 mM (cited in Ref. [20]). In our example, the crabs were able to detect and consume more of the high Ca diet.

Ca net flux during postmolt has been studied before in crayfish [1,21] and there are existing reports of first day postmolt fluxes in *Carcinus maenas* [22] and in *Callinectes sapidus* [23]. Fluxes range from 3200 μmol kg^{-1} h^{-1} for the marine species *Carcinus* and *Callinectes* to values as low as 1000 μmol kg^{-1} h^{-1} for the crayfish *Cherax destructor* living in freshwater containing Ca at around 0.2 mmol L^{-1}. Results presented here suggest that although it is expected that terrestrial crabs do not rely heavily on water sources for calcification, they do utilize available Ca in the water under the experimental conditions presented here. The results also suggest that calcification in these animals can last longer than expected compared to their aquatic counterparts.

Acknowledgments

We would like to thank FAPESP (96/09756-9) and Universidade Presbiteriana Mackenzie for the financial support and NSF grant IBN 0076035 to MGW.

References

[1] F.P. Zanotto, M.G. Wheatly, The effect of ambient pH on electrolyte regulation during the postmoult period in freshwater crayfish *Procambarus clarkii*, J. Exp. Biol. 178 (1993) 1–19.

[2] F.P. Zanotto, M.G. Wheatly, Calcium balance in crustaceans: nutritional aspects of physiological regulation, Comp. Biochem. Physiol. 133 (3 A) (2002) 645–660.

[3] P. Greenaway, Ion and water balance, in: W.W. Burggren, B.R. McMahon (Eds.), Biology of the Land Crabs, Cambridge University Press, Cambridge, 1988, pp. 211–248.

[4] H.Y. Chen, C.F. Chang, Quantification of vitamin C requirements for juvenile shrimp (*Penaeus monodon*) using polyphosphorylated L-ascorbic acid, J. Nutr. 124 (10) (1994) 2033–2038.

[5] S.Y. Shiau, C.W. Hsu, Dietary pantothenic acid requirement of juvenile grass shrimp, *Penaeus monodon*, J. Nutr. 129 (3) (1999) 718–721.

[6] S.Y. Shiau, Y.H. Chin, Dietary biotin requirement for maximum growth of juvenile grass shrimp, *Penaeus monodon*, J. Nutr. 128 (12) (1998) 2494–2497.

[7] S.Y. Shiau, J.S. Liu, Quantifying the vitamin K requirement of juvenile marine shrimp (*Penaeus monodon*) with menadione, J. Nutr. 124 (2) (1994) 277–282.

[8] H.Y. Chen, F.C. Wu, S.Y. Tang, Thiamin requirement of juvenile shrimp (*Penaeus monodon*), J. Nutr. 121 (12) (1991) 1984–1989.

[9] G. Cuzon, J. Guillaume, C. Cahu, Composition, preparation and utilization of feeds for Crustacea, Aquaculture 124 (1994) 253–267.

[10] C.F.A. Pantin, Notes on Microscopical Technique for Zoologists, Cambridge University Press, Cambridge, 1948.

[11] P. Greenaway, Calcium and magnesium balance during molting in land crabs, J. Crustac. Biol. 13 (2) (1993) 191–197.

[12] P. Greenaway, S. Raghaven, Digestive strategies in two species of leaf-eating land crabs (Brachyura:Gecarcinidae) in a rain forest, Physiol. Zool. 71 (1) (1998) 36–44.

[13] T.D. Steinke, A. Rajh, A.J. Holland, The feeding-behavior of the red mangrove crab *Sesarma meinerti*-De Man, 1887 (Crustacea, Decapoda, Grapsidae) and its effect on the degradation of mangrove leaf-litter, S. Afr. J. Mar. Sci.-Suid-Afrikaanse Tydskrif Vir Seewetenskap 13 (1993) 151–160.

[14] L.C. Kucharski, R.S.M. Da Silva, Effect of diet composition on the carbohydrate and lipid metabolism in an estuarine crab, *Chasmagnathus granulata* (Dana, 1851), Comp. Biochem. Physiol. 99 (A) (1991) 215–218.

[15] S.C. Pennings, et al., Feeding preferences of a generalist salt–marsh crab: relative importance of multiple plant traits, Ecology 79 (6) (1998) 1968–1979.

[16] D.L. Wolcott, T.G. Wolcott, Food quality and cannibalism in the red land crab, *Gecarcinus lateralis*, Physiol. Zool. 57 (3) (1984) 318–324.

[17] T.G. Wolcott, D.L. Wolcott, Availability of salts is not a limiting factor for the land crab *Gecarcinus lateralis* (Freminville), J. Exp. Mar. Biol. Ecol. 120 (1988) 199–219.

[18] T.G. Wolcott, D.L. Wolcott, Ion conservation by reprocessing of urine in the land crab *Gecarcinus lateralis* (Freminville), Physiol. Zool. 64 (1) (1991) 344–361.

[19] K.A. Mesce, Calcium-bearing objects elicit shell selection behavior in a hermit crab, Science 215 (1982) 993–995.

[20] K.A. Mesce, Morphological and physiological identification of chelar sensory structures in the hermit-crab *Pagurus hirsutiusculus* (Decapoda), J. Crust. Biol. 13 (1) (1993) 95–110.

[21] S. Zare, P. Greenaway, Ion transport and the effects of moulting in the freshwater crayfish *Cherax destructor* (Decapoda:Parastacidae), Aust. J. Zool. 45 (1997) 539–551.

[22] P. Greenaway, Uptake of calcium at the postmoult stage by the marine crabs *Callinectes sapidus* and *Carcinus maenas*, Comp. Biochem. Physiol. 75 (2 A) (1983) 181–184.

[23] J.N. Cameron, Post-moult calcification in the blue crab (*Callinectes sapidus*): relationship between apparent net H+ excretion, calcium and bicarbonate, J. Exp. Biol. 119 (1985) 275–285.

International Congress Series 1275 (2004) 96–103

ELSEVIER

www.ics-elsevier.com

Integrative aspects of renal epithelial calcium transport in crayfish: temporal and spatial regulation of PMCA

Michele G. Wheatly*, Yongping Gao, Minal Nade

Department of Biological Sciences, Wright State University, Dayton, OH 45435-0001, USA

Abstract. The molting cycle of the freshwater (FW) crayfish, *Procambarus clarkii*, has been used as a model to study the cellular physiology and molecular biology of proteins (channels, exchangers and pumps) that effect epithelial Ca transport (ECT). Specifically, periods of net Ca flux (typically postmolt influx or premolt efflux) have been compared with periods of net Ca balance (intermolt). In the present study, we further explore the spatial and temporal regulation of plasma membrane Ca ATPase (PMCA) in the antennal gland (kidney). Crayfish are uniquely adapted to produce dilute urine through reabsorption of filtered Ca at the nephridial canal; reabsorption increases in pre/postmolt to compensate for the freshwater absorbed at ecdysis to elicit shedding. Prior work has suggested that PMCA mRNA and protein increase in pre- and postmolt stages compared with intermolt at the antennal gland. In the present paper, we used state-of-the-art techniques to increase the spatial and temporal resolution of this observation. Real-time PCR indicated that the PMCA mRNA expression increased 10-fold in premolt with a further doubling in postmolt. In situ hybridization confirmed that the PMCA mRNA was expressed primarily within the nephridial canal and labyrinth of the antennal gland, and that labelling increased in pre- and postmolt. Immunolocalization with confocal visualization confirmed that the PMCA protein is primarily membrane associated in the nephridial canal cells (basolateral but also apical). © 2004 Elsevier B.V. All rights reserved.

Keywords: Plasma membrane Ca ATPase; PMCA; Antennal gland; Calcium; Crayfish

* Corresponding author. Tel.: +1 937 775 2611; fax: +1 937 775 3068.
E-mail address: michele.wheatly@wright.edu (M.G. Wheatly).

0531-5131/ © 2004 Elsevier B.V. All rights reserved.
doi:10.1016/j.ics.2004.08.077

1. Introduction

Crustaceans have emerged as ideal animal models to study epithelial Ca transport (ECT) by virtue of their exoskeleton, mineralized with $CaCO_3$ that must be shed and replaced to permit incremental growth (the molting cycle [1,2,3]). The associated cyclical nature of cuticular demineralization (premolt)/mineralization (postmolt) requires the primary Ca transporting epithelia (gills, hepatopancreas, antennal gland, hypodermis) to operate alternately in absorptive or secretory mode; this is in stark contrast with the intermolt period when ECT is minimal. By providing a predictable "light switch" for activating/deactivating impressive vectorial ECT, the model is enabling researchers to study the proteins involved in ECT and the genes that encode them.

The freshwater (FW) crayfish possesses the relatively unique ability to produce dilute urine, through reabsorption of ions primarily in the nephridial canal of the paired antennal (green) glands. Routinely during intermolt they reabsorb 92% of Ca in urinary filtrate [4,5,6] and unidirectional Ca influx at the antennal gland ($\sim$40 μmol kg^{-1} h^{-1}) exceeds influx at the gill or digestive epithelium. In epithelial cells, active basolateral Ca efflux involves the plasma membrane Ca ATPase (PMCA) which has been physiologically characterized using isolated membrane vesicles [7]. In vitro Ca uptake capacity was virtually identical to in vivo Ca influx in intermolt (Table 1). However in postmolt, in order to correct a hemodilution caused by FW loading at ecdysis, renal Ca reabsorption must increase by as much as 40%, which would necessitate proliferation of PMCA pumps. Our laboratory recently cloned and sequenced the PMCA3 (one of four isoforms) from crayfish antennal gland, and demonstrated increased expression of mRNA (Northern analysis) and protein (Western analysis, Fig. 1) in pre- and postmolt compared with intermolt [8]. In the present study, we sought to use the tools of modern molecular and cellular biology to further explore this expression pattern at the temporal (real-time PCR) and spatial levels (in situ hybridization for mRNA and confocal microscopy for protein). In so doing, we hoped to better understand ECT in crustacean cells.

2. Materials and methods

Crayfish, *Procambarus clarkii* (Girard), were obtained/maintained and molting stage was determined using procedures routinely employed in our laboratory [7].

Table 1
Capacity for ATP-dependent unidirectional Ca influx at the crayfish antennal gland as a function of molting stage

Molting stage	Approach	Ca influx (μmol h^{-1}animal^{-1})
Intermolt	in vitro	3.7[a]
	in vivo	3.4
Postmolt	in vitro	[b]
	in vivo	4.8 (estimate)

[a] Data taken from Ref. [7].
[b] Not determined.

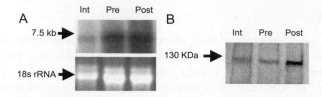

Fig. 1. (A) Northern analysis of PMCA3 in crayfish antennal gland in intermolt (Int), premolt (Pre) and postmolt (Post). Upper: total RNA (20 μg) was loaded in each lane and the membrane was hybridized to a 1164 bp crayfish PMCA3 probe and exposed to X-ray film for 24 h. Lower: to normalize the signal, 18S rRNA was run on a corresponding formaldehyde–agarose gel and visualized by ethidium bromide staining under UV light before being transferred to the membrane. (B) Western analysis of PMCA3 in crayfish antennal gland in different molting stages. Total membrane protein (30 μg) was loaded in each lane and the membrane was hybridized to a PMCA3 polyclonal antibody. (Data taken from Ref. [8].)

2.1. Quantifying PMCA mRNA expression through real-time PCR analysis

Total RNA was reverse transcribed with random hexamers to create cDNA (Taqman Reverse Transcription kit, Applied Biosystems) that was employed in PCR amplifications optimized with gene-specific primers containing a fluorescent reporter molecule (SYBR Green PCR core reagents Kit, PE AB). Oligonucleotide primers for the PMCA3 gene (sense 5'-GCAAGTGGTGGCTGTAACTGGT-3'; antisense 5'-GGCCTCCTTTGCAACAT-CAGTA-3') were chosen using Primer Express TM software (PE AB) using published sequence information [8]. A number of controls were performed to ensure proper PCR amplification. Negative controls consisting of no template controls and PCR performed on samples not subjected to reverse transcription were run on every plate. Dissociation curves were run on all PCR products to ensure that only a single PCR product was produced in each reaction. In addition, efficiency controls to show that the target sequence amplified at the same efficiency as the endogenous control (in this case 18S rRNA) was performed for each primer set. This was done to demonstrate that the slope of the difference in the cycle of threshold was under 0.01 as required for the $\Delta\Delta$Ct method that was used to quantitate the relative levels of PMCA3. Quantitative real-time PCR reactions were performed in a 96-well microtiter plate format on an ABI prism 7900HT sequence detection system (PE AB). Each cDNA sample was analyzed in triplicate and fold change relative to untreated control was calculated based on the $\Delta\Delta$Ct method assuming a primer efficiency of two and normalized to the endogenous control RNA levels.

2.2. Localization and visualization of PMCA mRNA through in situ hybridization

In situ hybridization was used to localize and visualize PMCA3 mRNA sequence in antennal gland by hybridizing a complementary nucleotide probe. The technique was adapted from Ref. [9] for crayfish (Nade, personal communication). Tissue was fixed in pre-chilled 4% paraformaldehyde (4% PFA [w/v], 0.1 M sodium acetate, pH 6.5–7.5) for 1 day and then placed in 4% PFA/20% sucrose for 3–6 days at 4 °C. Serial transverse sections (20 μm) were taken in a cryostat (−20 °C Cm3050 Leica), transferred on 0.2% gelatin coated slides, and stored in −80 °C until use.

A 42 bp oligonucleotide probe was designed for crayfish antennal gland PMCA3 against a region in the loop between transmembrane regions 4–5 (5' to 3', GGA AGG

AAA AGA ATT TAA TAG GAG AGT TAG AGA TGA GTC GGG). A sense probe was used as a negative control for nonspecific hybridization. The probe (20 pM) was ^{35}S labelled using a terminal deoxynucleotidyl transferase (TdT) kit and unincorporated radiolabel was removed in a Mini Quick-Spin DNA column. The probe was diluted in hybridization buffer [$4\times$ SSC, 50% formamide [v/v], $1\times$ Denhardt, 250 μg ml^{-1} yeast tRNA, 10% dextran sulfate [v/v], 10 mM DTT, 500 μg ml^{-1} boiled salmon sperm DNA] to yield approximately 0.5×10^6 cpm 100 μl^{-1} and stored at -20 °C.

Slides were prewashed (0.01 M PBS, 15 min, room temperature (RT) and then $2\times$ SSC 30 min, RT). Sections were then hybridized with the sterile ^{35}S-labelled probe (30 μl probe per section, overnight at 37 °C) and postwashed ($1\times$ SSC, 1 h at RT, $1\times$ SSC 15 min at RT thrice, and finally $1\times$ SSC 30 min at 50°C).

Slides were dried and placed in a Fujifilm BAS cassette with a BAS-IIIs imaging plate along with high and low standards to convert intensity to μCi. The Fujifilm was scanned after 1 day on a Fuji FLA-2000 scanner attached to a Power Macintosh 7300/200 computer with Image Gauge v3.3 software. Specific labelling was measured as intensity of signal mm^{-2} less background (to correct for nonspecific labelling). Sections were subsequently examined with standard histology (staining with cresyl violet) or emulsion autoradiography (coating with photographic emulsion) so that radioactive labelling could be correlated with cellular structure.

2.3. Immunolocalization of PMCA3 protein with confocal visualization

Subcellular expression of PMCA3 in antennal gland was examined using immunolocalization with confocal visualization [10] using polyclonal homologous antisera for crayfish PMCA3 raised in rabbits [11]. Antisera specificity has been confirmed previously through immunoblotting [8] and immunohistochemistry [11].

Briefly, cryostat sections (20 μm thick) were collected. Following washing and blocking with normal horse serum, sections were incubated with primary PMCA3 antibody. Immunoreactivity was visualized with appropriate secondary antibody namely donkey-anti-rabbit IgGs coupled to Cy3 (1-h incubation). Sections were mounted and coverslipped with Vectashield. Single immunofluorescence was analyzed on an Olympus Fluoview laser-scanning confocal microscope using air-cooled krypton/argon lasers (krypton 568 laser lines for Cy3 excitation). Emission light from the fluorochromes was separated using a dichroic mirror (EDM570) and emission filters with longpass of 585 nm (Cy3 channel, red emission). Cell nuclei were visualized with fluorescent nucleic acid stains as appropriate, to define cellular organization. Optical sections were obtained through each section at 0.5 μm separation in the Z-axis, using a $\times100$ oil immersion objective (NA 1.4) or a $\times60$ dry objective (NA 0.9). Image analysis employed ImagePro Plus (version 4.1; Media Cybernetics) and CorelDRAW.

3. Results

3.1. Quantifying PMCA3 mRNA expression through real-time PCR analysis

Real-time PCR data (Table 2) revealed dynamic upregulation of transcription of PMCA3 mRNA (relative to 18S rRNA) in pre- and postmolt antennal gland compared

Table 2
Real-time PCR expression of PMCA3 mRNA in crayfish antennal gland during molting stages

Molting stage	Fold changes of expression
Intermolt	1.00
Premolt	10.17±2.30
Postmolt	18.02±3.54

with intermolt. PMCA3 gene expression increased significantly (10-fold) in premolt with a further doubling in postmolt.

3.2. Localization and visualization of PMCA3 mRNA through in situ hybridization

In situ hybridization revealed that PMCA3 was ubiquitously expressed in all regions of the antennal gland, but was most abundant in the labyrinth and the nephridial canal as opposed to the coelomosac and bladder (see Fig. 2). Quantitation of the hybridization signal indicated that expression increased significantly in premolt (compared with intermolt) with a further increase in postmolt stage.

3.3. Immunolocalization of PMCA3 protein with confocal visualization

Confocal visualization (Fig. 3) clearly revealed PMCA3 protein immunolocalization in nephridial canal cells of the crayfish antennal gland. Labelling was prominent at the cell membrane, particularly the apical membrane adjoining the lumen; however, labelling was also apparent in the cytoplasm and the basolateral membrane. In premolt, the intensity of labelling was clearly increased.

4. Discussion

The crayfish has long been heralded as a model for hyperionic regulation because of its ability to maintain extracellular fluid (ECF) concentration significantly above ambient freshwater. The antennal gland (kidney) has emerged as the key transporting epithelium enabling this to occur. It was discovered some time ago that the crayfish antennal gland produces dilute urine, which is a major adaptation for evolution into FW, since it enables elimination of a water load without commensurate ion loss. Under routine (intermolt) conditions above 90% of the major EC ions are reabsorbed from the primary filtrate. In fact unidirectional influxes of Na, Cl and Ca at the antennal gland exceed the rates measured at the gill [12]. Confirming the relative importance of the antennal gland in ion reabsorption, specific activities of key ion motive enzymes (Na and Ca pumps) were greater in antennal gland than in gill. The ability of the crayfish to produce a dilute urine [13] has been correlated with the morphologically distinct distal nephridial tubule, a region not present in marine species that produce isoionic urine. That region was shown to be the site of active Na and Cl reabsorption [14] and presumably is also the site of Ca reabsorption.

ECT at the antennal gland has become a focus of study in our laboratory. Renal Ca reabsorption, which is impressive in intermolt, is believed to increase around ecdysis, as the animal corrects a hemodilution. A myriad of Ca channels, pumps and exchangers are involved in ECT and the emerging model of transcellular Ca flux is complex. For this reason, in the present study, we elected to present data on a single isoform of the Ca pump, PMCA3.

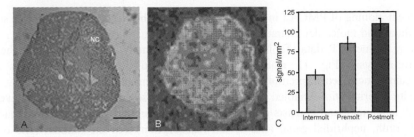

Fig. 2. (A) Histology of antennal gland section (bar, 100 µm; NC, nephridial canal; L, labyrinth; B, bladder). (B) Digitized computer image of in situ hybridization for PMCA3 mRNA in the same section (red/orange indicates greater expression). (C) Quantification of in situ hybridization as a function of molting stage.

PMCA is the ATP-dependent mechanism located on the plasma membrane that, along with Na/Ca exchanger, is believed to play a role in active renal unidirectional Ca flux. In Ca absorptive mode (as occurs at the antennal gland), its location is presumed to be basolateral, and it works to pump Ca against a concentration gradient from the cytoplasm into the hemolymph. Physiological characterization in vitro in inside-out basolateral membrane vesicles [7] confirmed ATP-dependence, and demonstrated that the transporter was inhibitable by vanadate and the Ca ionophore A_{23187}; kinetics and temperature coefficients were established.

As in vertebrates, PMCA in crustaceans is encoded by four genes [8]. Some isoforms may be housekeeping while expression of others distinctly responds to changes in ECT.

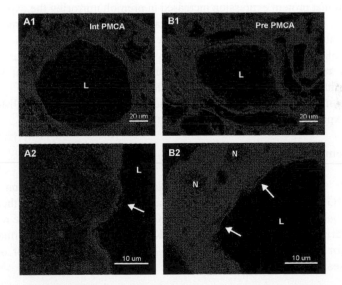

Fig. 3. Projected stacks of optical sections through crayfish antennal gland nephridial canal region (1, low magnification; 2, high magnification) showing PMCA protein labelling (red, arrows) in intermolt (A) and premolt stages (B). (L, lumen of nephridial tubule; N, nucleus.) Punctate membrane labelling is especially prominent at the luminal surface of the cells as well as in the cytoplasm and basal membrane; labelling appears more intense in premolt compared to intermolt.

The recent cloning of PMCA3 in our laboratory has enabled us to further explore some of the cellular and molecular characteristics of this isoform.

The real-time PCR data (Table 2) presented in this study confirmed our Northern and Western analysis (Fig. 1), namely that expression of PMCA3 mRNA was indeed significantly increased in premolt with a further doubling in postmolt.

In situ hybridization enabled us to translate this observation to the tissue level. The crayfish antennal gland consists of a coelomosac (where ultrafiltration occurs) leading to the labyrinth, nephridial canal (site of ion reabsorption) and the bladder (site of urine storage). These sequential regions become coiled upon each other, so that, in cross section, the nephridial canal is positioned at the periphery of the green gland. While PMCA3 was ubiquitously expressed in sections through the intact antennal gland, abundance was greatest at the periphery (Fig. 2). Corresponding histological analysis revealed this to be the location of the nephridial canal and labyrinth. Again, this would confirm that the nephridial canal/labyrinth is the site of Ca reabsorption. Quantitation of the in situ hybridization (performed on a whole section basis) revealed that PMCA3 mRNA expression increased in premolt with a further increase in postmolt, again reinforcing the trend obtained with real-time PCR data. Had the in situ analysis been restricted only to the nephridial canal region, presumably the increase in PMCA expression would have been quantitatively greater. An increase in PMCA mRNA during increased Ca flux has also been shown in the hypodermal mineralizing epithelium of a terrestrial isopod [15].

The availability of a PMCA3 antibody [11] has enabled us to focus on the subcellular distribution of this protein in distal nephridial canal cells (recognized by their columnar shape, see Fig. 3A2). Confocal visualization confirmed that PMCA3 is indeed membrane associated and that protein expression increased in premolt mirroring the expression profile of the mRNA. Interestingly the protein was associated with both plasma membranes. Models have always positioned PMCA on the basolateral membrane as it functions in apical to basolateral ECT. Several studies in the literature have suggested an apical placement in readiness to effect Ca secretion [16,17,18]. The present study clearly demonstrates that the PMCA3 is not restricted to the basolateral domain.

In conclusion, the present study has convincingly demonstrated that PMCA3 mRNA and protein expression increase with levels of renal Ca reabsorption.

Acknowledgements

This study was supported by the U.S. National Science Foundation (Grant IBN 0076035 to MGW). The authors gratefully acknowledge the following for their assistance: Dr. Steve Berberich, Director of the Center for Genomics Research, for the real-time PCR data; Dr. Mariana Morris and Ms. Mary Key, Department of Pharmacology and Toxicology, for the in situ hybridization; and Dr. Robert Fyffe, Director of the Center for Brain Research for the confocal imaging.

References

[1] P. Greenaway, Calcium balance and moulting in the crustacean, Biol. Rev. 60 (1985) 425–454.
[2] M.G. Wheatly, An overview of calcium balance in crustaceans, Physiol. Zool. 69 (1996) 351–382.

[3] M.G. Wheatly, Crustacean models for studying calcium transport: the journey from whole organisms to molecular mechanisms, J. Mar. Biol. Assoc. UK 77 (1997) 107–125.

[4] P. Greenaway, Calcium regulation in the freshwater crayfish *Austropotamobius pallipes* (Lereboullet): I. Calcium balance in the intermoult animal, J. Exp. Biol. 57 (1972) 471–487.

[5] P. Greenaway, Total body calcium and haemolymph calcium concentrations in the crayfish *Austropotamobium pallipes* (Lereboullet), J. Exp. Biol. 61 (1974) 19–26.

[6] M.G. Wheatly, T. Toop, Physiological responses of the crayfish *Pacifastacus leniusculus* (Dana) to environmental hyperoxia: II. The role of the antennal gland, J. Exp. Biol. 143 (1989) 53–70.

[7] M.G. Wheatly, R.C. Pence, J.R. Weil, ATP-dependent calcium uptake into basolateral vesicles from transporting epithelia of intermolt crayfish, Am. J. Physiol. 276 (1999) R566–R574.

[8] Y. Gao, M.G. Wheatly, Characterization and expression of plasma membrane Ca^{2+} ATPase (PMCA) in crayfish *Procambarus clarkii* antennal gland during molting, J. Exp. Biol. 207 (2004) 2991–3002.

[9] M. Key, et al., Quantitative in situ hybridization for peptide mRNAs in mouse brain, Brain Res. Protoc. 8 (2001) 8–15.

[10] E.A.L. Muennich, R.E.W. Fyffe, Focal aggregation of voltage-gated, Kv2.1 subunit-containing, potassium channels at synaptic sites in rat spinal motoneurones, J. Physiol. 554 (2003) 673–685.

[11] M.G. Wheatly, et al., Novel subcellular and molecular tools to study Ca transport mechanisms during the elusive moulting stages of crustaceans: flow cytometry and polyclonal antibodies, J. Exp. Biol. 204 (2001) 959–966.

[12] M.G. Wheatly, A.T. Gannon, Ion regulation in crayfish: freshwater adaptations and the problem of molting, Am. Zool. 35 (1995) 49–59.

[13] J.A. Riegel, Comparative Physiology of Renal Excretion, Oliver & Boyd, Edinburgh, 1972.

[14] D.R. Peterson, R.F. Loizzi, Ultrastructure of the crayfish kidney coelomosac, J. Morph. 142 (1974) 241–263.

[15] A. Ziegler, et al., Expression of Ca^{2+} ATPase and Na/Ca exchanger is upregulated during epithelial Ca^{2+} transport in hypodermal cells of the isopod *Porcellio scaber*, Cell Calcium 32 (2002) 131–141.

[16] P. Greenaway, R.M. Dillaman, R.D. Roer, Quercitin-dependent ATPase activity in the hypodermal tissue of *Callinectes sapidus* during the moult cycle, Comp. Biochem. Physiol. 111 (1995) 303–312.

[17] T.A. Reinhardt, et al., Ca^{2+}-ATPase protein expression in mammary tissue, Am. J. Physiol. 279 (2000) C1595–C1602.

[18] S.J. DeMarco, M.C. Chicka, E.E. Strehler, Plasma membrane Ca^{2+} ATPase isoform 2b interacts preferentially with the Na^+/H^+ exchanger regulatory factor 2 in apical plasma membranes, J. Biol. Chem. 277 (2002) 10506–10511.

www.ics-elsevier.com

The Cl⁻ ATPase pump

G.A. Gerencser[a,*], J. Zhang[b]

[a]Department of Physiology and Functional Genomics, College of Medicine, University of Florida, United States
[b]Department of Medicine, College of Medicine, University of Florida, United States

Abstract. Seven widely documented mechanisms of chloride transport across plasma membranes are anion-coupled antiport, sodium symport, sodium potassium chloride symport, potassium chloride symport, proton-coupled symport, an electrochemical coupling process, and chloride channels. No direct genetic evidence has yet been provided for primary active chloride transport despite numerous reports of cellular Cl⁻-stimulated ATPases coexisting in the same tissue with uphill chloride transport that could not be accounted for by the four common active chloride transport processes. Cl⁻-stimulated ATPases are a common property of practically all biological cells with the major location being of mitochondrial origin. It also appears that plasma membranes are sites of Cl⁻-stimulated ATPase activity. Recent studies of Cl⁻-stimulated ATPase activity and chloride transport in the same membrane system, including liposomes, suggest a mediation by the ATPase in net movement of chloride up its electrochemical gradient across plasma membranes. Further studies, especially from a molecular biological perspective, are required to confirm a direct transport role to plasma membrane-localized Cl⁻-stimulated ATPases. © 2004 Elsevier B.V. All rights reserved.

Keywords: Cl⁻-stimulated ATPase; Cl⁻ pump; Primary active transporter

1. Introduction

Seven mechanisms of Cl⁻ transport across plasma membranes have been widely documented and they are Na^+/Cl^- symport, $Na^+/K^+/2Cl^-$ symport, K^+/Cl^- symport, H^+/Cl^- symport, Cl^-/anion antiport Cl^- channels, and a passive electrochemical coupling process [1]. Although there have been numerous reports of primary active transporters for Cl⁻ (Cl⁻ ATPase) existing in numerous tissues, the evidence for their actual existence and functional role(s) have been, for the most part, indirect and suspect. This review will

* Corresponding author. Tel.: +1 352 392 4482; fax: +1 352 846 0270.
E-mail address: gag@phys.med.ufl.edu (G.A. Gerencser).

0531-5131/ © 2004 Elsevier B.V. All rights reserved.
doi:10.1016/j.ics.2004.09.033

highlight relatively new evidence supporting the hypothesis that Cl^- ATPase exists and that it mediates the transport of Cl^- across animal plasma membranes by the hydrolysis of ATP. Since the time Durbin and Kasbekar [2] first observed anion-stimulated ATPase activity in a microsomal fraction of frog gastric mucosa in the mid-1960s, there has been little question as to the existence of, at least, the biochemical manifestation of this enzyme. The distribution of anion-stimulated ATPase activity appears to be as widely distributed throughout biology as the number of different plants and animals studied [3–5]. DeRenzis and Bornancin [6] demonstrated the existence of a Cl^-/HCO_3^--stimulated ATPase in goldfish gill epithelia. It was not until this documentation in 1977 that Cl^--stimulated ATPase activity was linked with possible primary active Cl^- transport because Cl^- stimulation of this enzyme had not been previously demonstrated.

1.1. Anatomical site

As stated, one of the most controversial issues regarding Cl^--stimulated ATPase activity is its site or anatomical localization within the microarchitecture of cells. Without question, the primary location of anion (specifically Cl^-)-stimulated ATPase activity within animal cells appears to be in the mitochondria, i.e., a property of the mitochondrial H^+ ATPase [7]. However, Gerencser and Lee [8] presented strong evidence for the existence of Cl^- ATPase activity in a plasma membrane system free from any possible mitochondrial contaminant ATPase. They presented evidence which indicated that purified basolateral membranes (BLM) of *Aplysia* foregut absorptive cells contained Cl^- ATPase activity. The failure of oligomycin to inhibit Cl^- ATPase activity in the BLM subcellular membrane fraction had a high specific activity in (Na^++K^+) ATPase but had no perceptible cytochrome c oxidase activity nor succinic dehydrogenase activity. The failure of oligomycin to inhibit Cl^- ATPase activity in the BLM fraction was also consistent with the nonmitochondrial origin of the Cl^- ATPase. Supporting this contention was the corollary finding that oligomycin inhibited *Aplysia* mitochondrial Cl^--stimulated ATPase activity. The finding that efrapeptin, a direct inhibitor of mitochondrial F_1 ATPase activity, significantly inhibited Mg^{2+} ATPase activity in the mitochondrial and not in the BLM fraction [8] unequivocally supported the notion that the plasma membrane fraction was pure and was free from mitochondrial contamination. Additionally, Gerencser and Lee [8] showed that vanadate, an inhibitor of only "P-type ATPases" [9], inhibited Cl^- ATPase activity in the purified BLM fraction and not in the mitochondrial fraction. This result is consistent with the others inasmuch as mitochondrial H^+ ATPase is an F-type ATPase [7,9]. Taken together, all of these observations strongly supported the hypothesis that Cl^--stimulated ATPase activity exists in at least one subcellular locus other than mitochondria. It appears that, in algae, sea hare, and rat motoneuron cells, which transport Cl^-, Cl^--stimulated ATPase activity forms an integral part of the plasma membrane as a separate system [1,10,11].

1.2. Functionality

To assign a direct role of Cl^- transcellular transport to an ATPase, the enzyme should be shown to be an integral component of the plasma membrane. The energy for active transport of Cl^- can, in principle, thus be obtained from the hydrolysis of ATP. Therefore, the following question can be asked. Is the anion-stimulated ATPase identical with a primary active transport mechanism (pump) for anions? The following discussion deals with this controversial question [3,12].

2. Physiological characteristics of *Aplysia* gut

2.1. Tissue

Aplysia californica foregut (crop) bathed in a Na^+-containing seawater medium elicits a spontaneous transepithelial potential difference (Ψ_{ms}) (0.5–3.0 mV) such that the serosal surface is negative relative to the mucosal surface [4,11,13]. The SCC across *A. californica* gut was accounted for by active absorptive mechanisms for both Na^+ and Cl^-, the net absorptive Cl^- transport exceeding the net aborptive Na^+ transport.

However, past observations suggested that Cl^- absorption was independent of Na^+ absorption [13]. Therefore, Cl^- absorption would be independent of Na^+–K^+-dependent ATPase activity. The Ψ_{ms} measured in a Na^+-free seawater medium was stable for 3–5 h, and the electrical orientation of Ψ_{ms} was serosa-negative relative to the mucosal solution. In the absence of Na^+ in the bathing medium, the SCC was identical to the net mucosal to serosal Cl^- flux [13,14]. In the absence of an electrochemical potential gradient for Cl^- across the tissue, these observations suggested that there was an active transport mechanism for Cl^-. However, these observations delineated neither location nor type of mechanism for the Cl^- active transport.

2.2. Cellular

Reports of intracellular Cl^- activity (a_{Cl}^i) in vertebrate enterocytes demonstrated that Cl^- was accumulated across the mucosal membrane such that the a_{Cl}^i was two to three times that predicted for electrochemical equilibrium across that membrane [15,16]. These studies concluded that Cl^- uphill movement across the mucosal membrane was coupled to the simultaneous downhill movement of Na^+, and it was this extracellular to intracellular Na^+ electrochemical gradient across the mucosal membrane that was the driving force responsible for intracellular Cl^- accumulation.

The mean a_{Cl}^i determined in *A. californica* gut epithelial cells bathed in a NaCl seawater medium devoid of substrate was 10.1 ± 0.5 mM [14,17]. The mean a_{Cl}^i significantly increased after mucosal glucose addition to 14.2 ± 0.6 mM. The a_{Cl}^i values both before and after D-glucose addition were significantly less than those predicted by the electrochemical equilibrium for Cl^- across the mucosal membrane. In the absence of Na^+ in the extracellular bathing solution, the mean a_{Cl}^i was 9.1 mM, which is also less than that predicted for electrochemical equilibrium for Cl^- across the mucosal membrane [18,19]. Thus, one need not postulate an active transport mechanism for Cl^- in the apical or mucosal membrane of the *Aplysia* foregut absorptive cell because Cl^- transport across this membrane could be driven by the downhill mucosal to cytosol electrochemical potential gradient for Cl^-. However, once the Cl^- was in the cytosol, it faced a very steep electrochemical potential gradient in its transit across the basolateral membrane into the serosal solution [4,18,20]. Therefore, thermodynamically, the active transport mechanism for Cl^- exhibited in the tissue studies had to exist in the basolateral membrane (BLM) of the *Aplysia* foregut absorptive cell.

3. Biochemistry and transport activity of the Cl⁻ ATPase

3.1. ATPase activity

Gerencser and Lee [8,21] presented evidence which indicated that the BLM, and only the BLM, of *Aplysia* foregut absorptive cells contains true Cl⁻ ATPase activity. Biochemical properties of the *Aplysia* foregut absorptive cells BLM-localized Cl⁻-stimulated ATPase include the following: (1) pH optimum=7.8; (2) ATP being the most effective nucleotide hydrolyzed; (3) also stimulated by HCO_3^-, SO_3^{-2}, and $S_2O_3^{-2}$ but inhibited by NO_2^- and no effect elicited by NO_3^- or SO_4^{-2}; (4) apparent K_m for Cl⁻ is 10.3 mM, while the apparent K_m for ATP is 2.6 mM; and (5) an absolute requirement for Mg^{2+} which has an optimal concentration of 3 mM [8,21]. Coincidentally, Cl⁻ has an intracellular activity [17] in the *Aplysia* foregut epithelial cell approximating its apparent K_m for the Mg^{2+}-dependent Cl⁻ ATPase, which supports the interrelationship of its physiological and biochemical activities.

3.2. Transport activity

To elucidate both the nature and electrogenicity of the ATP-dependent Cl⁻ transport process, several experimental maneuvers were performed by Gerencser [22] as follows. First, an inwardly directed valinomycin-induced K^+ diffusion potential, making the BLM inside-out vesicle interior electrically positive, enhanced ATP-driven Cl⁻ uptake compared with vesicles lacking the ionophore. Second, an inwardly directed FCCP-induced H^+ electrodiffusion potential, making the BLM inside-out vesicle interior less negative, increased ATP-dependent Cl⁻ uptake compared to control. Third, ATP increased intravesicular negativity measured by lipophilic cation distribution across the vesicular membrane. Both ATP and Cl⁻ appeared to be necessary for generating the negative intravesicular membrane potential because substituting a nonhydrolyzable ATP analog for ATP in the presence of Cl⁻ in the extravesicular medium did not generate a potential above that of control.

Likewise, substituting NO_3^- for Cl⁻ in the extra- and intravesicular media in the presence of extravesicular ATP caused no change in potential difference above that of control. These results also suggested that hydrolysis of ATP is necessary for the accumulation of Cl⁻ in the vesicles. Furthermore, vanadate and thiocyanate inhibited both the (ATP+Cl⁻)-dependent intravesicular negativity and ATP-dependent Cl⁻ uptake. In addition, it had been demonstrated that the pH optimum of the Cl⁻-stimulated ATPase [21] coincided exactly with the pH optimum of 7.8 of the ATP-dependent Cl⁻ transport in the *Aplysia* foregut absorptive cell BLM vesicles [8]. Bafilomycin had no effect on either ATP-dependent potential change or ATP-dependent Cl⁻ transport, supporting the notion that this transporter was a P ATPase and not a V ATPase as bafilomycin is an inhibitor of V ATPase activity [23]. Further buttressing this observation was the observation that DCCD, an inhibitor of P, V, or F ATPase proton pumps [9], had no effect on the ATP-dependent transport parameters: Cl⁻ transport or vesicular membrane potential change. These results negated a proton-recycling mechanism [23] as the means for net Cl⁻ uptake in BLM vesicles.

Finally, all three aspects of the BLM-localized Cl⁻ pump (ATPase, ATP-dependent Cl⁻ transport, and ATP-dependent vesicular membrane potential change) have the same pH optimum and have the same Mg^{2+} and Cl^- kinetic parameters [24,25], which suggests that these properties are part of the same molecular mechanism.

3.3. Reconstitution of the Cl^- pump

Reconstitution of a membrane protein into a liposome provides one of the few methods needed to rigorously demonstrate the existence of a separate and distinct biochemical and physiological molecular entity. This method also provides evidence that all components of the solubilized protein have been extracted intact. With this premise in mind, Gerencser [26] reconstituted both aspects of the Cl^- pump; i.e., the catalytic (ATPase) and transport components from the BLM of *Aplysia* gut absorptive cells. Cl^--stimulated ATPase activity existed significantly above Mg^{2+}-stimulated ATPase activity found in the proteoliposome population extracted and generated with digitonin. Vanadate abolished this Cl^--stimulated ATPase activity. From this digitonin-generated proteoliposome population, there is a significant ATP-dependent Cl^- uptake into these proteoliposomes above that of control, and that this ATP-dependent Cl^- uptake was also abolished by vanadate.

These data suggested that these two major observations are manifestations of one molecular mechanism: the Cl^- pump. Support of this contention rested with the findings that vanadate (an inhibitor of P-type ATPases) inhibited both Cl^--stimulated ATPase activity and ATP-dependent Cl^- transport in the digitonin-based proteoliposomes. Krogh [27] first coined the term "Cl^- pump" in 1937, it was not until the reconstitution of all of its components into an artificial liposomal system through the study mentioned above [26] that the existence of this mechanism (primary active transport mechanism) was proven. Similar reconstitutions of Cl^- pump activity have since been reported in bacteria [28], algae [29], and rat brain [30,31]. However, the alga studies [29] are somewhat ambiguous as Cl^- inhibited the Mg^{2+} ATPase activity despite there being an ATP-dependent Cl^- uptake into the proteoliposomes.

3.4. Molecular weight

The approximate molecular weight of the Cl^- pump was ascertained [32] utilizing electrophoretic techniques to digitonin-generated proteoliposomes containing the Cl^- pump protein from *Aplysia* gut absorptive cells, as shown previously [26]. Inasmuch as both aspects of the Cl^- pump were inhibited by vanadate, it was surmised that the approximate molecular weight of the Cl^- pump of *Aplysia* should be around 100 kDa as vanadate only inhibited "P" type ATPases and not "F" or "V" type ATPases [9]. The alpha-subunit or catalytic unit of all "P" type ATPases approximates 100 kDa in molecular weight. One major protein band was eluted through PAGE, and its molecular weight was found to be 110 kDa [32]. Recently, similar molecular weights have been obtained for Cl^- pump catalytic subunits in alga [29,33] and rat brain [31,34], confirming the possible E_1–E_2 or P nature of the ATPase, although the authors of these studies postulate these structural subunits to be part of a V-type ATPase assembly. These conclusions were reached despite the ATPases being partially inhibited by vanadate, a specific inhibitor of P ATPases [9].

3.5. Reaction mechanism

The semipurified protein (Cl^- pump) had been subjected to phosphorylation within the proteoliposome, and the reaction sequence and kinetics of the reaction sequence of the enzyme have been determined: Mg^{2+} causing phosphorylation, Cl^- causing dephosphor-ylation, and all in a time frame consistent with an aspartyl phosphate linkage [11,32]. Hydroxylamine and high pH destablized this phosphorylation, confirming an acyl phosphate bond as an intermediate in the reaction sequence [35]. Vanadate almost completely inhibited the Mg^{2+}-driven phosphorylation reaction, which corroborates the protein catalytic subunit molecular weight of 110 kDa, and it also defines the protein as a P-type ATPase because vanadate is a transition state competitive inhibitor of phosphate [9].

More recently, Gerencser and Zhang [36] have shown that E_1–P formation was 26 s^{-1}. This approximated E_1–P rate constant values for other electrogenic uniport P-type ATPases, and therefore, it was concluded from these results that the Cl^- ATPase phosphorylation kinetics did not greatly differ from cation ATPase phosphorylation kinetics. Fig. 1 is an operational model of the reaction sequence of the *Aplysia* Cl^- pump [32].

3.6. Stoichiometry

The stoichiometry of ATP hydrolyzed to Cl^- transported during a single cycle of the reaction sequence was ascertained through thermodynamic means [37]. Intracellular concentrations of ATP, ADP, and inorganic phosphate were determined and, coupled with an estimate of the standard free energy of hydrolysis for ATP, the operant free energy for ATP hydrolysis was calculated. Because the operating free energy of the Cl^- pump (electromotive force) was approximately one-half the energy (140 mV) obtained from the total free energy of ATP hydrolysis (270 mV), the only possible integral stoichiometries were one or, at the most, two Cl^- transported per cycle per ATP hydrolyzed.

Physiologically, the electrogenic Cl^- pump [22] most likely transports one Cl^- per ATP hydrolyzed per reaction cycle. This increased electrochemical driving force created by the electrogenic nature of the pump could fuel secondary electrophoretic (or electroneutral) transport processes such as the nutritional uptake of sugars and/or amino acids [38].

3.7. Kinetics

Utilizing a purified BLM vesicle preparation containing Cl^- ATPase from *Aplysia* gut, it was demonstrated that ATP and its subsequent hydrolysis stimulated both intravesicular Cl^- accumulation and intravesicular negativity with almost identical kinetics [24].

Reaction Sequence of Cl⁻ Pump

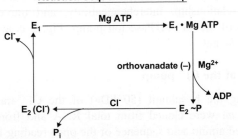

Fig. 1. Working model of reaction sequence for Cl^- pump. E_1 and E_2 are assumed to be different conformational states of the enzyme as it has been demonstrated that all P-type ATPases have at least two major conformational states [5]. (–) represents inhibition by orthovanadate of the Mg^{2+}-driven phosphorylation reaction. Taken from Ref. [32] with permission.

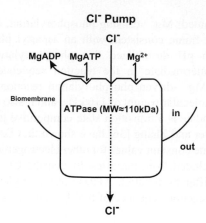

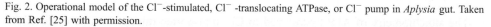

Fig. 2. Operational model of the Cl⁻-stimulated, Cl⁻-translocating ATPase, or Cl⁻ pump in *Aplysia* gut. Taken from Ref. [25] with permission.

Additionally, in the proteoliposomal preparation the apparent K_ms of Cl⁻ concentration for ATP-dependent Cl⁻ uptake, ATP-dependent membrane potential change, and Cl⁻-stimulated ATPase activity were almost identical to each other [25]. These values were similar to what had been reported for Cl⁻ ATPase activity in the *Aplysia* BLM preparation [8] and in rat brain motoneurons [31].

Similarly, the apparent K_ms of ATP for ATP-dependent Cl⁻ uptake, ATP-dependent membrane potential change, and Cl⁻-stimulated ATPase in the proteoliposomal preparation were similar to each other [25] and to the apparent K_m for ATP found for Cl⁻ ATPase in the BLM of *Aplysia* [11,39] and for ATP-induced phosphorylation of Cl⁻ ATPase in the same proteoliposomal preparation of *Aplysia* [11,39]. These kinetic experiments demonstrate the correspondence between overall ATPase activity, Cl⁻ ATPase phosphorylation, ATP-dependent Cl⁻ transport, ATP-dependent membrane potential change, and Cl⁻ ATPase activity which are similar to those characteristics detected in cation-activated and cation-motive ATPases [9].

These kinetics are uniquely significant not only because they are the first and only results obtained with an isolated protein anion transporter ATPase but also because they demonstrate the interrelationship, interchangeability, and universality between both transport and catalysis of the Cl⁻ ATPase ion pump. Fig. 2 is an operational model of the Cl⁻ pump in *Aplysia* gut.

4. Molecular biology of the Cl⁻ pump

The genes encoding the b subunit (50 kDa) of the Cl⁻ translocating ATPase of *Acetabularia acetabulum* were cloned from total RNA and from poly(A)⁺ RNA and sequenced. The deduced amino acid sequence of the open reading frame consisted of 478 amino acids and showed high similarity to the β subunit of chloroplast F_{1-} ATPases [33]. Gene fragments encoding the putative β subunit of chloroplast F_{1-} (273 bp) and mitochondrial F_{1-} ATPases (332 bp) were also cloned from *A. acetabulum* and sequenced, respectively. The deduced amino acid sequence of the chloroplast F_{1-} ATPase showed

92.5% identity to the primary structure of the b subunit of the Cl⁻-translocating ATPase, while the nucleotide sequences were 79.9% identical. The deduced amino acid sequence was 79.9% identical. The deduced amino acid sequence of the latter was 77.3% identical to that of the b subunit of the Cl⁻-translocating ATPase, and the nucleotide sequences were 67.5% identical.

Reverse transcriptase polymerase chain reaction was used to detect the mRNA of the *A. californica* foregut Cl⁻ pump. The Cl⁻ pump RNA had a high homology relative to mRNAs of subunits of Na^+/K^+ ATPase and other P-type ATPases. The cDNA sequence of the *A. californica* Cl⁻ ATPase was cloned, and the resulting 200-base-pair sequence was shown to be 76% identical to regions of alpha-subunits of P-type ATPases [36].

Recently, the DNA of a 55-kDa protein derived from a 520-kDa Cl⁻ ATPase complex was cloned from rat brain [34]. Sequences of nucleic acids in the cDNA and the deduced amino acids were not homologous with any known ion-translocating ATPases [9], and the application of its antisense oligonucleotides induced increases in Cl⁻ concentrations in primary cultured rat hippocampal neurons, suggesting that the 55-kDa protein acts as a catalytic subunit of the Cl⁻ ATPase pump.

5. Conclusions and thoughts

In contrast to most higher animals, the *Aplysia* gut has evolved a double-salt pump system. It has a Na^+ pump (Na^+/K^+ ATPase) and a Cl⁻ pump (Cl⁻ ATPase) which, upon first view, leads one to think how inefficient salt absorption by these cells are in terms of ATP utilization. One can easily envision the Na^+ pump generating the intracellular electrochemical asymmetry needed for Na^+-coupled entry of energetic and structural equivalents. These equivalents (e.g., sugars, amino acids, etc.) are needed for the continued maintenance and survival of the organism. However, a Cl⁻ pump that utilizes more ATP than the Na^+ pump appears to be a frivolous vestigium of a gone-awry evolutionary process. Not necessarily so if one considers the environment that the *Aplysia* gut cells are bathed in each and every second of their existence! These cells are surrounded by seawater, a medium so rich in Cl⁻ that the Cl⁻ concentration is at least 100 mEq l^{-1} higher than any other ion in this medium. The *Aplysia* gut cells had to adapt to survive the onslaught of Cl⁻ rushing into their internal environment, thereby causing the demise of these cells and therefore the animal itself. The Cl⁻ pump is a survival mechanism intended to prevent osmotic lysis of the *Aplysia* gut cells. The survival instinct through evolutionary adaptation, in the case of *Aplysia*, has helped maintain the existence of this species for millions and millions of years.

Acknowledgements

The first author wishes to acknowledge his gratitude to his technologists, students, and collaborators for their able contributions to the studies reviewed and performed herein. These studies were supported by D.S.R. Seed Award (No. 229K15) in Whitehall Foundation Grant (No. 78-156 ck-1), D.S.R. Award (No. 122101010) and the Eppley Foundation for Research.

References

[1] G.A. Gerencser, The chloride pump: a Cl⁻-transport locating P-type ATPase, Critical Reviews in Biochemistry and Molecular Biology 31 (1996) 303–337.

[2] R.P. Durbin, D.K. Kasbekar, Adenosine triphosphate and active transport by the stomach, Federation Proceedings 24 (1965) 1377–1381.

[3] J.J.H.H.M. DePont, S.L. Bonting, Anion-sensitive ATPase and (K⁺+H⁺)-ATPase, in: S.L. Bonting, J.J.H.H.M. Depont (Eds.), Membrane Transport, Elsevier/North Holland Biomedical Press, 1981, pp. 209–222.

[4] G.A. Gerencser, Primary electrogenic chloride transport across the Aplysia gut, in: J. Durham, M. Hardy, (Eds.), Bicarbonate, Chloride and Proton Transport Systems, Annual New York Academy of Science, vol. 574, pp. 1–10.

[5] F. Schuurmanns Stekhoven, S.L. Bonting, Transport adenosine triphosphatases: properties and functions, Physiological Reviews 61 (1981) 1–76.

[6] G. DeRenzis, M. Bornancin, Cl⁻/HCO₃⁻ATPase in the gills of Carassius auiratus: its inhibition by thiocyanate, Biochimica et Biophysica Acta 467 (1977) 192–207.

[7] E. Racker, ATPase and oxidative phosphorylation, Federation Proceedings 21 (1962) 54.

[8] G.A. Gerencser, S.H. Lee, Cl⁻/HCO3⁻-stimulated ATPase in intestinal mucosa of Aplysia, American Journal of Physiology 248 (1985) R241–R248.

[9] P.L. Pedersen, E. Carafoli, Ion motive ATPases: I. Ubiquity, properties, and significance to cell function, Trends in Biochemical Sciences 12 (1987) 146–150.

[10] G.A. Gerencser, Properties and functions of Cl⁻-stimulated ATPase, Trends in Life Science 1 (1986) 1–18.

[11] G.A. Gerencser, B. Zelezna, Existence of a chloride pump in mollusks, in: G.A. Gerencser (Ed.), Electrogenic Cl⁻ Transporters in Biological Membranes, Advances in Comparative and Environmental Physiology, vol. 19, 1994, pp. 39–58.

[12] G.A. Gerencser, Invertebrate epithelial transport, American Journal of Physiology 244 (1983) R127–R129.

[13] G.A. Gerencser, Thiocyanate inhibition of active chloride absorption in Aplysia intestine, Biochimica et Biophysica Acta 775 (1984) 389–394.

[14] G.A. Gerencser, Electrogenic and electrically coupled chloride transport across molluscan intestine, in: G.A. Gerencser (Ed.), Chloride Transport Coupling in Biological Membranes and Epithelia, Elsevier, Amsterdam, 1984, pp. 183–203.

[15] W.McD. Armstrong, W. Wojtkowski, W.R. Bixenman, A new solid-state microelectrode for measuring intracellular chloride activities, Biochimica et Biophysica Acta 465 (1977) 165–170.

[16] W.McD. Armstrong, et al., Energetics of coupled Na⁺ and Cl⁻ entry into epithelial cells of bullfrog small intestine, Biochimica et Biophysica Acta 551 (1979) 207–212.

[17] G.A. Gerencser, J.F. White, Membrane potentials and chloride activities in epithelial cells of Aplysia intestine, American Journal of Physiology 239 (1980) R445–R449.

[18] G.A. Gerencser, Electrophysiology of chloride transport in Aplysia (mollusk) intestine, American Journal of Physiology 244 (1983) R143–R149.

[19] G.A. Gerencser, Transport across the invertebrate intestine, in: G. Gilles, M.G. Gilles-Baillien (Eds.), Transport Processes Iono- and Osmoregulation, vol. II, Springer, Berlin, 1985, pp. 251–264.

[20] G.A. Gerencser, Transport energetics of the Cl⁻ pump in Aplysia gut, Biochimica et Biophysica Acta 1330 (1997) 110–112.

[21] G.A. Gerencser, S.H. Lee, Cl⁻-stimulated adenosine triphosphatase: existence, location and function, Journal of Experimental Biology 106 (1983) 142–161.

[22] G.A. Gerencser, Electrogenic ATP-dependent Cl⁻ transport by plasma membrane vesicles from Aplysia intestine, American Journal of Physiology 254 (1988) R127–R133.

[23] H. Wieczorek, The insect V-ATPase, a plasma membrane proton pump energizing secondary active transport: molecular analysis of electrogenic potassium transport in the tobacco hornworm midgut, Journal of Experimental Biology 172 (1992) 335–343.

[24] G.A. Gerencser, K.R. Purushotham, A novel Cl⁻ pump: intracellular regulation of transport activity, Biochemical and Biophysical Research Communications 215 (1995) 994–1000.

[25] G.A. Gerencser, K.R. Purushotham, Reconstituted Cl⁻ pump protein: a novel ion (Cl⁻)-motive ATPase, Journal of Bioenergetics and Biomembranes 28 (1996) 459–469.

[26] G.A. Gerencser, Reconsitution of a chloride-translocating ATPase from *Aplysia californica* gut, Biochimica et Biophysica Acta 1030 (1990) 301–303.

[27] A. Krogh, Osmotic regulation in the frog (*R. esculenta*) by active absorption of chloride ions, Skandinavica Archives of Physiology 76 (1937) 60–74.

[28] L. Zimanyi, J. Lanyi, Halorhodopsin: a light-driven active chloride transport system, in: J. Durham, M. Hardy (Eds.), Bicarbonate, Chloride and Proton Transport Systems, Ann. N.Y. Acad. Sci., 1989, pp. 11–19.

[29] M. Keda, D. Oesterhelt, A Cl⁻-translocating adenosinetriphosphatase in *Acetabularia acetabulum*: 2. Reconstitution of the enzyme into liposomes and effect of net charges of liposomes on chloride permeability and reconstitution, Biochemistry 29 (1990) 2065–2070.

[30] X.T. Zeng, M. Hara, C. Inagaki, Electrogenic and phosphatidylinositol-4-monophosphate-stimulated Cl⁻ transport by Cl⁻ pump in the rat brain, Brain Research 641 (1994) 167–170.

[31] C. Inagaki, M. Hara, M. Inoue, Transporting Cl⁻-ATPase in rat brain, in: G.A. Gerencser (Ed.), Electrogenic Cl⁻ Transporters in Biological Membranes, Advances in Comparative and Environmental Physiology, vol. 19, 1994, pp. 59–79.

[32] G.A. Gerencser, B. Zelezna, Reaction sequence and molecular mass of a Cl⁻-translocating P-type ATPase, Proceedings of the National Academy of Sciences 90 (1993) 7970–7974.

[33] C. Moritani, et al., Purification and characterization of a membrane-bound ATPase from *Acetabularia cliftoni* that corresponds to a Cl⁻-translocating ATPase in *Acetabularia acetabulum*, Bioscientific and Biotechnical Biochemistry 58 (1994) 2087–2089.

[34] X.T. Zeng, et al., Antiserum against Cl⁻ pump complex recognized 51 kDa protein, a possible catalylic unit in the rat brain, Neuroscience Letters 258 (1998) 85–88.

[35] F. Vara, R. Serrano, Phosphorylated intermediate of the ATPase of plant plasma membranes, Journal of Biological Chemistry 257 (1982) 12826–12830.

[36] G.A. Gerencser, J. Zhang, The Cl⁻ pump in mollusks: a Cl⁻-translocating P-type, Comparative Biochemistry and Physiology 126A (2000) S59.

[37] G.A. Gerencser, Stoichiometry of a Cl⁻-translocating ATPase, Federation of European Biochemical Societies Letters 333 (1993) 133–140.

[38] G.A. Gerencser, et al., Is there a Cl⁻ pump? American Journal of Physiology 255 (1988) 677–692.

[39] G.A. Gerencser, A novel P-type Cl⁻-stimulated ATPase: phosphorylation and specificity, Biochemical and Biophysical Research Communications 196 (1993) 1188–1194.

ELSEVIER

www.ics-elsevier.com

Organelle-specific zinc ATPases in Crustacean ER and lysosomal membranes

Gregory A. Ahearn*, Prabir K. Mandal, Anita Mandal

Department of Biology, 4567 St. Johns Bluff Road, S., University of North Florida, Jacksonville, Florida 32224, United States

Abstract. In crustaceans, the hepatopancreas is the major organ system responsible for heavy metal detoxification, and within this structure the endoplasmic reticulum (ER) and lysosomes are two organelles that regulate cytoplasmic metal concentrations by selective sequestration processes. This study compares the physiological properties of purified membranes from hepatopancreatic ER and lysosomes for zinc uptake from the cytoplasm and its sequestration in these organelles. The endoplasmic reticulum is a cellular organelle that sequesters calcium in many types of cells through the action of a calcium ATPase transporter (SERCA), maintaining a low cytoplasmic activity of the cation as a result of this ATP-dependent carrier function. The present investigation showed that $^{45}Ca^{2+}$ and $^{65}Zn^{2+}$ were transported by the same ATP-dependent, vanadate and thapsigargin-sensitive, ER carrier system displaying substrate binding cooperativity. In contrast, lysosomes, known centers for metal and calcium sequestration and complex formation with a variety of inorganic and organic anions, transferred $^{65}Zn^{2+}$ across their membranes by ATP-dependent, vanadate- and divalent cation-inhibited, thapsigargin-insensitive, carrier processes that illustrated Michaelis–Menten influx kinetics. These results suggest that two distinct types of carrier-mediated ATPases may be involved in the sequestration and detoxification of heavy metals in the two hepatopancreatic organelles. © 2004 Elsevier B.V. All rights reserved.

Keywords: Zinc transport; Lysosomes; Endoplasmic reticulum; ATPase; SERCA

1. Introduction

Environmental and dietary heavy metals are required by crustaceans and other organisms as essential cofactors in many enzymatically catalyzed reactions and must be

---

* Corresponding author. Tel.: +1 904 620 1806; fax: +1 904 620 3885.
  E-mail address: gahearn@unf.edu (G.A. Ahearn).

0531-5131/ © 2004 Elsevier B.V. All rights reserved.
doi:10.1016/j.ics.2004.08.067

provided to cells by membrane transport systems in low concentrations so that metabolic activities will be optimized [1]. However, as metal concentrations increase beyond organismic physiological and biochemical needs, they may become toxic to cells potentially leading to death of the organism [2,3]. Crustaceans, and other invertebrates, have developed a number of heavy metal detoxification mechanisms for reducing intracellular concentrations of heavy metals by sequestering them in specific organelles [4–7] or binding them to cytoplasmic proteins called metallothioneins that can be genetically upregulated in response to elevated concentrations of cellular xenobiotics [5,8,9]. Besides metallothioneins and other metal-binding proteins that reduce the concentrations of soluble cytoplasmic metals, mitochondria [10–13], endoplasmic reticulum (ER) [14–16], and lysosomes [17,18] are organelle centers of heavy metal sequestration that use membrane transport carrier proteins and channels to accumulate cytoplasmic cationic metals, and in some cases, complex them with organic and inorganic anions delivered to the organelles from the cytoplasm by their own complement of membrane transfer systems. Once the cationic metals and anions are accumulated to a sufficient concentration within these centers of sequestration, a precipitate is formed that isolates the metal from the rest of the organism and reduces its potentially deleterious effects on cells and tissues [19].

This study compares the physiological transport properties for calcium and zinc of lobster hepatopancreatic endoplasmic reticulum and lysosomes, two known centers for metal sequestration and detoxification. Findings suggest that different ATPase transport systems with dissimilar kinetic properties may be present on the membranes of these two organelles for isolating and sequestering metals from the cytoplasm.

2. Materials and methods

2.1. Animals

Live Atlantic lobsters (*Homarus americanus*) with a body mass of 500–700 g, were purchased from local commercial dealers in Jacksonville, Florida and maintained in a seawater holding tank at 15 °C until needed for experimentation. Intermolt (molt stage estimated by gastrolith weight/carapace length ratio) lobsters were used for all experiments. Lobsters were provided with mussel meat for up to 15–20 days and all experiments were conducted only on animals that had not been fed for approximately 24 h to ensure an evacuated hepatopancreas.

2.2. Isolation of hepatopancreatic endoplasmic reticulum (ER) vesicles

Methods used to isolate and purify hepatopancreatic ER vesicles followed the procedure described previously [16]. Briefly, hepatopancreatic ER vesicles were prepared from fresh organs of individual lobsters. Hepatopancreatic tissue was quickly placed in Solution 1 consisting of 250 mM sucrose and 10 mM MOPS, pH 7.2 and left in ice. The tissue was excised and homogenized in a glass hand homogenizer and centrifuged at $15,000 \times g$ for 20 min. The supernatant was centrifuged at $100,000 \times g$ for 40 min. The resulting supernatant was decanted and the pellet resuspended with the hand homogenizer in Solution 2 consisting of 250 mM sucrose, 10 mM MOPS–Tris, and KCl (0.9 g in 20 ml), pH 7.2 and left on ice for 40 min. This mixture was centrifuged at $15,000 \times g$ for 20 min. The resulting supernatant was centrifuged at 100,000×g for 40 min and the pellet resuspended in 50–100 µl of Solution 1.

2.3. Isolation of hepatopancreatic lysosomal membrane vesicles

Methods used to isolate and purify hepatopancreatic lysosomal membrane vesicles followed the protocols developed by Thamotharan et al. [20] and Zhou et al. [21] for mammals which were modified for crustacean tissues by Chavez-Crooker et al. [18]. Briefly, whole hepatopancreas was minced into small pieces and homogenized in Buffer A containing PMSF (250 mM sucrose, 20 mM HEPES, 1 mM EDTA, 300 µl/100 ml of a 100 mM PMSF solution, pH 7.0). The homogenate was diluted 10-fold in Buffer A and centrifuged at 750×g for 10 min. The resulting pellet was discarded and centrifugation was repeated. The supernatant from the second centrifugation was collected and centrifuged at 20,000×g for 10 min and the resulting pellet resuspended in Buffer B (250 mM sucrose, 20 mM Hepes, adjusted to pH 7.0 with Tris base). The suspension was mixed with isotonic Percoll in the ratio of 9:11 (pellet suspended in Buffer B: isotonic Percoll) and centrifuged at 40,000×g for 90 min. The brownish dense lysosomal band near the bottom of the gradient was removed, diluted with Buffer B, and centrifuged at 20,000×g for 10 min. The resulting pellet was incubated in freshly prepared Buffer B containing 5 mM methionine methyl ester, 2 mg/ml bovine serum albumen, and 2 mM MgCl$_2$, for 20 min at 37 C. An equal volume of ice-cold isotonic Percoll was added to the incubation mixture and centrifuged at 35,000×g for 30 min. A brownish band at the top of the gradient, which was purified lysosomal membrane vesicles, was resuspended in preloading transport buffer and allowed to equilibrate for 15 min before starting an experiment.

The enrichments of NADPH–cytochrome c reductase (endoplasmic reticulum enzyme marker) and alkaline phosphatase (brush border enzyme marker) were used to show the purification of the ER membrane samples used in the present investigation. While the brush border enzyme marker, alkaline phosphatase, was not significantly enriched ($p > 0.05$) in the ER membrane fraction compared to the original tissue homogenate, the ER enzyme, NADPH–cytochrome c reductase, was purified by greater than a factor of 13 in the final vesicle suspension used in subsequent transport studies [16].

Similarly, enzyme characterization of lobster hepatopancreatic lysosomal membrane vesicles produced by the methods described above compared the relative enrichments of alkaline phosphatase with a lysosomal enzyme marker, acid phosphatase in the original tissue homogenate with the final purified lysosomal vesicles. As before, alkaline phosphatase was not significantly ($p > 0.05$) enriched in the final lysosomal membrane vesicle fraction, but the lysosome-specific membrane marker, was purified by more than a factor of 10.0 in the final vesicle sample used for the transport experiments that follow. These results suggest that the ER and lysosomal vesicle fractions used in this investigation were relatively pure and had a minimal membrane contamination from other parts of the cell such as the plasma membrane.

2.4. $^{45}Ca^{2+}$ and $^{65}Zn^{2+}$ transport experiments

Characteristics of $^{45}Ca^{2+}$ and $^{65}Zn^{2+}$ transport by isolated vesicles from hepatopancreatic ER and lysosomes were studied at room temperature (23 °C). Experiments were initiated by diluting a vesicle suspension into a medium containing trace amounts of $^{45}Ca^{2+}Cl_2$ or ^{65}Zn-sulfate and unlabelled calcium gluconate or zinc sulfate, respectively. The composition of the final vesicle suspension solutions (inside vesicles) and incubation media are described separately for each experiment. Uptake of radiolabelled substrates were initiated by rapidly mixing 20 µl of cell suspension (150 µg of protein), preloaded with buffer (pH 7.2), with 180 µl of transport medium (described separately for each experiment) and incubating for appropriate time periods. Transport was terminated by addition of 2 ml (10-fold dilution) ice-cold buffer (stop solution) and the suspension was immediately collected under vacuum on a Millipore filter (HAWP, 45 µm pore size), utilizing the Millipore filtration technique developed by Hopfer et al. [32]. Filters were then dissolved in liquid scintillation cocktail (Ecolume) and the radioactivity counted in a Beckman Coulter LS 6500 Multipurpose scintillation counter. Isotope uptake was expressed as pmol/mg protein x sec and the protein content of the vesicle suspension was determined according to Bradford's procedure (BioRad), using bovine serum albumin as a standard. Displayed calcium and zinc activities were achieved using appropriate concentrations of calcium or zinc, NTA (nitriloacetic acid; N,N-bis[carboxymethyl]glycine), magnesium, and EGTA using Winmax Chelator 2.0 software [33]. Isotope uptake into cells was corrected for nonspecific isotope binding by injecting an aliquot of cells and isotope directly into ice-cold stop solution without prior mixing. The resulting cell suspension was then filtered, rinsed, and counted as described previously. Resulting values for nonspecific isotope binding were subtracted from total isotope uptake in each experiment, providing an index of transmembrane transport of the respective radiolabelled cation. Time points are presented as means of 3–5 replicates and their associated standard errors. Experiments were repeated at least once. Statistical comparisons were made using Student's t-test where a value of $p < 0.05$ was considered significant. Curve fitting procedures were accomplished using Sigma Plot 7.101 software (Jandel).

2.5. Chemicals

$^{45}CaCl_2$ and ^{65}Zn-sulfate were obtained from DuPont New England Nuclear, Boston, MA. Vanadate, thapsigargin, tetramethylammonium hydroxide (TMA-OH), Na- and Ca-gluconate, Zn-sulfate, EGTA, TRIS, D-mannitol, and other reagent grade chemicals were purchased from Sigma (St. Louis, MO), Fisher (Pittsburgh, PA), or Bio-Rad Laboratories, Hercules, CA.

3. Results

3.1. Time course of $^{45}Ca^{2+}$ and $^{65}Zn^{2+}$ uptake by hepatopancreatic ER vesicles

The time course of 25 µM $^{45}Ca^{2+}$ and $^{65}Zn^{2+}$ uptake into ER vesicles was studied in the presence and absence of 1 mM ATP and in the presence and absence of 100 or 250 µM vanadate. Calcium uptake was initially rapid for the first 30 s followed by equilibration by 300 s, while zinc uptake by the same vesicle preparation was considerably slower over the entire 300 s incubation and did not reach equilibrium during this interval [16]. The time courses of both $^{45}Ca^{2+}$ and $^{65}Zn^{2+}$ uptakes were proportionally stimulated by the presence of 1 mM ATP in the incubation medium and in each case this stimulation was significantly ($p < 0.01$) inhibited by 100 or 250 µM vanadate, suggesting the presence of a P-type ATPase in this organelle that was capable of transporting both cations.

3.2. Effects of ATP, vanadate, and thapsigargin on $^{45}Ca^{2+}$ influx kinetics in hepatopancreatic ER vesicles

The kinetics of $^{45}Ca^{2+}$ influx into hepatopancreatic ER was evaluated by incubating purified ER vesicles in external buffer containing varying activities of calcium and either 1 mM ATP, 250 μM vanadate, or 10 μM thapsigargin for 8 s. Fig. 1 shows that in the absence of either inhibitor, $^{45}Ca^{2+}$ influx was a sigmoidal function of calcium activity over the range of 0.5–25 μM and followed the Hill Equation for multisite cooperativity:

$$J_{Ca} = \left(J_{max}[Ca]^n / K_m^n + [Ca]^n\right)$$

where J_{Ca} is total calcium influx, J_{max} is maximal calcium entry, K_m^n is an apparent affinity constant of the transporter for calcium, [Ca] is the calcium activity in the medium, and n is the Hill Coefficient that is an index of the apparent number of ions transported across the membrane per transport cycle. The kinetic constants for $^{45}Ca^{2+}$ influx under control conditions are displayed in Table 1. The Hill Coefficient for $^{45}Ca^{2+}$ influx under control conditions, approximating two, suggests that two calcium ions were apparently transported for each transport cycle in the absence of ATP or inhibitors. Addition of 1 mM ATP to the incubation medium significantly ($p < 0.01$) elevated the rate of $^{45}Ca^{2+}$ influx at all calcium activities used and retained the sigmoidal nature of the transport relationship (Fig. 1). The kinetic constants for $^{45}Ca^{2+}$ influx in the presence of 1 mM ATP are shown in Table 1 and suggest that ATP increased the maximal transport velocity by almost a factor of two, but had no significant effect ($p > 0.05$) on either K_m^n or n. When either 10 μM thapsigargin or 250 μM vanadate were added individually to the incubation medium in the presence of 1 mM ATP during the measurement of calcium influx, the sigmoidal nature of the uptake curve was

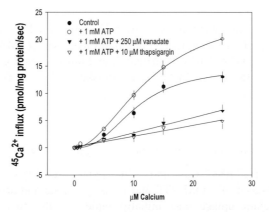

Fig. 1. Effects of 1 mM ATP, 250 μM vanadate, and 10 μM thapsigargin on the influx kinetics of $^{45}Ca^{2+}$ by lobster hepatopancreatic endoplasmic reticulum. Vesicles were collected, washed, and resuspended in a medium containing 450 mM KCl, 20 mM HEPES at pH 7.2 and were incubated for 8 s in a medium containing $^{45}Ca^{2+}$-gluconate activities ranging from 0 to 25 μM, 0.5 NTA, 20 mM HEPES/Tris and 450 mM KCl at pH 7.2. Values are means±1 S.E.M. ($n = 3$–5 replicates/mean). Lines were drawn through data using Jandel Sigma Plot curve fitting software, 7.101 version.

Table 1
Effect of ATP on $^{45}Ca^{2+}$ and $^{65}Zn^{2+}$ influx kinetic constants in hepatopancreatic ER membrane vesicles

Ion	Treatment	K_m (µM)	J_{max} (pmol/mg protein×s)	Hill Coefficient (n)
Ca	control	10.38±1.01	14.75±1.27	2.53±0.46
Ca	+1 mM ATP	12.76±0.91	25.46±1.46*	1.96±0.15
Zn	control	38.63±0.52	19.36±0.17	1.81±0.13
Zn	+ 1 mM ATP	43.85±3.68	29.28±1.43*	1.58±0.19

Values are means±1 S.E.M. Kinetic constants were obtained using Sigma Plot software. Each constant was obtained using 3–5 replicates per point. In addition, the experiment was repeated once with similar qualitative results.
* Significantly different than controls ($p<0.05$).

abolished and replaced by linear relationships between the variables. These results suggest that either inhibitor blocked calcium transport by the sigmoidal, ATP-dependent, carrier-mediated transfer process, leaving a residual uptake that may have occurred by simple diffusion.

3.3. Effects of ATP, vanadate, and thapsigargin on the kinetics of $^{65}Zn^{2+}$ influx by hepatopancreatic ER vesicles

Fig. 2 is a kinetic analysis of ER $^{65}Zn^{2+}$ influx in the presence and absence of 1 mM ATP, 250 µM vanadate, and 10 µM thapsigargin. As found with $^{45}Ca^{2+}$ influx described in Fig. 1, zinc influx in ER vesicles was a sigmoidal function of zinc concentration and illustrated a Hill Coefficient similar to that found for calcium entry (Table 1). Addition of 1 mM ATP enhanced $^{65}Zn^{2+}$ influx at each zinc activity, but the overall sigmoidal nature of the kinetic relationship was still maintained. As shown in Table 1, the effect of adding 1 mM ATP on $^{65}Zn^{2+}$ influx was primarily on increasing the maximal transport velocity of the metal without significantly altering the apparent binding affinity or the Hill Coefficient of transport. As with calcium transport by ER vesicles (Fig. 1), the addition of either 250

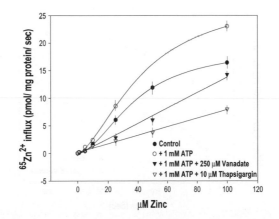

Fig. 2. Effects of 1 mM ATP, 250 µM vanadate, and 10 µM thapsigargin on $^{65}Zn^{2+}$ influx by lobster hepatopancreatic endoplasmic reticulum. Vesicles were collected, washed, and resuspended in a medium containing 450 mM KCl and 20 mM HEPES at pH 7.2 and were incubated for 8 s in a medium containing $^{65}Zn^{2+}$-sulfate activities ranging from 0 to 100 µM, 0.5 mM NTA, 20 mM HEPES/Tris and 450 mM KCl at pH 7.2. Values are means±1 S.E.M. (n=3 replicates/mean). Lines were drawn through data using Jandel Sigma Plot curve fitting software, 7.101 version.

μM vanadate or 20 μM thapsigargin abolished the sigmoidal nature of $^{65}Zn^{2+}$ influx and replaced it with a linear influx process similar to diffusion.

3.4. Time course of $^{65}Zn^{2+}$ uptake by hepatopancreatic lysosomal vesicles

Fig. 3 illustrates the effect of 250 μM vanadate on the time course of 25 μM $^{65}Zn^{2+}$ uptake into purified hepatopancreatic lysosomal vesicles. Zinc uptake into vesicles purified from this organelle more rapidly approached equilibrium than did ER vesicles, but vanadate was not as effective an inhibitor of metal accumulation in membranes derived from lysosomes as it was for those from ER. Whereas 250 μM vanadate abolished $^{65}Zn^{2+}$ uptake into ER vesicles [16], only about half of metal uptake was inhibited in the lysosomal preparation by this compound (Fig. 3). Similarly, Fig. 4 shows the effects of 25 μM Ca^{2+} or Cu^{2+} on the uptake time course of 25 μM $^{65}Zn^{2+}$, and in this instance approximately half of the metal uptake was eliminated by the presence of the inhibiting divalent cations. These two figures suggest that only approximately half of zinc uptake by lysosomal vesicles was sensitive to inhibition by drugs or cations and the similarity in percent inhibition by these factors suggest that they may be abolishing metal uptake by a common process.

3.5. Effects of ATP, vanadate, and thapsigargin on the kinetics of $^{65}Zn^{2+}$ influx in hepatopancreatic lysosomal vesicles

Fig. 5 illustrates the effects of 1 mM ATP, 250 μM vanadate, and 10 μM thapsigargin on the kinetics of $^{65}Zn^{2+}$ influx into purified hepatopancreatic lysosomal vesicles. Zinc influx under control conditions was a hyperbolic function of external zinc concentration, following the Michaelis–Menten equation:

$$J_{Zn} = J_{max}[Zn]/K_m + [Zn]$$

where J_{Zn} is carrier-mediated zinc influx, J_{max} is maximal carrier transport, K_m is an apparent affinity constant, and [Zn] is the external zinc concentration. The kinetic constants

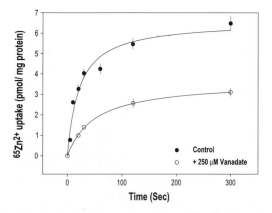

Fig. 3. Effect of 250 μM vanadate on the time course of 25 μM $^{65}Zn^{2+}$ uptake by lobster hepatopancreatic lysosomal membrane vesicles. Vesicles were collected, washed and resuspended in a medium containing 450 mM KCl and 20 mM HEPES/Tris at pH 7.0 and were incubated in a medium containing 25 μM $^{65}Zn^{2+}$-sulphate, 450 mM K-gluconate, and 20 mM HEPES/Tris at pH 7.0. Values are means±1 S.E.M. (n=3–5 replicates/mean). Lines were drawn through data using Jandel Sigma Plot curve fitting software 7.101 version.

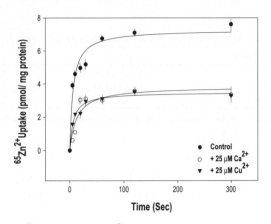

Fig. 4. Effects of 25 μM Ca^{2+}-gluconate and Cu^{2+}-sulfate on the time course of 25 μM $^{65}Zn^{2+}$ uptake by hepatopancreatic lysosomal membrane vesicles. Vesicles were collected, washed and resuspended in a medium containing 450 mM K-gluconate and 20 mM HEPES/Tris at pH 7.0 and were incubated in a medium containing 25 μM $^{65}Zn^{2+}$-sulphate, 450 mM K-gluconate, and 20 mM HEPES/Tris at pH 7.0. Values are means±1 S.E.M. (n=3–5 replicates/mean). Lines were drawn through data using Jandel Sigma Plot curve fitting software, 7.101 version.

obtained under control conditions are displayed in Table 2. Addition of 1 mM ATP enhanced $^{65}Zn^{2+}$ influx at each [Zn], but maintained the hyperbolic nature of the influx curve. Table 2 shows that the effect of adding ATP was to significantly (p<0.05) increase J_{max}, without affecting K_m. Addition of 10 μM thapsigargin slightly reduced $^{65}Zn^{2+}$ influx (Table 2), but this effect was not significant (p>0.05). Lastly, 250 μM vanadate abolished the hyperbolic nature of the influx relationship and replaced it by a slow linear process that resembled diffusion. These results suggest that zinc transport by lysosomal membrane vesicles likely occurred by an ATP-dependent, vanadate-inhibited, thapsigargin-insensitive,

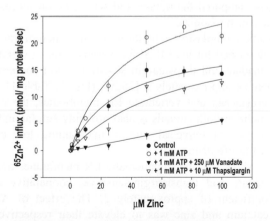

Fig. 5. Effects of 1 mM ATP, 250 μM vanadate, and 20 μM thapsigargin on the kinetics of $^{65}Zn^{2+}$ influx by hepatopancreatic lysosomal membrane vesicles. Vesicles were collected, washed and resuspended in a medium containing 450 mM K-gluconate and 20 mM HEPES/Tris at pH 7.0 and were incubated in a medium containing variable activities of $^{65}Zn^{2+}$-sulphate, 450 mM K-gluconate, and 20 mM HEPES/Tris at pH 7.0. Values are means±1 S.E.M. (n=3–5 replicates/mean). Lines were drawn through data using Jandel Sigma Plot curve fitting software, 7.101 version.

Table 2
Effect of 1 mM ATP and 10 μM thapsigargin on $^{65}Zn^{2+}$ influx in hepatopancreatic lysosomal vesicles

Ion	Treatment	K_m (μM)	J_{max} (pmol/mg protein×s)
Zn	control	32.26±10.76	20.65±2.61
Zn	+ATP	35.89±10.58	31.94±3.72*
Zn	+thap	72.87±42.75	22.86±7.03

Values are means±1 S.E.M. Kinetic constants were obtained using Sigma Plot software. Each constant was obtained using 3–5 replicates per point.
　*Significant difference from control condition at $p < 0.05$.

transport system that illustrated hyperbolic influx kinetics and therefore deviated from the cooperative zinc transport system characterized for ER vesicles (Fig. 2).

4. Discussion

The crustacean hepatopancreas has a multitude of functions including digestion, emulsification, and absorption of dietary nutrients, regulation of cellular and hemolymph ion concentrations through absorption and secretion processes, storage of ions, carbohydrates, lipids, and proteins, synthesis of hemocyanin, and sequestration and detoxification of a wide variety of xenobiotics including heavy metals [22,23]. Many of the processes performed by the hepatopancreas, as an organ system, are localized within specific organelles in one of the four kinds of cells found in this structure [5,6,24]. Dietary heavy metals that cross hepatopancreatic epithelial brush border membranes enter the cytoplasm and may undergo one of several potential regulatory fates: (1) complexation with cytoplasmic metallothioneins, (2) uptake and sequestration in mitochondria, (3) uptake and sequestration in endoplasmic reticulum (ER), (4) uptake and sequestration into lysosomes, or (5) export from the cell via transport across the basolateral membrane to the blood. This study has compared the uptake and sequestration mechanisms of $^{65}Zn^{2+}$ by hepatopancreatic ER and lysosomes.

The hepatopancreatic endoplasmic reticulum exhibits calcium transport properties that are similar to those described for the ER SERCA transporter in vertebrate cells including ATP dependency, vanadate and thapsigargin sensitivity, and cooperative influx kinetics with a Hill Coefficient of approximately 2 [25,26] (Fig. 1; Table 1). Given the transport similarity between crustacean and vertebrate ER membranes, the calcium sequestering function of this organelle in both animals is also probably similar and it is likely that this structure plays an important universal role in maintaining low cytoplasmic calcium activities for most of the life of the cell.

Fig. 2 and Table 1 show that hepatopancreatic ER membranes transported zinc by an ATP-dependent, vanadate and thapsigargin-sensitive, cooperative carrier process that exhibited a Hill Coefficient of approximately 2. The effect of ATP addition on the transports of both calcium and zinc was to elevate their respective maximal transport velocities without affecting either their K_m- or n-values (Table 1). Vanadate and thapsigargin each abolished the sigmoidal character of both calcium and zinc influx, replacing it with an apparent diffusion process. (Figs. 1, 2). Because thapsigargin is a specific SERCA inhibitor, it can be concluded that both calcium and zinc were transported by a SERCA analogue in hepatopancreatic ER in the present investigation.

Figs. 3, 4 and Table 2 show that hepatopancreatic lysosomes possessed a distinctly different type of zinc uptake process than was displayed for this metal and for calcium by the ER in the same organ. While zinc was transported by an ATP-dependent, vanadate-inhibited, uptake mechanism in both organelles (Figs. 2, 3, 5), zinc transfer in lysosomes was insensitive to the ER-specific inhibitor, thapsigargin, while this compound completely abolished the carrier transport of both calcium and zinc in ER membranes (Figs. 1, 2). In addition, zinc and calcium transport in ER was cooperative, displaying sigmoidal influx kinetics (1,2), while the transfer of zinc by lysosomes occurred by a carrier exhibiting hyperbolic, Michaelis–Menten kinetics (Fig. 5). These dissimilarities in transport properties for the two hepatopancreatic organelles suggest that while an ATP-dependent SERCA analogue might be operative in ER for divalent cation uptake from the cytoplasm and its sequestration, a different ATP-dependent transporter was likely to be present in lysosomal membranes and was responsible for accumulation of metals in that location.

Zinc transport by cells is generally regulated by members of the ZIP or ZnT gene families [27]. Whereas members of the ZIP family increase intracellular zinc activity by transport into a cell from the environment, the ZnT members lead to a decrease in cytoplasmic metal activity as a result of efflux from the cell or transfer into organelles or vesicles. In both families, the transport proteins function as facilitated diffusion or secondary active transport processes without the direct use of ATP to transfer the metal across a membrane. Because $^{65}Zn^{2+}$ transport by hepatopancreatic lysosomes was significantly stimulated by the addition of ATP (Fig. 5), it is unlikely that a zinc transport system of the ZIP or ZnT families was responsible for metal accumulation in the present investigation.

In a recent study of copper transport by lobster hepatopancreatic lysosomes, the presence of a calcium-stimulated, vanadate-inhibited, copper ATPase was proposed to occur in the organelle [18]. Fig. 3 of the present investigation suggests that copper was an effective inhibitor of $^{65}Zn^{2+}$ uptake by hepatopancreatic lysosomes, implying the potential competitive interaction between zinc and copper during metal transport. In vertebrate cells copper is accumulated within the Golgi and other vesicular bodies, including lysosomes, by either the Menkes ATPase (ATP7A) (non-liver cells) or the Wilson's ATPase (ATP7B) (liver cells) [28–31]. A likely candidate for the identity of the lysosomal zinc ATPase characterized in the present study may be an isoform of one or both of these vertebrate copper transport systems disclosed in human disease. Future molecular sequencing information of the lysosomal transport system will be needed to clarify this issue.

Acknowledgements

This study was supported by National Science Foundation grant IBN99-74569.

References

[1] T. Watanabe, V. Kiron, S. Satoh, Trace minerals in fish nutrition, Aquaculture 151 (1997) 185–207.
[2] A. Viarengo, Heavy metals in marine invertebrates: mechanisms of regulation and toxicity at the cellular level, Rev. Aquat. Sci. 1 (1989) 295–317.
[3] A. Viarengo, J.A. Nott, Mechanisms of heavy metal cation homeostasis in marine invertebrates, Comp. Biochem. Physiol. 404C (1993) 355–372.

[4] S.G. George, Heavy metal detoxification in the mussel *Mytilis edulis*: composition of Cd-containing kidney granules (tertiary lysosomes), Comp. Biochem. Physiol. 76C (1983) 53–57.

[5] S.Y. Al-Mohanna, J.A. Nott, The accumulation of metals in the hepatopancreas of the shrimp, *Penaeus semisulcatus* de Haan (Crustacea: Decapoda) during the moult cycle, in: R. Halwagy, D. Clayton, M. Behbehani (Eds.), Marine Environment and Pollution, Kuwait University, 1985, pp. 195–209.

[6] S.Y. Al-Mohanna, J.A. Nott, R-cells and the digestive cycle in *Penaeus semisulcatus* (Crustacea: Decapoda), Mar. Biol. 95 (1987) 129–137.

[7] S.P. Hopkin, Ecophysiology of metals in terrestrial invertebrates, Appl. Sci., Elsevier, London, 1989.

[8] M. Brouwer, D.R. Winge, W.R. Gray, Structural and functional diversity of copper-metallothioneins from the American lobster *Homarus americanus*, J. Inorg. Biochem. 35 (1989) 289–303.

[9] M. Brouwer, et al., Metal-specific induction of metallothionein isoforms in the blue crab *Callinectes sapidus* in response to single- and mixed-metal exposure, Arch. Biochem. Physiol. 294 (1992) 461–468.

[10] G.L. Becker, J.D. Termine, E.D. Eanes, Comparative studies of intra- and extramitochondrial calcium phosphates from the hepatopancreas of the blue crab (*Callinectes sapidus*), Calcif. Tissue Res. 21 (1976) 105–113.

[11] N.E. Saris, K. Niva, Is Zn^{2+} transported by the mitochondrial calcium uniporter? Fed. Eur. Biochem. Soc. Lett. 356 (1994) 195–198.

[12] M.J. Klein, G.A. Ahearn, Calcium transport processes of lobster hepatopancreatic mitochondria, J. Exp. Zool. 283 (1999) 147–159.

[13] P. Chavez-Crooker, N. Garrido, G.A. Ahearn, Copper transport by lobster (*Homarus americanus*) hepatopancreatic mitochondria, J. Exp. Biol. 205 (2002) 405–413.

[14] G.P. Borrelly, et al., Surplus zinc is handled by Zym1 metallothionein and Zhf endoplasmic reticulum transporter in *Schizosaccharomyces pombe*, J. Biol. Chem. 277 (33) (2002) 30394–30400.

[15] S. Clemens, et al., A transporter in the endoplasmic reticulum of *Schizosaccharomyces pombe* cells mediates zinc storage and differentially affects transition metal tolerance, J. Biol. Chem. 277 (20) (2002) 18215–18221.

[16] P.K. Mandal, A. Mandal, G.A. Ahearn, Physiological characterization of $^{45}Ca^{2+}$ and $^{65}Zn^{2+}$ transport by lobster hepatopancreatic endoplasmic reticulum, J. Exp. Zool. (2004).

[17] A.C. Havelaar, et al., Characterization of a heavy metal ion transporter in the lysosomal membrane, FEBS Lett. 436 (1998) 223–227.

[18] P. Chavez-Crooker, et al., Copper transport by lobster (*Homarus americanus*) heptopancreatic lysosomes, Comp. Biochem. Physiol. 135C (2003) 107–118.

[19] G. Vogt, E.T. Quinitio, Accumulation and excretion of metal granules in the prawn, *Penaeus monodon*, exposed to water-borne copper, lead, iron and calcium, Aquat. Toxicol. 28 (1994) 223–241.

[20] M. Thamotharan, et al., An active mechanism for completion of the final stage of protein degradation in the liver, lysosomal transport of dipeptides, J. Biol. Chem. 272 (1997) 11786–11790.

[21] X. Zhou, et al., Characterization of an oligopeptide transporter in renal lysosomes, Biochim. Biophys. Acta 1466 (2000) 372–378.

[22] P.B. Van Weel, Processes of secretion, restitution, and resorption in gland of mid-gut (glandula media intestini) of *Atya spinipes* Newport (Decapoda–Brachyura), Physiol. Zool. 28 (1955) 40–54.

[23] P.B. Van Weel, Hepatopancreas? Comp. Biochem. Physiol. 47A (1974) 1–9.

[24] S.Y. Al-Mohanna, J.A. Nott, Functional cytology of the hepatopancreas of *Penaeus semisulcatus* (Crustacea: Decapoda) during the moult cycle, Mar. Biol. 101 (1989) 535–544.

[25] D.L. Stokes, T. Wagenknecht, Calcium transport across the sarcoplasmic reticulum. Structure and function of Ca^{2+}-ATPase and the ryanodine receptor, Eur. J. Biochem. 267 (2000) 5270–5274.

[26] F. Wuytack, L. Raeymaekers, L. Missiaen, Molecular physiology of the SERCA and SPCA pumps, Cell Calcium 32 (2002) 279–305.

[27] J.P. Liuzzi, R.J. Cousins, Mammalian zinc transporters, Annu. Rev. Nutr. (2004) 151–172.

[28] C.D. Vulpe, S. Packman, Cellular copper transport, Annu. Rev. Nutr. 15 (1995) 293–322.

[29] M. Suzuki, J.D. Gitlin, Intracellular localization of the Menkes and Wilson disease proteins and their role in intracellular copper transport, Pediatr. Int. 41 (1999) 436–442.

[30] E.D. Harris, Cellular copper transport and metabolism, Annu. Rev. Nutr. 20 (2000) 291–310.

[31] M.C. Linder, Biochemistry and molecular biology of copper in mammals, in: E.J. Massaro (Ed.), Handbook of Copper Pharmacology and Toxicology, Humana Press, New Jersey, 2002, pp. 3–32.

[32] U. Hopfer, et al., Glucose transport in isolated brush border membrane from rat small intestine, J. Biol. Chem. 248 (1973) 25–32.
[33] D.M. Bers, C.W. Patton, R. Nuccitelli, A practical guide to the preparation of Ca^{2+} buffers, in: Methods in Cell Biology, vol. 40, Academic Press, United States, 1994, pp. 3–29.

International Congress Series 1275 (2004) 126–133

www.ics-elsevier.com

Unity and diversity in chemical signals of arthropods: the role of neuropeptides in crustaceans and insects

Heather G. Marco*

Zoology Department, University of Cape Town, Private Bag, Rondebosch, ZA-7701, South Africa

Abstract. Neuropeptides can function as hormones, transmitters and modulators. These chemical signals have been well researched in certain arthropod groups, where many physiological processes are regulated by neuropeptides. This contribution will provide a comparative overview of a selection of neuropeptide families that are used as chemical signals in the two sister groups, Insecta and Crustacea, and will look at the extent of conservation/diversity of function, primary structure and where possible, also the mode of action. The following peptide families will be discussed: crustacean hyperglycaemic-like hormones, allatostatins, red pigment-concentrating hormone/adipokinetic hormone and pigment-dispersing hormone/pigment-dispersing factor. © 2004 Elsevier B.V. All rights reserved.

Keywords: Neuropeptide; Crustacea; Insecta; Crustacean hyperglycaemic hormone; Allatostatin; Adipokinetic hormone, Red pigment-concentrating hormone; Pigment-dispersing hormone; Receptor; Mode of action

1. Introduction

The nervous and the endocrine systems are classically known as systems of communication between cells, tissues and organs of some metazoan phyla. In this way, cellular and behavioural responses are coordinated, and biochemical and physiological processes are regulated in animals. Another form of communication in animals is provided by the so-called neuroendocrine system which is already present in the Cnidaria and persists up to the Vertebrata: modified neurons synthesise peptides (=neuropeptides) which are transported along the axons, stored in a neurohaemal organ and released into the circulatory

* Tel.: +27 21 650 3606; fax: +27 21 650 3301.
E-mail address: hmarco@botzoo.uct.ac.za.

0531-5131/ © 2004 Elsevier B.V. All rights reserved.
doi:10.1016/j.ics.2004.08.053

system. These peptides can function as hormones, transmitters or neuromodulators. In arthropods, specifically insects and crustaceans, neuropeptides have long been scientifically investigated to understand their role(s) in regulating important physiological and developmental processes; some of the information may be useful in combatting pest insect species [1], aquaculture ventures [2] and in assigning phylogenetic relationships [3]. For the comparative physiologist and biochemist, it is interesting to learn how two sister groups have successfully used their neuropeptides as chemical signals and how these bioregulators effect their function(s). This paper presents an overview of what is currently known about a selection of neuropeptide families that are common to insects and crustaceans, with respect to primary structure, prohormone structure, biological function, receptors and mode of action; the selected examples will illustrate unity and diversity regarding the use of neuropeptides as chemical signals in two phylogenetically related groups.

2. The adipokinetic hormone(AKH)/red pigment-concentrating hormone (RPCH) family

Structurally, members of the AKH/RPCH family are characterised by a chain length of 8–10 amino acids; blocked N-terminus (pGlu) and C-terminus (amide) and some invariant residues [4]. RPCH was first completely sequenced in 1972 from crustacean tissue extracts of the shrimp *Pandalus borealis* and is so named because of its concentrating effect on pigments in epidermal chromatophores of crustaceans [5]; RPCH has also been shown to modulate the stomatogastric system of crustaceans [6]. AKH was sequenced from locusts a few years after RPCH and it was shown to have a hyperlipaemic effect in locusts [7]; AKHs in other insect species may regulate the mobilisation or synthesis of carbohydrates and/or proline [4].

In all the crustacean species studied to date, there is only one RPCH (octapeptide) which is identical in all infraorders [8]. In contrast, most of the insect orders have more than one (up to three) AKH peptides with amino acid substitutions and even a difference in chain length [4]. Recently, RPCH was isolated and sequenced from an insect, viz. the stinkbug *Nezara viridula*, in which it mobilises lipids [9]. Thus, conservation of peptide structure and functional cross-activity of RPCH and AKH peptide across the two phylogenetic groups have been demonstrated. Additionally, the preprohormones share a similar general organisation: a signal peptide, the AKH/RPCH sequence, the signal for amidation (glycine), a dibasic cleavage signal and a "precursor-related peptide". The purpose of the latter is still unknown and, although the AKH- and RPCH-precursor related peptides have no homology to each other, there is considerable similarity among the precursor-related peptides within a taxonomic group [4]; it will be interesting to see whether the structure of the AKH precursor-related peptide of *N. viridula* resembles that of other insects or crustaceans. Nevertheless, information on the AKH/RPCH family indicates that genes and preprohormone processing mechanisms have been conserved during the evolution of insects and crustaceans, and furthermore, that the receptor structure has remained virtually unchanged (at least, in the ligand-binding region), albeit that the receptor is located on different tissues (epidermal chromatophores of crustaceans versus fat body of insects).

Thus far, receptors for AKH have been cloned from insects only, largely thanks to the completely sequenced genome of some insects; the G-coupled receptors are similar in structure to receptors for the gonadotropin-releasing hormone of vertebrates, with the highest identity in the seven transmembrane regions [10].

Much is known with respect to the signal transduction cascade of AKHs in insects and the reader is referred to a recent review for details [11]. Briefly, with those AKHs that elicit hyperlipaemia: adenylate cyclase (AC) is stimulated, cAMP is produced and an influx of Ca^{2+} ions stimulates lipase. For a hypertrehalosaemic effect of AKH, glycogen phosphorylase must be activated; in this case, phospholipase C (PLC) is stimulated and two second messengers, inositol trisphosphate (IP_3) and diacylglycerol are produced which mobilise intracellular Ca^{2+} ions. In crustaceans, pigment aggregation is thought to involve a similar signalling pathway as AKHs that effect hypertrehalosaemia, i.e. via activation of PLC, IP_3, diacylglycerol and internal Ca^{2+} ions [12].

3. The pigment-dispersing hormone (PDH)/pigment-dispersing factor (PDF) family

PDH was first isolated from crustaceans in 1976; it is antagonistic to RPCH by having a dispersing effect on pigments in chromatophores of the epidermis, thus, having a darkening effect [13]. PDF, isolated from insects much later, is so named because it is structurally related to PDH and because it has a dispersing effect on epidermal pigment in crustaceans, although it has no effect on pigmentation in insects [6]. Instead, from evidence based on the immunocytochemical localisation of PDH cells, experiments with induced lesions and transplantation of these cells, and the effect of injected PDH on locomotor activity rhythms, it is thought that PDH/F acts as a neurotransmitter on the circadian pacemaker cells of insects; in some cases, the PDH immunoreactive cells also express proteins that are essential in the pacemaker function [14]. In crustaceans, some PDH-immunoreactivity is also associated with non-secretory neurons and thus, PDH may also serve as a neurotransmitter or modulator in crustaceans in addition to its blood-borne pigmentary effect [6].

PDH/PDF is an octadecapeptide with a free N-terminus, an amidated C-terminus and several conserved residues. The preprohormone sequences also show the same basic organisation: signal peptide, a "precursor-related peptide" of unknown function and of variable sequence and length, a cleavage site, and the PDH/PDF sequence followed by the amidation signal [6]. In crustaceans, up to three different PDHs may be present in one species, indicating that the gene has undergone duplication and point mutations [6]. To date, a PDH/PDF receptor has not been sequenced but it has been suggested that a G protein-coupled receptor may be involved with AC, cAMP and a cAMP-dependant protein kinase (PKA) being part of the signalling cascade for eliciting pigment dispersion (see Ref. [12]). It seems that, as with the AKH/RPCH peptide family, genes, preprohormone processing mechanisms and receptor structure (based only on cross-activity of PDF in crustaceans) are conserved for members of the PDH/PDF family, despite the peptide itself being used in a different functional context.

4. The A-allatostatin family of peptides

The first allatostatins were sequenced from the cockroach, *Diploptera punctata* [15,16], the name of the peptide is derived from its function (as assayed in vitro), viz. it acts negatively on the corpora allata of certain insects (cockroach, cricket, moth), inhibiting the biosynthesis of juvenile hormone (JH) [17]. JH maintains larval characters of insects during development and suppresses metamorphosis into the adult form but it also plays a role in reproduction by stimulating the synthesis of vitellogenin in the fat body of cockroach females and by promoting oocyte growth [18]. JH is a species-specific acyclic sesquiterpenoid epoxide which is not present in crustaceans, although a non-epoxidated precursor molecule, methyl farnesoic acid (MF), does occur in crustaceans and seems to play a role in crustacean larval development [19].

In insects there are three major structural forms of allatostatins (called A-, B- and C-types according to features of their primary sequence); the A-type allatostatins are common to both insects and crustaceans and are discussed in this overview. Several isoforms of these A-allatostatin peptides occur in individual crustacean/insect species, e.g. 14 in *Periplaneta americana* and 40 in the prawn *Penaeus monodon*; these peptides are characterised by a common C-terminal pentapeptide of YXFGLamide and range in length from 5 to 30 amino acids [20]. Isolated from brains, corpora cardiaca and antennal pulsatile organs of insects, these peptides, in most insect species, do not affect the biosynthesis of JH, but are myoinhibitory, vitellogenesis-inhibiting or modulate the activity of certain enzymes in the midgut [17]. A-allatostatins that were isolated from crustacean tissues (brain and ventral nerve cord) also display a myoinhibitory function on crustacean hindgut and inhibit the hormonally induced contractions of cockroach hindgut [21]; thus, there is functional cross-activity. Immunocytochemical studies have shown A-allatostatin immunoreactivity in nerve fibres innervating neurohaemal release sites and muscles in crustaceans and insects, suggesting that the allatostatins may also play a role as neurotransmitter and/or neuromodulator [20,21], in addition to their role as neurohormone.

The A-type allatostatin precursor is, thus far, known only from insects. It is characterised by a signal peptide, a "precursor-related peptide" of unknown function, clusters of the various allatostatin sequences separated by "acidic spacers" and, finally, a "tail peptide" whose action is also not known [17]. It is enigmatic why as many as 40 isoforms of a peptide should be synthesised and released in one organism to effect the same biological task. It has been speculated that the primary function of the peptides is myoinhibitory and that the different isoforms may either have different target tissues in the organism or have different potencies on the same target [20]. It may also be that the different isoforms have the same target and function, and the simultaneous release ensures a vital (high) concentration of the ligand. It remains to be seen whether the allatostatin precursor of crustaceans is organised in a similar way to that of the insects or whether several genes encode only a selection of the isoforms.

Sequence data of receptors that bind the A-type allatostatins are now known from a few insect species, thanks to molecular biological techniques. The first receptor was cloned from *Drosophila melanogaster*; this G protein-coupled receptor has homology to the mammalian receptors for galanin [22]. In receptor binding assays using the cloned cockroach receptor and expressing it in frog oocytes, the binding of the allatostatin peptides to the receptor was measured by means of electrophysiological techniques; such assays showed that the C-terminal core pentapeptide sequence is sufficient for receptor binding and that all of the 14 cockroach allatostatins can bind to the cockroach receptor [G. Gäde, H.G. Marco, R. Weaver and D. Richter, unpublished]. On the other hand, two putative allatostatin receptors have been cloned from *D. melanogaster* and from the prohormone, four allatostatin isoforms are deduced to be present in this species [23].

Future research will show whether there are more than one specific receptor for the different allatostatin isoforms of insects and crustaceans. Recently, antiserum to the second allatostatin receptor of *D. melanogaster* was used to localise a putative receptor in eyestalks of the prawn, *P. monodon*, and the sinus gland was identified [24]; further confirmation is needed that this is indeed the site of an allatostatin receptor in crustaceans and perhaps may lead to the first sequence data of such a receptor in crustaceans.

5. The CHH peptide family

For a very long time it was thought that peptides belonging to this hormone family occurred only in crustaceans. Relatively recently, though, homologous structures were shown in other arthropods, including insects. The peptide family is named after the first member to be sequenced, viz. crustacean hyperglycaemic hormone (CHH).

CHH is a neuropeptide of 72 amino acids that was first isolated and sequenced from sinus glands of the shore crab, *Carcinus maenas*, and shown to mobilise glucose from the hepatopancreas [25]. Since then, peptides with CHH bioactivity have been structurally characterised from many other decapod crustacean species [8]. In all the decapod infraorders studied to date, CHH has conserved structural features: chain length of 72 amino acids, 6 Cys residues in conserved positions with three intramolecular disulfide bridges (highly conserved; the first two Cys residues are separated by 15 amino acids) and an amidated C-terminus. Overall interspecies identity of CHHs ranges from around 40–99% (highest identity is generally found between species of the same infraorder) [26] due to several homologous motifs; mostly present as two or more isoforms per species, the N-terminus of the major CHH isoform in astacideans and brachyurans is blocked by a pGlu residue, whereas a free N-terminus is characteristic of all CHHs from other crustaceans. Interestingly, the N-terminal state does not seem to affect biological activity nor the rate of peptide degradation in the haemolymph [26], whereas the C-terminus is important for hyperglycaemic bioactivity and is also implicated in group-specific receptor binding [27].

Apart from the CHH peptides with the classical function of mobilising glucose from the hepatopancreas, similar peptides with other bioactivity, e.g. inhibiting the synthesis of moulting hormones and MF, and inhibiting vitellogenesis, have also been characterised, biochemically sequenced or cloned from the X organ-sinus gland complex in decapod crustaceans [8,26]. These neuropeptides are named after their corresponding biological activity: moult-inhibiting hormone (MIH), mandibular organ-inhibiting hormone (MOIH) and vitellogenesis-inhibiting hormone (VIH), and show structural similarity to cHH: chain length ranges from 74 to 78 amino acids, the N-terminus is a free Arg, while the C-terminus is mostly free and amidation is reported for a few species only [8]. In MIH, MOIH and VIH, although 6 Cys residues are also present with the characteristic conserved disulfide linkages, the first 2 Cys are separated by 16 residues.

The insect representative of the CHH family is a neuropeptide that was first structurally elucidated by means of a combination of peptide sequencing and molecular cloning and named ion transport peptide (ITP) because it stimulates the transport of Cl^- across the insect ileum [28]; several ITP structures have since been deduced from cDNA sequences of other insects and comparisons show that ITP is more homologous to cHH than to MIH-type peptides [8]. A difference in the organisation of the preprohormones has also justified the division of the CHH peptide family into two types, viz. the CHH/ITP subfamily and the MIH/VIH/MOIH subfamily. In the former, the preprohormone consists of: a signal peptide, a so-called "CHH precursor-related peptide" (CRPR; 17–41 amino acids; a peptide with sequence homology to CPRPs of other crustacean species but of unknown function), a dibasic cleavage site, the cHH/ITP sequence, followed by the signal for amidation; whereas the preprohormone of the MIH/VIH/MOIH subfamily does not have a "precursor-related peptide" [29].

Of all the members of the CHH peptide family, CHH is by far the most intriguing in terms of functional significance/ability. In the first place, it has been shown in several crustacean species that CHH is a multifunctional peptide; in the spiny lobster Jasus lalandii, for example, it (a) raises the circulating glucose levels homospecifically, (b) significantly suppresses the ecdysteroid synthesis in conspecific Y-organs and (c) acts as a putative VIH by inhibiting protein synthesis heterospecifically in ovaries of the prawn *Penaeus semisulcatus* [30–32]. In the spider crab *Libinia emarginata*, a peptide that clearly belongs to the CHH/ITP subfamily (based on preprohormone organisation and sequence homology) functions as MOIH [33]. Although not rigorously tested, it is apparent that this multifunctionality is limited to CHH; neither MIH, nor VIH and MOIH can effect hyperglycaemia in conspecific bioassays [8]. Is this significant and what does it imply w.r.t receptors and receptor binding of CHH family peptides? The implications are: (a) CHH receptors are not restricted to the hepatopancreas (where glucose is stored in the form of glycogen) but are also found on other tissues (e.g. Y-organ, mandibular organ, ovary) or (b) there is sufficient homology between the CHH molecule and the ligand-binding region of the MIH/VIH/MOIH receptors that CHH can bind and elicit a physiological response and, (c) specific receptors for MIH/VIH/MOIH may be more restricted in their distribution and therefore, these peptides may not be multifunctional or, (d) there may be too little similarity between the ligand-binding region of the CHH specific receptor and the other family members, hence MIH/VIH/MOIH cannot interact with the CHH receptor. Unfortunately, there is no report on the structure of receptors for the CHH peptide family. Using the classical membrane-binding approach, it was demonstrated that CHH can bind to receptors on hepatopancreas, heart muscle, epidermis and Y-organs, whereas MIH could only bind to receptors on the Y-organs and these seemed to be a different set of receptors than the CHH-binding ones (see Ref. [8]). With improved molecular biological techniques available, we may soon have structural information about receptors for the CHH peptide family and this could be used, in turn, to study the distribution and expression of the receptors during specific physiological/developmental events.

Information about interspecies receptor structures would certainly also shed some light on another intriguing aspect of CHHs, viz. that, despite relatively high structural homology, the hyperglycaemic effect of CHH seems to be group- or infraorder-specific [34]. This was also demonstrated at the receptor level by membrane binding experiments (see Ref. [8]). It is, therefore, not wholly surprising, that functional cross-activity could not be demonstrated between CHH and the insect ITP (see Ref. [8]). These results may imply that the ligand-binding region of the CHH receptor or the receptor-activating region of CHH must be highly conserved and specific to infraorders (or phylogenetic groups) to prevent interspecies binding and consequent hyperglycaemia. Does this also imply that the receptor and its ligand have "co-evolved" or how (and why) did this come about?

When the CHH sequences from different decapod crustaceans and the insect ITPs are aligned, the greatest variation can be seen in the C-terminus (for primary sequences see Table 3 in Ref. [8]), perhaps this part of the peptide is involved in ligand binding? We do know that the C-terminus of cHH/ITP is important for biological activity, especially the amidated end [8,26]; why is it then that so many of the MIH-type peptides are non-amidated and still have biological activity (albeit not in a hyperglycaemic capacity)?

Another puzzle (and yet another motivation for closing the huge gap in our information about crustacean receptors) is the demonstrated fact that CHH elicits an interspecific biological VIH effect (see Ref. [32]), i.e. CHH binds to receptors on the ovaries of other crustacean species (infraorders) to affect protein synthesis. This may mean that a different region of the CHH peptide is involved in the receptor-binding and activation (not the group-conserved part of the peptide) of the receptor on the ovary.

A further challenge to our understanding of the role of the CHH peptide family is the fairly recent demonstration of extra-eyestalk sources of CHH, notably, from transient gut paraneurons (involvement in water uptake to facilitate ecdysis), pericardial organs and suboesophageal ganglion (see Refs. [8,26]). Also, there is not much known about the signal transduction pathways that are activated by the CHH family of peptides (see Ref. [8] for information).

In conclusion then, the large CHH family of peptides demonstrates unity in its primary structures but there is diversity at the level of prohormones, biological effects, receptor-ligand interactions and perhaps also the mode of action. Much remains to be done to have a clearer picture of the role of any one of the CHH family peptides in a particular crustacean or insect species, but at the same time, this challenge also heightens the excitement around research into arthropod neurohormones.

References

[1] G. Gäde, G.J. Goldsworthy, Insect peptide hormones: a selective review of their physiology and potential application for pest control, Pest Manag. Sci. 59 (2003) 1063–1075.

[2] H. Laufer, W.J. Biggers, J.S.B. Ahl, Stimulation of ovarian maturation in the crayfish Procambarus clarkii by methyl farnesoate, Gen. Comp. Endocrinol. 111 (1998) 113–118.

[3] G. Gäde, The hypertrehalosaemic peptides of cockroaches: a phylogenetic study, Gen. Comp. Endocrinol. 75 (1989) 287–300.

[4] G. Gäde, The revolution in insect neuropeptides illustrated by the adipokinetic/red pigment-concentrating hormone family of peptides, Z. Naturforsch., C 51 (1996) 607–617.

[5] P. Fernlund, L. Josefsson, Crustacean color-change hormone: amino acid sequence and chemical synthesis, Science 177 (1972) 173–175.

[6] K.R. Rao, Crustacean pigmentary-effector hormones: chemistry and functions of RPCH, PDH, and related peptides, Am. Zool. 41 (2001) 364–379.

[7] J.V. Stone, et al., Structure of locust adipokinetic hormone, a neurohormone that regulates lipid utilisation during flight, Nature 263 (1976) 207–211.

[8] G. Gäde, H.G. Marco, Structure, function and mode of action of select arthropod neuropeptides, in: A. Ur-Rahmann (Ed.), Studies in Natural Product Chemistry (Bioactive Natural Products), 2004, in press.

[9] G. Gäde, et al., Red pigment-concentrating hormone is not limited to crustaceans, Biochem. Biophys. Res. Commun. 309 (2003) 967–973.

[10] F. Staubli, et al., Molecular identification of the insect adipokinetic hormone receptors, Proc. Natl. Acad. Sci. U. S. A. 99 (2002) 3446–3451.

[11] G. Gäde, L. Auerswald, Mode of action of neuropeptides from the adipokinetic hormone family, Gen. Comp. Endocrinol. 132 (2003) 10–20.

[12] L.E. Nery, A.M.L. Castrucci, The Crustacean Nervous System, in: K. Wiese (Ed.), Springer-Verlag, Berlin, 2002, pp. 98–112.

[13] P. Fernlund, Structure of a light-adapting hormone from the shrimp, *Pandalus borealis*, Biochim. Biophys. Acta 439 (1976) 17–25.

[14] B. Petri, M. Stengl, Presumptive insect circadian pacemakers in vitro: immunocytochemical characterization of cultured pigment-dispersing hormone-immunoreactive neurons of *Leucophaea maderae*, Cell Tissue Res. 296 (1999) 635–643.

[15] A.P. Woodhead, et al., Primary structure of four allatostatins: neuropeptide inhibitors of juvenile hormone synthesis, Proc. Natl. Acad. Sci. U. S. A. 86 (1989) 5997–6001.

[16] G.E. Pratt, et al., Identification of an allatostatin from adult *Diploptera punctata*, Biochem. Biophys. Res. Commun. 163 (1989) 1243–1247.

[17] G. Gäde, Allatoregulatory peptides—molecules with multiple functions, Invertebr. Reprod. Dev. 41 (2002) 127–135.

[18] C.G.H. Steel, K.G. Davey, Integration in the insect endocrine system, in: G.A. Kerkut, L.I. Gilbert (Eds.), Comprehensive Insect Physiology, Biochemistry and Pharmacology, vol. 8, Pergamon Press, Oxford, 1985, pp. 1–35.

[19] H. Laufer, et al., Methyl farnesoate: its site of synthesis and regulation of secretion in a juvenile crustacean, Insect Biochem. 17 (1987) 1129–1131.

[20] H. Duve, et al., Allatostatins of the tiger prawn, *Penaeus monodon* (Crustacea: Penaeidea), Peptides 23 (2002) 1039–1051.

[21] H. Dircksen, et al., Structure, distribution, and biological activity of novel members of the allatostatin family in the crayfish *Orconectes limosus*, Peptides 20 (1999) 695–712.

[22] N. Birgül, et al., Reverse physiology in *Drosophila:* identification of a novel allatostatin-like neuropeptide and its cognate receptor structurally related to the mammalian somatostatin/galanin/opioid receptor family, EMBO J. 18 (1999) 5892–5900.

[23] C. Lenz, et al., Identification of four *Drosophila allatostatins* as the cognate ligands for the *Drosophila* orphan receptor DAR-2, Biochem. Biophys. Res. Commun. 286 (2001) 1117–1122.

[24] N. Panchan, et al., Immunolocalization of allatostatin-like neuropeptides and their putative receptor in eyestalks of the tiger prawn *Penaeus monodon*, Peptides 24 (2003) 1563–1570.

[25] G. Kegel, et al., Amino acid sequence of the crustacean hyperglycaemic hormone (CHH) from the shore crab, *Carcinus maenas*, FEBS Lett. 255 (1989) 10–14.

[26] D. Soyez, Recent data on the crustacean hyperglycaemic hormone family, in: M. Fingerman, R. Nagabhushanam (Eds.), Recent Advances in Marine Biotechnology, vol. 10, Science Publishers, Plymouth, UK, 2003, pp. 279–301.

[27] H. Katayama, et al., Significance of a carboxyl-terminal amide moiety in the folding and biological activity of crustacean hyperglycaemic hormone, Peptides 23 (2002) 1537–1546.

[28] J. Meredith, et al., Locust ion transport peptide (ITP): primary structure, cDNA and expression in a baculovirus system, J. Exp. Biol. 199 (1996) 1053–1061.

[29] C. Lacombe, P. Greve, G. Martin, Overview on the sub-grouping of the crustacean hyperglycaemic hormone family, Neuropeptides 33 (1999) 71–80.

[30] H.G. Marco, W. Brandt, G. Gäde, Elucidation of the amino acid sequence of a crustacean hyperglycaemic hormone from the spiny lobster, *Jasus lalandii*, Biochem. Biophys. Res. Commun. 248 (1998) 578–583.

[31] H.G. Marco, et al., Characterization and sequence elucidation of a novel peptide with molt-inhibiting activity from the South African spiny lobster, *Jasus lalandii*, Peptides 21 (2000) 1313–1321.

[32] H.G. Marco, et al., In search of a vitellogenesis-inhibiting hormone from the eyestalks of the South African spiny lobster, *Jasus lalandii*, Invertebr. Reprod. Dev. 41 (2002) 143–150.

[33] L. Liu, et al., A neurohormone regulating both methyl farnesoate synthesis and glucose metabolism in a crustacean, Biochem. Biophys. Res. Commun. 237 (1997) 694–701.

[34] R.S.E.W. Leuven, et al., Species or group specificity in biological and immunological studies of crustacean hyperglycaemic hormone, Gen. Comp. Endocrinol. 46 (1982) 288–296.

International Congress Series 1275 (2004) 134–140

ELSEVIER

www.ics-elsevier.com

Flight or fight—the need for adipokinetic hormones

Gerd Gäde*

Zoology Department, University of Cape Town, Rondebosch, South Africa

Abstract. An attempt is made to show similarities in function and mode of action of mammalian adrenaline and the adipokinetic hormone (AKH) of insects. As specific case studies, the elucidation of primary structures of AKHs of heteropteran Hemiptera are presented and their function in flight metabolism in this taxon of insects is discussed in detail. All investigated species, representing the families Pentatomidae, Coreidae and Notonectidae, apparently rely (mainly) on lipid oxidation to provide energy for flight and, where measured, for swimming as well. In another case study, beetles which use proline as a fuel for flight, e.g., *Pachnoda sinuata*, need to oxidize fatty acids in order to produce acetyl CoA which will combine with alanine to resynthesise proline. Recent studies demonstrate that the injection of the endogenous AKH of *P. sinuata* and flight (upon which AKH is released) are able to activate the enzyme triacylglycerol lipase. The second messengers in this process are cAMP and Ca^{2+}. © 2004 Elsevier B.V. All rights reserved.

Keywords: Mammalian adrenaline; Insect adipokinetic hormone; Flight metabolism; Flight substrates; Glycogenolysis; Lipolysis; Second messengers; Lipase activation

1. Adrenaline and the "fight and flight reaction"

The adrenal gland of mammals consists of two distinct endocrine tissues: (a) the medulla with chromaffin cells which produce the catecholamines, adrenaline and noradrenaline and (b) the cortex with adrenocortical cells producing the glucocorti-coids, cortisol and corticosterone, in addition to the mineralocorticoid, aldosterone. In the context of the present work, I want to draw the attention of the reader to the action of adrenaline [1]. It is especially well-known for its involvement in what is called the "fight and flight reaction". Upon sudden, mostly threatening, changes in the

---

* Tel.: +27 21 6503615; fax: +27 21 6503301.
E-mail address: ggade@botzoo.uct.ac.za.

0531-5131/ © 2004 Elsevier B.V. All rights reserved.
doi:10.1016/j.ics.2004.08.094

environment, the autonomous sympathetic nervous system is activated. Those neurons that innervate the medulla release their neurotransmitter acetylcholine which, in turn, activates the release of adrenaline into the blood. Adrenaline results in a number of changes in the body which are all aimed at gearing the organism to either a fight or flight decision. The major effects of adrenaline are an increase of the heart rate and cardiac output accompanied by splanchnic vasoconstriction and increase of blood flow through skeletal muscles. Adrenaline is responsible for an increase in respiratory rate and it also inhibits the food passage through the alimentary tract by relaxing the smooth muscles. Metabolically, muscular and hepatic glycogenolysis is increased resulting in a rise in blood sugar levels; in addition, lipolysis is activated in adipose tissue causing an increase of free fatty acids in the blood. In both instances, cAMP is the second messenger involved and phosphorylase and lipase, respectively, are activated. Mediation of the biological actions of adrenaline is via a number of different subtypes of adrenergic receptors. There is a pleptora of information available on such adrenergic receptors which are all coupled to G-proteins [2,3]. The most important information in the context discussed here is that, at least some, α-adrenergic receptors signal via a $G_{q/11}$ G-protein and activate a phospholipase C (PLC) which results in the production of two second messengers, viz. inositol 1,4,5 trisphosphate (IP_3) which is responsible for intracellular Ca^{2+} mobilisation, and diacylglycerol (DAG) which activates a protein kinase C (PKC). On the other hand, certain β-adrenergic receptors signal via a G_s G-protein causing adenylate cyclase (AC) activation and production of the single second messenger, cAMP (see Fig. 1).

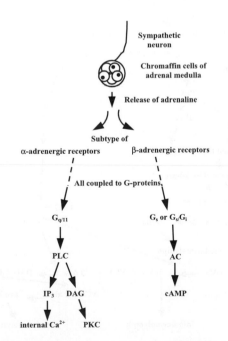

Fig. 1. The mammalian adrenergic system. For abbreviations, see text.

2. The insect peptidergic "equivalent" to the mammalian "fight and flight" adrenaline

In all major orders of insects, including the newly discovered order Mantophasmatodea (Gäde et al., unpublished results), short peptides of the so-called adipokinetic hormone/red pigment-concentrating hormone family (AKH/RPCH) have been found to be present [4]. These peptides have a variety of functions that overlap in a number of actions with those of adrenaline in mammals. The effects of AKHs span from metabolic control by regulating the mobilisation of different fuels for flight such as carbohydrates, lipids and proline, to myotropic actions (especially stimulating the heartbeat), inhibition of the synthesis of RNA, fatty acids and protein in the fat body, stimulation of the biosynthesis of mitochondrial cytoheme a+b, stimulation of general locomotory activity, and even stimulatory effects on the locust's immune system [5,6]. Because a number of these effects, especially metabolic effects such as activation of phosphorylase and lipase, are similar to those achieved by adrenaline, it may be justified to view part of the actions of AKH's as "equivalent" to the adrenaline-induced "fight and flight reactions" (Fig. 2). Of course, aminergic communication with such effects is well known in insects but is not the subject of this short presentation.

The AKH peptides are synthesised and stored in endogenous neurosecretory cells of the corpora cardiaca (CC) and in most insect species they are the most abundant

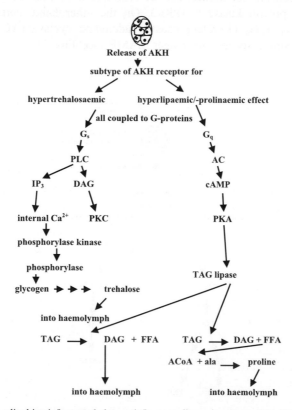

Fig. 2. The insect adipokinetic/hypertrehalosaemic/hyperprolinaemic system. For abbreviations, see text.

peptides of this neurohaemal organ. Therefore, AKHs can be separated and purified from other peptidic components with relative ease in a single HPLC step; because Trp is a characteristic amino acid in each member of the AKH family, detection is facilitated and sensitivity is increased by monitoring Trp fluorescence during purification [7]. Sequences have been determined by Edman degradation after the enzymatic cleavage of the N-terminal pGlu residue, and various mass spectrometric [fast atom bombardment (FAB), matrix-assisted laser desorption/ionisation (MALDI), electrospray ionisation (ESI)] methods have been used successfully to confirm AKH sequences [8,9]. Today, mass spectrometric techniques can also be performed on crude extracts of single CCs to obtain sequence data [10,11]. The primary structures of AKH peptides are typically characterised by a chain length of 8 to 10 amino acids, blocked termini (pGlu at the N-terminus, amide at C-terminus), aromatic amino acids at least at positions 4 (mostly Phe or Tyr) and 8 (always Trp), positions 3 and 5 are either Asn/Thr or Thr/Ser, respectively, and position 9 is always Gly. Most of the variability is found at position 7, including an acidic amino acid (Asp) in the otherwise always noncharged AKHs (see Refs. [5,8,12] for comprehensive tables with primary structures and species names in which they have been found).

The newest examples of AKH structures have been found by "mining" the data of the complete genome of the malaria mosquito *Anopheles gambiae* (Brown, personal communication), and by a combination of classical purification, Edman degradation and ESI mass spectrometry to fully elucidate a posttranslationally modified AKH, an additional, phosphorylated peptide in a cetoniid beetle (Gäde et al., unpublished results).

Genes of some AKHs are known, the preprohormones deduced or even isolated and sequenced; the general organisation of AKH precursors is: signal peptide, AKH peptide, amidation and processing sites, AKH-related peptide of unknown function and variable length [5,8].

One of the main functions of AKHs is the regulation of metabolic events, specifically mobilisation of stored fuels which can be used during intense muscular work, such as flight or running. There are a number of studies known which investigate the role of AKH peptides during flight in locusts, grasshoppers, moths, beetles, bees and flies [13–15].

3. Case studies

In this short overview, I mainly want to present case studies on the involvement of AKHs in flight metabolism in a group of insects that are mostly underrepresented in physiological work, viz. the heteropteran *Hemiptera*.

Firstly, we have established that the stinkbug *Nezara viridula* (Family Pentatomidae) contains an AKH that is structurally identical to the red pigment-concentrating hormone (RPCH) which, up to then, had never been found in insects and is the only member of the AKH family represented in a wide variety of crustaceans [10]. This distribution pattern of RPCH may be cautiously interpreted as one more indication of the sister–group relationship between Hexapoda and Crustacea, which is also suggested by molecular and morphological data [16]. Although I have observed *N. viridula* flying for several meters and minutes in nature, they could not be induced to fly in the laboratory. Nevertheless, injection of the synthetic endogenous peptide resulted in an increase in the concentration of total lipids in the haemolymph. This indicates that lipid oxidation will be used to power the contraction of their flight muscles.

Secondly, we analysed the metabolism of another terrestrial heteropteran insect, the twig wilter *Holopterna alata* (Family Coreidae) which was more amenable to flight experiments in the laboratory. Our preliminary results can be summarised as follows (Gäde et al., unpublished results): adult specimens of *H. alata* have a higher concentration of lipids in the haemolymph than carbohydrates. Injection of a conspecific extract of the corpus cardiacum or of a low dose of the endogenous AKH peptide causes a significant increase in the concentration of lipids but not carbohydrates in the haemolymph. A short flight of about 3-min duration results in a significant decrease in the concentration of the carbohydrates, but not of lipids in the haemolymph. However, if lipids are measured in the haemolymph 1 h after cessation of flight, there is a significant increase in concentration which is indicative of lipid mobilisation by AKH during the phase of activity. Because of the strenuous activity, however, an accumulation of lipids can only be demonstrated after cessation of the activity when no further lipids are used. Further support for the usage of mainly lipids for flight comes from results demonstrating significant changes in the composition of various lipid classes in the thorax (decrease of triacylglycerols) and haemolymph (increase of diacylglycerols).

Thirdly, a lipid-based metabolism was also established in the water bug *Notonecta glauca* (Family Notonectidae) [11]: the concentration of lipids in the haemolymph is high, whereas only a very small amount of carbohydrates is present. Injection of extract from the bug's own corpus cardiacum, as well as of a low dose of the endogenous AKH octapeptide (Anaim-AKH as in the Emperor dragonfly *Anax imperator*) elicits a clear hyperlipaemic response, but the carbohydrate concentration in the haemolymph stays constant. Further experiments demonstrated that *N. glauca* uses lipids for flight and for the exercise of forced swimming for 1 h. Although the lipid concentration in the haemolymph was unchanged after a 5-min period of flight, the concentration doubled when those individuals were allowed to rest for 1 h after flight. Forced swimming of 1 h duration also increased the level of lipids in the haemolymph significantly, demonstrating that both modalities of movement in this bug are supported by the oxidation of lipids. Despite the low amounts of free carbohydrates (in haemolymph) and stored glycogen (in thorax), significant decreases were measured upon flight; thus, carbohydrate metabolism is contributing to flight.

4. Lipase activation is necessary for hyperprolinaemia caused by AKH

My research group has extensively studied flight metabolism of the fruit beetle *Pachnoda sinuata* [15,17]. For flight purposes, this species oxidises two substrates, carbohydrates and proline, at about equal amounts. An AKH peptide, apparently, can activate different receptor subtypes to achieve hypertrehalosaemia and hyperprolinaemia. To mobilise carbohydrates, it is clear that PLC is activated via a G protein-coupled receptor; this generates two second messengers IP_3 and DAG, endogenous Ca^{2+} is then released from internal stores (and external Ca^{2+} is also involved), glycogen phosphorylase is activated, glycogenolysis is initiated and, finally, trehalose is produced via a number of intermediates (see Fig. 2). For the AKH-controlled synthesis of proline, alanine (the product of the partial oxidation of proline during flight) combines with acetyl CoA which is generated from the breakdown of lipids in β-oxidation of fatty acids. It is, therefore, postulated that the primary action of AKH to cause hyperprolinaemia is on a triacylglycerol lipase and should be similar to the action of AKH in moth to cause hyperlipaemia [18]. Recently, we investigated the activation state of lipase in the fat body of *P. sinuata* in response to the endogenous AKH of the beetle and upon flight; we were able to measure an activation of the enzyme in both cases, indicating that the AKH is released upon the flight stimulus (Auerswald et al., unpublished results). Thus, also during the regulation of proline synthesis, lipolysis is stimulated by AKH. The second messengers in this process are cAMP and intracellular Ca^{2+} (from IP_3-insensitive stores) and extracellular Ca^{2+} (see Fig. 2).

I hope that I have conclusively shown a number of parallels between the vertebrate adrenergic "fight and flight" system and the AKH system in insects. Especially the mode of action of AKH for the dual substrate system in the fruit beetle, its postulated subtypes of receptors, its activation of glycogenolysis and lipolysis and the different second messengers involved, are all reminiscent of the adrenergic system. Recently, it was even shown that AKH and the immune response in the migratory locust are intimately related [19]. Again, interaction of the adrenergic system and the immune system are well known [1]. It would certainly be rewarding to closely study the literature on vertebrate adrenergic systems in order to model experiments on insects to achieve a better insight into the similarities and variations in these systems.

Acknowledgements

The author is indebted to post-docs, collaborating colleagues and technicians for contributing to the research discussed, to Dr H.G. Marco for improving the English and to the National Research Foundation (Pretoria, South Africa, gun number 2053806) and UCT Research Committee for partial financial support.

References

[1] L.J. DeGroot, J.L. Jameson (Eds.), Endocrinology, 4th edition, WB Saunders, Philadelphia, 2001.

[2] T. Koshimizu, et al., Recent advances in α_1-adrenoceptor pharmacology, Pharmacol. Ther. 98 (2003) 235–244.

[3] M. Philipp, L. Hein, Adrenergic receptor knockout mice: distinct functions of 9 receptor subtypes, Pharmacol. Ther. 101 (2004) 65–74.

[4] G. Gäde, The adipokinetic hormone/red pigment-concentrating hormone peptide family: structures, interrelationships and functions, J. Insect Physiol. 36 (1990) 1–12.

[5] G. Gäde, K.H. Hoffmann, J.H. Spring, Hormonal regulation in insects. Facts, gaps, and future directions, Physiol. Rev. 77 (1997) 963–1032.

[6] G. Gäde, Regulation of intermediary metabolism and water balance of insects by neuropeptides, Annu. Rev. Entomol. 49 (2004) 93–113.

[7] G. Gäde, Extraction, purification and sequencing of adipokinetic/red pigment-concentrating hormone-family peptides, in: A.R. McCaffery, D.I. Wilson (Eds.), Chromatography and Isolation of Insect Hormones and Pheromones, Plenum Press, New York, 1990, pp. 165–182.

[8] G. Gäde, The revolution in insect neuropeptides illustrated by the adipokinetic hormone/red pigment-concentrating hormone family of peptides, Z. Naturforsch. 51c (1996) 607–617.

[9] G. Gäde, The explosion of structural information on insect neuropeptides, in: W. Herz, G.W. Kirby, R.E. Moore, W. Steglich, Ch. Tamm (Eds.), Progress on the Chemistry of Organic Natural Products, Springer Verlag, Wien, 1997, pp. 1–128.

[10] G. Gäde, et al., Red pigment-concentrating hormone is not limited to crustaceans, Biochem. Biophys. Res. Commun. 309 (2003) 967–973.

[11] G. Gäde, et al., Substrate usage and its regulation during flight and swimming in the backswimmer, Notonecta glauca, Physiol. Entomol. 29 (2004) 84–93.

[12] G. Gäde, H.G. Marco, Structure, function and mode of action of select arthropod neuropeptides, in: Atta-Ur Rahmann (Ed.), Studies in Natural Product Chemistry (Bioactive Natural Products), 2004, in press.

[13] G. Gäde, The hormonal integration of insect flight metabolism, Zool. Jb. Physiol. 96 (1992) 211–225.

[14] G. Gäde, L. Auerswald, Insect neuropeptides regulating substrate mobilisation, S. Afr. J. Zool. 33 (1998) 65–70.

[15] G. Gäde, L. Auerswald, Beetles' choice—proline for energy output: control by AKHs, Comp. Biochem. Physiol. 132B (2002) 117–129.

[16] G. Giribert, G.D. Edgecombe, W.C. Wheeler, Arthropod phylogeny based on eight molecular loci and morphology, Nature 413 (2001) 157–161.

[17] G. Gäde, L. Auerswald, Mode of action of neuropeptides from the adipokinetic hormone family, Gen. Comp. Endocrinol. 132 (2003) 10–20.

[18] E.L. Arrese, et al., Lipid storage and mobilization in insects; current status and future directions, Insect Biochem. Mol. Biol. 31 (2001) 7–17.

[19] G.J. Goldsworthy, et al., Interactions between endocrine and immune systems in locusts, Physiol. Entomol. 28 (2003) 54–61.

International Congress Series 1275 (2004) 141–148

ELSEVIER

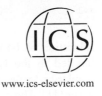

www.ics-elsevier.com

Multilocal expression of B-type allatostatins in crickets (*Gryllus bimaculatus*)

Junling Wang[a], Martina Meyering-Vos[a], Klaus H. Hoffmann[a,b,*]

[a]*Department of Animal Ecology I, University of Bayreuth, 95440 Bayreuth, Germany*
[b]*Zoology Department, University of Cape Town, Rondebosch 7701, South Africa*

Abstract. B-type allatostatins (AST) inhibit the biosynthesis of juvenile hormone (JH) in vitro in crickets, but are also present in other insects, where they may bare different functions. By means of one-step RT-PCR and in situ hybridization recently, we could show that the mRNA of the gene is expressed in various cells of the central nervous system, but also in endocrine cells of the gut. The latter results corroborated a function of these peptides in regulating gut motility. Here we report on the expression of the gene in the ovary, the fat body and the flight muscles of female adult crickets, which suggests further putative functions of the B-type allatostatins beyond their role as brain–gut peptides. © 2004 Elsevier B.V. All rights reserved.

Keywords: Allatostatin; Preprohormone; Gene expression; Ovary; Fat body; Flight muscle; Cricket

1. Introduction

Allatostatins (AST) were first isolated from the cockroach *Diploptera punctata* based on their ability to inhibit juvenile hormone (JH) biosynthesis by the corpora allata (CA) [1]. The peptides were characterized by a C-terminal pentapeptide sequence Y/FXFGLa and were designated FGLamides or A-type AST. The peptides inhibit JH biosynthesis from cockroaches and crickets [2–4]. A more general role of these peptides seems to be the inhibition of visceral muscle contractions [5–8]. Besides the A-type AST, two other peptide families with allatostatic function were reported. A single peptide (C-type AST) was first isolated from brains of *Manduca sexta* which strongly inhibited JH biosynthesis in vitro by CA of larvae and adults of the moth, but not of other insect orders [9].

* Corresponding author. Department of Animal Ecology I, University of Bayreuth, 95440 Bayreuth, Germany. Tel.: +49 921 552650; fax: +49 921 552784.
E-mail address: klaus.hoffmann@uni-bayreuth.de (K.H. Hoffmann).

0531-5131/ © 2004 Elsevier B.V. All rights reserved.
doi:10.1016/j.ics.2004.07.032

Inhibition of JH biosynthesis by extracts of the brains of crickets (*Gryllus bimaculatus*) has led to the isolation of a number of neuropeptides, which showed high sequence similarity to the myoinhibiting peptides isolated from *Locusta migratoria* [10] and *M. sexta* [11]. These peptides were designated Grybi-AST type B or W^2W^9amides [4,12]. The allatostatic activity of the peptides seems to be restricted to crickets (reviewed in Ref. [13]), but alternative roles in other insects are suggested. For example, in the silkworm *Bombyx mori* a member of this peptide family (Bommo-PTSP) inhibits the synthesis of ecdysteroids in the prothoracic glands [14]. In crickets, ovarian ecdysteroid biosynthesis in vitro is inhibited by B-type ASTs [4].

Neuropeptides are generally expressed as a precursor (preprohormone), including one to several putative peptides. So far, a B-type AST preprohormone has been identified only for *Drosophila melanogaster* [15]. Recently, we reported the identification of a partial sequence of the B-type preproallatostatin from *G. bimaculatus*. By PCR screening of a random primer cDNA library and by RACE, a 535-bp 3′ cDNA sequence was obtained, which encodes a putative translation product of 85 amino acids, containing six copies of B-type ASTs. By means of RNA dot blot and RT in situ PCR analyses we demonstrated the mRNA expression of the gene in the nervous system and the digestive tract of female and male adult crickets [16,17].

In this study, experiments were performed to localize the expression of the B-type AST precursor in the ovary of adult female crickets by RT in situ PCR, because it is well established that (neuro)peptides control the synthesis and release of juvenile hormones and ecdysteroids during ovarian development and vitellogenesis. In addition, expression was investigated in the fat body, thoracic muscle, and accessory reproductive glands of females and in accessory reproductive glands and testes of males in order to shed light on the multilocal distribution of the peptides and their putative functions in *G. bimaculatus*.

2. Materials and methods

Mediterranean field crickets, *G. bimaculatus* de Geer (Ensifera, Gryllidae) were reared as described [16,17]. Total RNA from the various tissues of 1-day-old females and males was extracted with the peqGOLD Trifast kit (Peqlab Biotechnologie) and the mRNA was extracted with the Oligotex ® mRNA Mini kit (Qiagen).

The Titanium one-step RT-PCR kit (Clontech) was used for one-step RT-PCR according to the instructions of the manufacturer, supplemented by 22 nM forward primer WJF2 (corresponding to nt 224–253 of the 3′ cDNA sequence in Ref. [17]) and 22 nM reverse primer WUR3 (corresponding to nt 421–459 in Ref. [17]). A control for genomic DNA contamination was done by performing a PCR in the presence of *Taq* DNA Polymerase (MBI Fermentas) under the same conditions as the RT-PCR reaction. One microliter of 20 ng/µl mRNA of various tissues was added to an aliquot of 9 µl master mix and the reaction carried out as described [17]. For RNA dot blot analyses, 100 ng mRNA was diluted into 50 µl DEPC water, mixed with 30 µl 20× SSC and 20 µl 37% (v/v) formaldehyde, heated to 65 °C for 15 min and then chilled on ice. The samples were transferred to a Nylon N+ membrane (Amersham) with the help of the dot blot manifold by vacuum. After crosslinking by UV irradiation, the membrane was hybridized with the DIG-labelled cRNA probe (corresponding to positions 1–199 of the 3' cDNA sequence of the cricket AST B-type gene [17]; EMBL Nucleotide Sequence Data Base, accession no. AJ704769) prepared with the DIG RNA labelling kit (SP6/T7)(Roche). The matched positive control was hybridized with the DIG-labelled cRNA probe for ß-actin of *G. bimaculatus* derived from the sequence submitted to GenBank (accession no. AB087882).

For RT in situ PCR, the tissues were dissected from 1-day-old females or males under Ringer [18] and immediately fixed in a fixation buffer [17]. The RT in situ PCR steps were derived from a method described by Nuovo [19] (for details, see also Ref. [17]) and the colour slides (10 μm) were examined using a Leitz Diaplan microscope provided with a digital camera (Cool SNAP RS Photometrics). Controls were done by leaving out the RNase inhibitor and additionally using RNase to digest the RNA.

3. Results

The mRNA samples from ovary, fat body, thoracic muscle and accessory reproductive glands of 1-day-old females and from accessory reproductive glands and testes of 1-day-old males were used for one-step RT-PCR and RNA dot blot analyses. For each tissue, RT-PCR amplification yielded a unique product of 236 bp (Fig. 1). When the same amount of mRNA from each tissue was used as template for PCR, but excluding the step of reverse transcription (control), no PCR product was detected (Fig. 1B). The results indicate that the Grybi-AST B gene is expressed in all these tissues, and this was confirmed by the RNA dot blot analyses shown in Fig. 2.

The cricket ovary is of the panoistic type and each of the ovarioles is composed of a terminal filament in which the oocytes are produced from the oogonia, and a vitellarium in which yolk is deposited into the growing oocytes. At the posterior end of the germarium, the oocytes are beginning to be surrounded by a monolayer of follicle cells. In the germarium, RT in situ PCR positive signals were detected in the nuclei of primary oocytes (Fig. 3A1,B1). Young primary oocytes located near the terminal filament contained highly

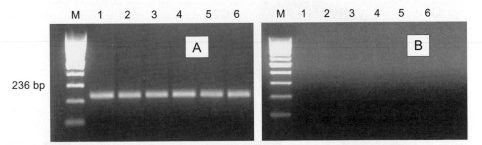

Fig. 1. The Grybi-AST type B expression analysis by RT-PCR. (A) Agarose gel electrophoresis of the RT-PCR products stained with ethidiumbromide. On the left, the 100-bp markers were run. The mRNA of (1) ovary, (2) fat body, (3) thoracic muscle, (4) accessory reproductive glands of 1 day-old females, and (5) accessory reproductive glands, (6) testes of 1-day-old males were used as templates. (B) Agarose gel electrophoresis of the control PCR amplification to test the genomic DNA contamination of the matched mRNA samples. Other details are as in panel (A).

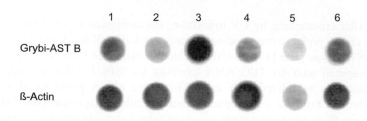

Fig. 2. RNA dot blot analyses of the Grybi-AST type B expression in different tissues. (1) Ovary, (2) fat body, (3) thoracic muscle, (4) accessory reproductive glands of 1-day-old females, and (5) accessory reproductive glands, (6) testes of 1-day-old males. β-Actin, matched positive controls (see Materials and methods).

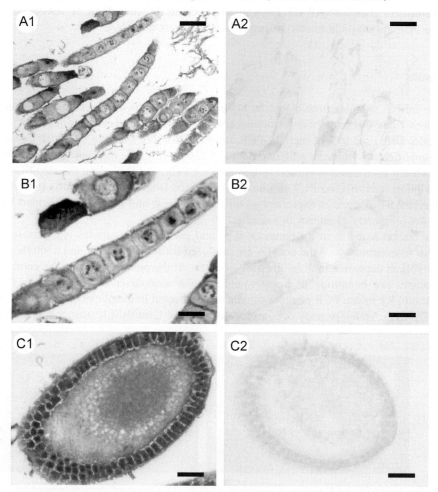

Fig. 3. Photomicrographs of Grybi-AST B expression by RT in situ PCR in sections of ovarioles of a 1-day-old female. (A1) Overview on the localization of expression in the germarium. (B1) Localization of the expression in primary oocytes during their development in the germarium. (C1) Localization of the expression in follicle cells enveloping the oocyte in the vitellarium. (A2, B2 and C2) Matched controls. Scale bars in A1, A2 = 100 μm; in B1, B2 = 40 μm; in C1, C2 = 20 μm.

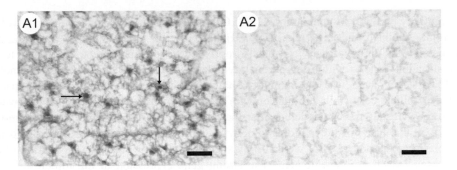

Fig. 4. Photomicrographs of Grybi-AST B expression by RT in situ PCR in sections of the fat body of a 1-day-old female. (A1) Expression in the nuclei (arrows) of the trophocytes. (A2) Matched control. Scale bars = 20 μm.

condensed signals, which appeared as more separated granules with weaker intensity during the ongoing development of the oocytes. No signals were found in the nuclei or in the cytoplasm of vitellogenic oocytes, but at this stage of development strong gene expression was observed in the follicle cells (Fig. 3C1). No signals were detected in the sections of the negative controls (Fig. 3A2–C2).

The fat body is mainly composed of trophocytes, which grow large in adults and become vacuolated. The vacuoles contain the reserves. RT in situ PCR positive signals were observed in the branched nuclei of the trophocytes (Fig. 4A1). In sections of the close-packed thoracic flight muscles, condensed RT in situ PCR positive signals were found in the nuclei of the muscle cells (Fig. 5A1). No signals were detected in the sections of the negative controls (Figs. 4A2 and 5A2).

4. Discussion

The results clearly demonstrate the expression of the Grybi-AST type B gene outside the nervous system and the gut, which suggests additional functions of the deduced peptides to those as brain/gut neurohormones. Moreover, the data confirm our earlier observations on the presence of B-allatostatin-like immunoreactivity in extracts of ovaries

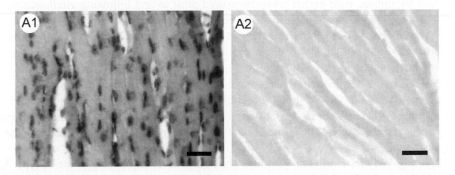

Fig. 5. Photomicrographs of Grybi-AST B expression by RT in situ PCR in sections of the thoracic flight muscle of a 1-day-old female. (A1) Expression in the nuclei of the muscle cells. (A2) Matched control. Scale bars = 20 μm.

and partially purified chromatographic (HPLC) fractions [20]. The immunopositive HPLC fractions inhibited the biosynthesis of JH in vitro in a homologous bioassay. B-allatostatin-like immunoreactivity was also observed in sections of ovaries from 0- to 4-day-old adult females within the cortical cytoplasm of the oocytes at the anterior poles [20]. However, there was no immunostaining in follicle cells, in intercellular spaces between follicle cells (in a terminal oocyte) or in any neural structure within the ovary. From these results we can conclude that the peptides deduced from the preprohormone mRNA in the nuclei of previtellogenic oocytes will be released, at least in part, into the cytoplasm of the oocytes, but we can only speculate on their putative function(s) at that early stage of oocyte development. The strong gene expression in the follicle cells of vitellogenic oocytes on the one side, but the lack of AST type B-immunoreactivity in the follicle cells on the other side, suggest that the deduced peptides may be quickly released from the follicle cells, either into the cytoplasm of the oocytes or into the haemolymph. Lorenz and coworkers [4,18] demonstrated that peptides of the AST B-type could effectively inhibit the biosynthesis of ecdysteroids in the ovary (follicle cells) of adult female crickets in vitro in a dose-dependent manner. In adult females of *G. bimaculatus*, the synthesis of ecdysteroids in the ovary [21,22] as well as the titer of ecdysteroids in the haemolymph increase during the first 4 days after imaginal moult but decrease thereafter. Whether B-type allatostatins from the ovary are directly involved in the regulation of ecdysteroid biosynthesis in the ovary of young adult females is still speculative, but the results from injection experiments strengthened this assumption [23]. Injection of B-type allatostatins into adult females during the first days after imaginal moult lowered the rate of ecdysteroid biosynthesis in the ovary as well as the titer of ecdysteroids in the haemolymph, whereas no effects of the injected peptides on haemolymph JH titers or the capacity of the CA to produce JH ex vivo was observed. Interestingly, the haemolymph titers of vitellogenins (Vg) were almost twice as high in allatostatin-injected animals as in Ringer-injected controls.

Members of the A-type AST family (FGLamides) have been identified from ovaries of various insect species [20, 24] and expression of their genes was also demonstrated [25,26]. In the cockroach *D. punctata*, A-type ASTs were expressed in the ovary as well as in the lateral and common oviducts, and the pattern of expression changed during the reproductive cycle. Specifically, expression was drastically reduced during the time of maximal Vg uptake, with higher levels measured prior to and following vitellogenesis. A supposed physiological parameter that A-type ASTs affect is the release of Vg from the fat body. Martin et al. [27,28] showed that the A-type ASTs inhibit Vg release by periovarian fat bodies of 4 day-old females of the cockroach *Blattella germanica* in vitro and that the effect is mediated by the glycosylation of Vg. These results suggest that allatostatins may be involved in the termination of vitellogenic cycles. Similar effects can be supposed for the B-type ASTs in the fat body of crickets. Recently, we have demonstrated the expression of A-type ASTs in the fat body of adult female crickets [26], and the present study localized the expression of the B-type AST preprohormone in the nuclei of the fat body trophocytes.

Meyering-Vos and Hoffmann [26] also showed distinct expression of the A-type AST preprohormone in the thoracic muscle of adult female crickets and the present study localized the expression of the B-type AST precursor within the nuclei of the muscle cells.

As yet, no true function of the allatostatins in skeletal/wing muscles is known, although Jansons et al. [29] suggested a role of the C-type AST (lepidopteran allatostatin type) prohormone gene expression in *Pseudaletia unipuncta* with the migratory flight of that species.

Further elucidation of predicted pleiotropic activities of allatostatins in crickets can be expected from the identification of the putative receptors as well as from functional knock out of the genes by using the RNA interference (RNAi) method. Such work is in progress.

Acknowledgements

This work was supported through a fellowship to JW by the Deutsche Forschungsgemeinschaft (Ho 631/15-4). We are grateful to Mr. Shih-long Yan for valuable suggestions and technical assistance with the RT in situ PCR method. We would like to thank Prof. Dr. F. Sehnal (Èeské Budìjovice) for offering the cDNA library and Prof. Dr. J. Woodring (Baton Rouge/Bayreuth) for a critical reading of the manuscript. The Alexander-von-Humboldt research award South Africa from the NRF to KHH is greatly acknowledged.

References

[1] A.P. Woodhead, et al., Primary structure of four allatostatins: neuropeptide inhibitors of juvenile hormone synthesis, Proc. Natl. Acad. Sci. U. S. A. 86 (1989) 5997–6001.

[2] B. Stay, S.S. Tobe, W.G. Bendena, Allatostatins: identification, primary structures, functions and distribution, Adv. Insect Physiol. 25 (1994) 267–337.

[3] K.H. Hoffmann, M. Meyering-Vos, M.W. Lorenz, Allatostatins and allatotropins: is the regulation of corpora allata their primary function? Eur. J. Entomol. 96 (1999) 255–266.

[4] M.W. Lorenz, Neuropeptides regulating developmental, reproductive, and metabolic events in crickets: structures and modes of action, J. Insect Biotechnol. Sericology 70 (2001) 69–93.

[5] A.B. Lange, K.K. Chan, B. Stay, Effect of allatostatin and proctolin on antennal pulsatile organ and hindgut muscle in the cockroach, *Diploptera punctata*, Arch. Insect Biochem. Physiol. 24 (1993) 789–792.

[6] H. Duve, A. Thorpe, Distribution and functional significance of Leu-callatostatins in the blowfly *Calliphora vomitoria*, Cell Tissue Res. 276 (1994) 367–379.

[7] H. Duve, P. Wren, A. Thorpe, Innervation of the foregut of the cockroach *Leucophaea maderae* and inhibition of spontaneous contractile activity by allatostatin neuropeptides, Physiol. Entomol. 20 (1995) 33–44.

[8] H. Duve, et al., Lepidopteran peptides of the allatostatin superfamily, Peptides 18 (1997) 1301–1309.

[9] S.J. Kramer, et al., Identification of an allatostatin from the tobacco hornworm *Manduca sexta*, Proc. Natl. Acad. Sci. U. S. A. 88 (1991) 9458–9462.

[10] L. Schoofs, et al., Isolation, identification and synthesis of Locusta-myoinhibiting peptide (Lom-MIP), a novel biologically active neuropeptide from *Locusta migratoria*, Regul. Pept. 36 (1991) 111–119.

[11] M.B. Blackburn, et al., Identification of four additional myoinhibiting peptides (MIPs) from the ventral nerve cord of *Manduca sexta*, Arch. Insect Biochem. Physiol. 48 (2001) 99–109.

[12] M.W. Lorenz, R. Kellner, K.H. Hoffmann, A family of neuropeptides that inhibit juvenile hormone biosynthesis in the cricket, *Gryllus bimaculatus*, J. Biol. Chem. 270 (1995) 21103–21108.

[13] G. Gäde, K.H. Hoffmann, J. Spring, Hormonal regulation in insects: facts, gaps and future directions, Physiol. Rev. 77 (1997) 963–1032.

[14] Y.-J. Hua, et al., Identification of a prothoracicostatic peptide in the larval brain of the silkworm, *Bombyx mori*, J. Biol. Chem. 274 (1999) 31169–31173.

[15] M. Williamson, et al., Molecular cloning, genomic organization, and expression of a B-type (cricket-type) allatostatin preprohormone from *Drosophila melanogaster*, Biochem. Biophys. Res. Commun. 281 (2001) 544–550.

[16] Wang J. Isolation and characterization of the B-type allatostatin gene of *Gryllus bimaculatus* de Geer (Ensifera, Gryllidae). PhD thesis, University of Bayreuth, Bayreuth, 2004.

[17] J. Wang, M. Meyering-Vos, K.H. Hoffmann, Cloning and tissue-specific localization of cricket-type allatostatin from *Gryllus bimaculatus*, Mol. Cell. Endocrinol. (2004) in press.

[18] J.I. Lorenz, M.W. Lorenz, K.H. Hoffmann, Factors regulating juvenile hormone synthesis in *Gryllus bimaculatus* (Ensifera: Gryllidae), Eur. J. Entomol. 94 (1997) 369–379.

[19] G.J. Nuovo, Nonradioactive analysis of biomolecules, in: C. Hessler (Ed.), In Situ PCR Amplification of cDNA, Springer, Berlin, 2000, pp. 343–355.

[20] G. Witek, K.H. Hoffmann, Immunological evidence for FGLamide- and W^2W^9-allatostatins in the ovary of *Gryllus bimaculatus* (Ensifera: Gryllidae), Physiol. Entomol. 26 (2001) 49–57.

[21] K. Weidner, et al., Developmental changes in ecdysteroid biosynthesis in vitro during adult life and embryogenesis in a cricket, *Gryllus bimaculatus* de Geer, Invertebr. Reprod. Dev. 21 (1992) 129–140.

[22] K.H. Hoffmann, M.W. Lorenz, The role of ecdysteroids and juvenile hormones in insect reproduction, Trends Comp. Biochem. Physiol. 3 (1997) 1–8.

[23] M.W. Lorenz, et al., In vivo effects of allatostatins in crickets, *Gryllus bimaculatus* (Ensifera: Gryllidae), Arch. Insect Biochem. Physiol. 38 (1998) 32–43.

[24] A.P. Woodhead, et al., Allatostatin in ovaries, oviducts, and young embryos in the cockroach *Diploptera punctata*, J. Insect Physiol. 49 (2003) 1103–1114.

[25] C.S. Garside, et al., Expression of allatostatin in the oviducts of the cockroach *Diploptera punctata*, Insect Biochem. Mol. Biol. 32 (2002) 1089–1099.

[26] M. Meyering-Vos, K.H. Hoffmann, Expression of allatostatins in the Mediterranean field cricket, *Gryllus bimaculatus* de Geer (Ensifera, Gryllidae), Comp. Biochem. Physiol., B 136 (2003) 207–215.

[27] D. Martin, M.D. Piulachs, X. Belles, Inhibition of vitellogenin production by allatostatin in the German cockroach, Mol. Cell. Endocrinol. 121 (1996) 191–196.

[28] D. Martin, M.D. Piulachs, X. Belles, Allatostatin inhibits vitellogenin release in a cockroach, Ann. N.Y. Acad. Sci. 839 (1998) 341–342.

[29] I.S. Jansons, et al., Molecular characterization of a cDNA from *Pseudaletia unipuncta* encoding the *Manduca sexta* allatostatin peptide (Mas-AST), Insect Biochem. Mol. Biol. 26 (1996) 767–773.

ELSEVIER

Inhibitor strategies to control coleopteran pests

B. Oppert*, T.D. Morgan, K.J. Kramer

USDA ARS Grain Marketing and Production Research Center, USDA ARS GMPRC,
1515 College Avenue, Manhattan, KS 66502, United States

Abstract. Enzyme inhibitors from plants are promising candidates for new biocontrol agents but are limited by the inherent compensatory responses to plant inhibitors by insects. We found that inhibitors targeting multiple proteinase classes were necessary to reduce cereal damage by the red flour beetle, *Tribolium castaneum*. We proposed that the multiple inhibitor approach was required for efficacy because *T. castaneum* larvae were able to compensate when fed individual proteinase inhibitors. To investigate the adaptive response, increasing levels of inhibitors that target cysteine and/or serine proteinases were fed to *T. castaneum* larvae, and the properties of digestive proteinases were examined in vitro. Under normal dietary conditions, *T. castaneum* larvae primarily used cysteine proteinases to digest food, with minor contributions from serine proteinases. When larvae were fed cysteine proteinase inhibitors, they responded with a dramatic shift from cysteine to serine proteinase-based digestion. A combination of cysteine and serine proteinase inhibitors in the diet prevented such a shift of dietary enzymes, resulting in a significant reduction in growth and increased mortality. These data suggest that by studying the complex of digestive proteinases in a target pest, combinations of proteinase inhibitors can be identified that overcome the adaptive response to inhibitors, thus providing a more effective control of insect pests by inhibitors. © 2004 Elsevier B.V. All rights reserved.

Keywords: Insect proteinase; Proteinase inhibitor; Coleopteran pests; *Tribolium castaneum*

1. Introduction

More than 15 years ago, we initiated a study to identify proteinase inhibitors for control of storage insect pests. At that time, various inhibitors had been used in insect bioassays with promising results. However, attempts to develop transgenic plants expressing protease inhibitor genes were largely unsuccessful (reviewed in Refs. [1,2]). By studying

* Corresponding author. Tel.: +1 91 785 776 2780; fax: +1 91 785 537 5584.
E-mail address: bso@ksu.edu (B. Oppert).

the biochemical and genetic expression of insect gut proteinases in response to inhibitors, researchers began to understand the adaptive response of insects to inhibitors. Insects respond to inhibitors with a variety of compensatory mechanisms, including the increased production of proteinases, production of new proteinases, or the neutralization of inhibitors through proteolytic degradation. These adaptive responses are an evolutionary result of the constant competition of insects for food sources and plant production of antinutritional defensive molecules.

The red flour beetle, *Tribolium castaneum*, is a major pest in the United States, causing damage to stored grain and grain products. *T. castaneum* is resistant to many synthetic and microbial pesticides. A major research project has been to develop new biologically based control methods for the control of *T. castaneum* larval damage to grains through the study of digestive enzymes and potential inhibitors.

The gut pH of *T. castaneum* was found to be generally acidic [3]. Acidic proteinases had been previously described in *T. castaneum* larvae [4,5]. However, cystatins and/or serine proteinase inhibitors effectively reduced the activity of *T. castaneum* gut proteinases in vitro [3,6–9]. Using this knowledge as background information, our goal was to develop new insect gut-targeted biologically based pesticides to be used in the integrated pest management of *T. castaneum*.

2. Materials and methods

Inhibitors used in this study included the microbial inhibitor L-trans-epoxysuccinyl-leucylamide [4-guanidino] butane (E-64) and soybean Kunitz trypsin inhibitor (Sigma, St. Louis, MO). Other proteinaceous inhibitors included equistatin from sea anemone and potato cysteine proteinase inhibitor (PCPI, both provided by Dr. Vito Turk, Ljubljana, Slovenia), and Job's Tear cysteine proteinase inhibitor (provided by Dr. Kohichi Yoza, Tsukuba, Japan). All other chemicals also were from Sigma unless otherwise noted.

2.1. Insect bioassay

T. castaneum larvae were reared in the laboratory on 95% wheat flour and 5% brewer's yeast. For bioassays, neonate larvae were placed on 85% toasted wheat germ, 10% flour, and 5% brewers yeast. Larvae were reared individually on 10 mg of inhibitor-treated or untreated diet in 200-μl microcentrifuge tubes, 28 °C and 75% relative humidity.

2.2. Insect gut dissection

Larvae were prechilled on ice, the posterior and anterior ends were removed with dissection scissors, and entire guts were isolated with forceps. Guts were pooled for each treatment group in deionized water (10 guts/25 μl) for proteinase assays and frozen at −20 °C. For microplate proteinase assays, samples were thawed, vortexed briefly, and the supernatant was collected following centrifugation at 15,000×g for 5 min.

2.3. Zymogram analysis

Sodium dodecyl sulphate–polyacrylamide electrophoresis (SDS–PAGE) gels with prestained casein (4–16% ZBC, Invitrogen, Carlsbad, CA) were used to analyze proteinases from gut extracts of *T. castaneum* larvae. Proteins (0.2 gut equivalents per well) were separated by electrophoresis, and gels were incubated in renaturation buffer (1% Triton X-100 in water) for 30 min on ice, washed twice in water, followed by incubation in the zymogram developing buffer (50 mmol l^{-1} Tris, pH 8.0, 200 mmol l^{-1} NaCl$_2$, 0.02% Brij 35; Invitrogen) with 5 mmol l^{-1} L-cysteine for 4 h.

2.4. Activity blot analysis

The procedure was as previously described [10]. Proteins in *T. castaneum* gut extracts were separated by non-reducing SDS–PAGE in precast 10–20% Tricine gels (Invitrogen). Separated proteins were transferred to nitrocellulose and were incubated in a solution of 0.5 mg/ml N-succinyl-ala-ala-pro-phe ρ-nitroanilide (SAAPFpNA) in 0.1 mol l^{-1} Tris–HCl, pH 8.1 and 0.02 mol l^{-1} CaCl$_2$. Liberated nitroanilide was visualized by subsequent incubations of 5 min each in 0.1% sodium nitrite in 1 mol l^{-1} HCl, 0.5% ammonium sulfamate in 1 mol l^{-1} HCl, and 0.05% N-(1-naphthyl)-ethylenediamine in 47.5% ethanol. Membranes were stored in heat-sealed bags at −20 °C.

2.5. Microplate proteinase assay

The effects proteinase inhibitors on gut proteolytic activity were evaluated by a previously described microplate assay [11]. Maximum activity of serine proteinases occurred in pH 8.4 Universal buffer containing acetate, phosphate, and borate salts [12]. This buffer was selected for the microplate proteinase assay to evaluate responses to serine and cysteine proteinase inhibitors. Inhibitors were added at the indicated concentration and incubated with gut extracts for 15 min at 37 °C prior to the addition of substrate. Fluorescently labelled casein (BODIPY-TR-X casein, Molecular Probes, Eugene, OR) was diluted according to the manufacturer's recommendation, and 10 μl (0.1 μg) was added to each well. Each sample was incubated in triplicate at 37 °C, and the fluorescence was measured (excitation wavelength of 584 nm and emission wavelength of 620 nm) and corrected by subtracting readings obtained from incubations of substrate only. Measurements of enzyme and buffer or buffer only produced negligible fluorescence and were not subtracted from readings.

3. Results

Different substrates were used to evaluate the relative activities of *T. castaneum* gut proteinases in vitro. A substrate for general proteinase activity, fluorescently labeled casein (BODIPY), was hydrolyzed more efficiently at acidic pH values in reducing buffers, with minor hydrolysis over the alkaline range (Fig. 1). These data suggested that cysteine proteinases with acidic pH optima were major digestive enzymes in *T. castaneum* larvae. In nonreducing buffers, trypsin (BApNA) and chymotrypsin (SAAPFpNA) substrates were hydrolyzed mostly in alkaline pH buffers. Two optima were observed with each pNA substrate, with maximal hydrolysis of BApNA at pH 4 and 9, and maximal hydrolysis of SAAPFpNA at pH 7 and 11. Overall, the amount of hydrolysis of SAAPFpNA was greater than that of BApNA, suggesting that chymotrypsin-like enzymes may be more important than trypsin-like serine proteinases as digestive enzymes in *T. castaneum* larvae.

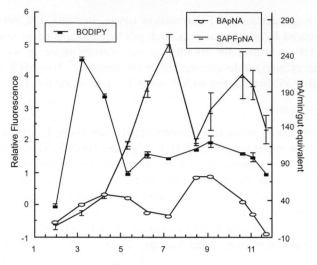

Fig. 1. The relative hydrolysis of casein (BODIPY, Relative Fluorescence) or BApNA and SAAPFpNA (mA min^{-1} gut^{-1} equivalent) by gut extracts of *T. castaneum* larvae.

A number of inhibitors were evaluated in vitro for the potential to decrease the activity of *T. castaneum* larvae. Based on the IC_{50} values, the most effective inhibitors were leupeptin and E-64 (Table 1). Other microbial inhibitors included antipain and chymostatin. Synthetic inhibitors of serine proteinases, TLCK and TPCK, also had activity against *T. castaneum* proteolytic activity. Effective proteinaceous inhibitors included equistatin, JCPI, PCPI, and STI. Some inhibitors, such as E-64, equistatin, JCPI, and PCPI have selective activity against cysteine proteinases. Other inhibitors, such as TLCK, chymostatin, TPCK, and STI are primarily active against serine proteinases. Inhibitors that reduce the activity of both cysteine and serine proteinases include leupeptin and antipain. The inhibitor patterns obtained demonstrated that inhibitors of both cysteine and serine proteinases were effective in reducing *T. castaneum* larval gut proteinase activity.

Table 1

Relative values for the concentration of inhibitor resulting in 50% inhibition (IC_{50}) of the hydrolysis of casein by *T. castaneum* gut extracts (adapted from Ref. [3])

In vitro inhibitor	IC_{50} (mmol l^{-1})
Leupeptin	0.05
E-64	0.11
Equistatin	0.24
TLCK	0.35
JCPI	0.43
PCPI	0.76
Antipain	0.83
Chymostatin	3.40
TPCK	24.0
STI	58.0

Selected inhibitors with in vitro activity were tested in bioassays with *T. castaneum* larvae. Results from those studies are summarized in Table 2. None of the proteinaceous inhibitors were as effective as E-64 in reducing growth and increasing mortality of *T. castaneum* larvae, especially in combinations with STI. A combination of 0.1% E-64 with 1.0% STI resulted in approximately 50% mortality, and 0.1% E-64 with 10% STI caused 100% mortality of *T. castaneum* larvae. Therefore, E-64 and STI were chosen for use in biochemical assays to evaluate the change in the proteolytic enzyme profile of *T. castaneum* larvae in response to dietary inhibitors.

T. castaneum larvae were fed increasing doses of E-64 and/or STI, and larvae were dissected at similar weights (~1.2–1.4 mg) to examine the digestive proteolyic enzyme patterns. Larvae fed inhibitors were older at the time of dissection when compared to control larvae fed a non-inhibitor treated diet. On control and STI diets, larvae were dissected around 14 days. However, larvae fed E-64 were dissected 2–3 days later, and larvae receiving the combination treatments were dissected at around 28–29 days of age, indicating an approximately twofold delay in development time. These delays in dissection time were consistent with the reduction in growth patterns observed in earlier bioassays [3,9]. Mortality was less than 4% for all treatments, except for the combination of 0.1% E-64 and 5% STI, for which mortality was 10%. Mortalities were not statistically different from the control, using the Fisher's exact test, $p < 0.05$. Proteolytic enzyme patterns in gut extracts from dissected larvae were compared in biochemical assays.

Gut extracts from *T. castaneum* larvae were incubated without inhibitor or with E-64 or STI to compare the effects of inhibitors in vitro on the caseinolytic activity of extracts from larvae fed different concentrations of inhibitor. When E-64 was added to the gut extracts, the ability of E-64 to reduce caseinolyic activity decreased as the dietary concentration of E-64 increased (Fig. 2). In diets treated with 0.5% E-64, there was a complete loss of E-64 inhibition in vitro. However, the amount of STI inhibition in the same extracts increased with increasing dietary E-64. In contrast, inhibition by E-64 or STI of extracts from larvae fed STI was similar at all concentrations. These data suggest that the inhibition of caseinolytic activity by dietary E-64 was more disruptive to overall proteolytic activity, emphasizing the importance of cysteine proteinases in *T. castaneum* digestion. In combination treatments, E-64 inhibited extracts obtained from larvae fed

Table 2
Percent reduction in the growth of *T. castaneum* larvae, as measured by weights at day 12 (summarized from Refs. [3,9])

Dietary inhibitor	Percent reduction in weight
0.1% E-64	38
1% STI	0
1% equistatin	43
1% PCPI	51
1% JCPI	47
0.1% E-64+1% STI	90
0.1% E-64+10% STI	94
1.0% equistatin+1% STI	53
1% PCPI+1% STI	72
1% JCPI+1% STI	25

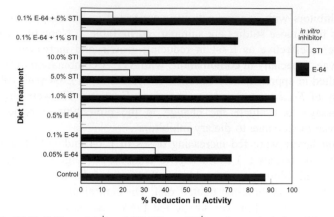

Fig. 2. The effect of E-64 (0.10 µmol l^{-1}) and STI (60 µmol l^{-1}) on the caseinolytic activity of gut extracts from *T. castaneum* larvae fed control or inhibitor-treated diets, as indicated.

0.1% E-64+1% STI approximately 10% less than control extracts but almost twice that of insects fed 0.1% E-64 only. When the amount of STI in the combination treatment was increased to 5%, the inhibition by E-64 was similar to the control, demonstrating compensation for E-64 in the diet. On the other hand, STI inhibition in the combination treatments decreased as the amount of dietary STI increased, suggesting the loss of serine proteinase activity.

The effect of dietary inhibitors on gut proteolytic activity was further demonstrated by casein zymograms (Fig. 3A). Extracts from control larvae had three major bands of caseinolytic activities, corresponding to proteins of approximately 15, 25, and 100 kDa in mass (Fig. 3Aa). When larvae were fed E-64, the 15 kDa activity was no longer detected, suggesting that this activity was due to cysteine proteinase(s) (Fig. 3Ab). However, in the

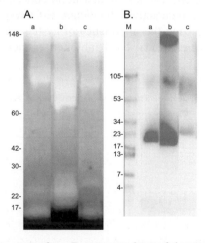

Fig. 3. Activity analyses of gut extracts from *T. castaneum* larvae fed untreated diets (Aa, Ba) or different concentrations of E-64 (0.5%: Ab, Bb) or STI (10%: Ac, Bc). (A) Zymogram analysis with casein gels; (B) activity blot analysis with SAAPpNA. M: molecular mass markers (denoted on the left of each figure).

same extract, the activities of the 25 and 100 kDa enzymes increased, suggesting that these were serine proteinases. These predictions were further corroborated by the analysis of extracts from STI-treated larvae, in which the 15 kDa activity was present, but the 25 and 100 kDa activities were decreased (Fig. 3Ac).

Activity blot analyses with the chymotrypsin substrate SAAPFpNA indicated that larvae fed control diets had a major chymotrypsin-like proteinase approximately 25 kDa in mass and a minor chymotrypsin-like proteinase of 100 kDa (Fig. 3Ba), similar to that observed in the previous zymogram. The activity of the 25 kDa proteinase was greatly stimulated in larvae fed E-64, as was the activity of ~100 kDa and larger proteinases (Fig. 3Bb). Larvae fed STI had a decreased a 25 kDa chymotrypsin-like activity, but the activity of the 100 kDa proteinase was slightly increased (Fig. 3Bc).

4. Discussion

Prior results demonstrated that serine or cysteine proteinase inhibitors fed individually to *T. castaneum* larvae have minimal effects on growth and mortality [9]. Our recent research has demonstrated further that a combination of serine and cysteine proteinase inhibitors is necessary to cause significant growth retardation and mortality in larvae of *T. castaneum* [3]. We proposed that cysteine proteinases were the major digestive enzymes in larvae fed normal untreated diets. However, when cysteine proteinase activity was inhibited, it appeared that larvae shifted to the production of more serine proteinases. Our data support this hypothesis.

As the amount of dietary E-64 increased, *T. castaneum* larvae produced enzymes that were less sensitive to inhibition by E-64. However, the loss of E-64 inhibition was accompanied by an increased STI sensitivity, as would be expected in larvae shifting from cysteine to serine proteinase-based digestion.

These results were further supported by the analysis of proteinase activity with a chymotrypsin substrate. At higher levels of dietary E-64, chymotrypsin-like activity increased, and at higher levels of dietary STI, chymotrypsin-like activity decreased. These data suggest that a selective and more potent inhibitor of a chymotrypsin-like enzyme may provide enhanced protection to the adaptive response to cysteine proteinase inhibitors in *T. castaneum* larvae.

A shift from cysteine to serine proteinase digestion would be more dramatic if the initial level of cysteine proteinase activity was high, as is the case in *T. castaneum* larvae. Therefore, larvae are much more sensitive to cysteine proteinase inhibitors under normal dietary conditions. However, serine proteinases become more crucial to digestion in larvae fed cysteine proteinase inhibitors. When this adaptive shift is prevented by a combination of inhibitors, larvae no longer are able to compensate, and thus mortality ensues.

With the completion of sequencing of the *T. castaneum* genome by researchers at the USDA-ARS, Kansas State University, and Baylor College of Medicine, sequences for proteinase genes will become available. Probes for *T. castaneum* proteinase genes are being developed to examine the genetic responses of larvae to dietary inhibitors. These data will help to design combinations of inhibitor genes in transgenic cereals to enhance protection against *T. castaneum* and probably other stored product insects.

Acknowledgements

Our thanks to Michele Zuercher for technical support, Dr. Vito Turk for equistain and PCPI, and Dr. Koichi Yoza for JCPI. This research was supported by the USDA ARS Agricultural Research Service. Mention of trade names or commercial products in this publication is solely for the purpose of providing specific information and does not imply recommendation or endorsement by the U.S. Department of Agriculture.

References

[1] B. Oppert, Transgenic plants expressing enzyme inhibitors and the prospects for biopesticide development, in: O. Koul, G.S. Dhaliwal (Eds.), Phytochemical Biopesticides, Harwood Academic, The Netherlands, 2000, pp. 83–95.

[2] C.R. Carlini, Grossi de Sa, Plant toxic proteins with insecticidal properties. A review on their potentialities as bioinsecticides, Toxicon 40 (2002) 1515–1539.

[3] B. Oppert, et al., Effects of proteinase inhibitors on growth and digestive proteolysis of the red flour beetle, *Tribolium castaneum* (Herbst) (Coleoptera: Tenebrionidae), Comp. Biochem. Physiol. 134C (2003) 481–490.

[4] J.E. Baker, Application of capillary thin layer isoelectric focusing in polyacrylamide gel to the study of alkaline proteinases in stored-product insects, Comp. Biochem. Physiol. 71B (1982) 501–506.

[5] A. Blanco-Labra, et al., Purification and characterization of a digestive cathepsin D proteinase isolated from *Tribolium castaneum* larvae (Herbst), Insect Biochem. Biol. 26 (1996) 95–100.

[6] Y. Birk, S.W. Applebaum, Effect of soybean trypsin inhibitors on the development and midgut proteolytic activity of *Tribolium castaneum* larvae, Enzymologia 22 (1960) 318–326.

[7] C. Liang, et al., Inhibition of digestive proteinases of stored grain Coleoptera by oryzacystatin, a cysteine proteinase inhibitor from rice seed, FEBS Lett. 2 (1991) 139–142.

[8] M.-S. Chen, et al., Rice cystatin: bacterial expression, purification, cysteine proteinase inhibiting activity and insect growth inhibiting activity of a truncated form of rice cystatin, Protein Expr. Purif. 3 (1992) 41–49.

[9] B. Oppert, et al., Dietary mixtures of cysteine and serine proteinase inhibitors exhibit synergistic toxicity toward the red flour beetle, *Tribolium castaneum*, Comp. Biochem. Physiol. 105C (1993) 379–385.

[10] B. Oppert, K.J. Kramer, Economical proteinase activity blot, Am. Biotechnol. Lab. 16 (1998) 20.

[11] B. Oppert, K.J. Kramer, W.H. McGaughey, Rapid microplate assay of proteinase mixtures, BioTechniques 23 (1997) 70–72.

[12] J.A.C. Frugoni, Tampone universale di Britton e Robinson a forza ionica costante, Gazz. Chim. Ital. 87 (1957) 403–407.

International Congress Series 1275 (2004) 157–164

ELSEVIER

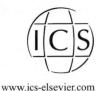

www.ics-elsevier.com

Oxygen uptake by convection and diffusion in diapausing moth pupae (*Attacus atlas*)

A. Wobschall, S.K. Hetz*

Department of Animal Physiology, Humboldt-Universität zu Berlin, Philippstrasse 13, D-10115 Berlin, Germany

Abstract. We investigated O_2 uptake of diapausing *Attacus atlas* pupae during the "fluttering" period of a DGC using plethysmometry and flow through respirometry in combination with tracheal pressure and tracheal PO_2 measurement. Within the initial phase of the fluttering period, convection of air during brief spiracle openings (<1 s) allowed oxygen uptake mainly by convection with certain amounts of air sucked into the highly compliant tracheal system. Pressure rise rates may reach 2200 Pa s^{-1} and maximum air flow rate into the tracheal system can thus be 50 μl s^{-1}. The total retention of CO_2 during the passive suction ventilation could be proved at maximum tracheal pressures below -6.27 Pa. Later in the fluttering period, the spiracular conductance increases, both with opening duration and frequency, leading to an O_2 uptake mainly by diffusion while CO_2 may be released in small peaks. Our results indicate a substantial contribution of the "passive suction ventilation" with its ability to conserve water to oxygen uptake only in the beginning of the fluttering period while diffusion is the dominating mechanism of gas exchange in the main proportion of the fluttering period. © 2004 Elsevier B.V. All rights reserved.

Keywords: Insect; Respiration; Oxygen uptake; Passive suction ventilation; Discontinuous carbon dioxide release

1. Introduction

Diapausing moth pupae are known to exchange respiratory gases discontinuously. While mostly people pay attention to the periodic or discontinuous discharge of carbon dioxide during an "opening"-period (O) of the spiracles, only few investigations have been

---

* Corresponding author. Tel.: +49 30 2093 6178; fax: +49 30 2093 6375.
E-mail address: stefan.k.hetz@rz.hu-berlin.de (S.K. Hetz).

0531-5131/ © 2004 Elsevier B.V. All rights reserved.
doi:10.1016/j.ics.2004.08.080

made so far on the oxygen uptake and spiracle behaviour during the "fluttering"-period (F) [1]. Like in diapausing silkmoth pupae [2–4], the discontinuous gas exchange cycle (DGC) in *Attacus atlas* mainly consist of a long "fluttering"-period, while the "constriction" (C) and "opening" periods are much shorter [5].

During the O-period, the air within the tracheal system is almost completely exchanged leading to an increase in oxygen content to nearly atmospheric levels [6]. Within the C-period, a sub-atmospheric pressure develops due to the oxygen uptake of the tissues from the tracheal system and due to extensive CO_2 buffering within hemolymph and tissues [7]. The oxygen partial pressure drops to a certain, usually low level, that is maintained throughout the F-period [6]. Oxygen uptake in the F-period repeatedly occurs during brief spiracle activity [8], so-called "microopenings" [9], when air enters the tracheal system by convection along the negative pressure gradient. This "passive suction ventilation" (PSV) is considered to protect the pupae from losing to much water via the tracheal system [10]. This is achieved by impeding an "anticurrent" (against the stream of inward flowing air) diffusion of H_2O and CO_2. The theoretical background of the PSV has been described in detail by Kestler [9].

Although the negative tracheal pressure will cause an inward air flow as soon as a spiracle opens, the air has to reach a certain flow rate through the spiracles in order to prevent the anticurrent diffusion of H_2O and CO_2 out of the tracheal system. However, to our knowledge, no direct measurements of opening duration and pressure rise or volume increase have been made in moth pupae to support that hypothesis. We therefore set up a plethysmometry system to record volume changes during the respiratory cycle in moth pupae and combined the data with flow through respirometry.

A main problem of the repeated oxygen uptake by convection is, that normal atmospheric air does only contain 21% of oxygen. Only the oxygen within the inspired air can be used to set up a sub-atmospheric pressure repeatedly. We therefore predict that, with time elapsing within the F-period, the mechanism of pure "passive suction ventilation" alone will not be able to maintain the oxygen partial pressure within the tracheal system and prevent the outward orientated diffusion of CO_2 and H_2O. Therefore, convection should be gradually substituted by diffusion.

2. Methods

In order to study the mechanisms of oxygen uptake during the F-period in detail, we used flow through respirometry and plethysmometry. We employed diapausing pupae of *A. atlas* for the experiments. The pupae were reared from eggs on *Ligustrum* sp. at temperatures between 22 and 28 °C. After pupation, a diapause stimulus (cool temperatures of 14 to 16 °C, dark environment) was applied to induce diapause with almost complete success. Diapausing pupae were stored in a container in complete darkness between 12 and 15 °C at a relative humidity of 80% to 90%. Diapause usually lasted longer than 9 months. Ten pupae were used for the flow through experiments (weight=8.169±0.648 g, $N=10$) while five pupae were used for the plethysmometry experiments (weight=8.252±0.555 g, $N=5$). From each data set of flow through experiments, 20 random flutter events were chosen for the analysis. All experiments were performed in complete darkness at 15 °C and a relative humidity of 60% to 90%.

A first set of experiments was performed using standard flow through respirometry combined with measurement of intratracheal pressure, CO_2 release rate, and abdomen movement as a measure for changes in tracheal volume. CO_2 free but moistened air was driven through the respirometer chamber with a pump (WISA 302, ASF Thomas, Wuppertal, Germany) regulated by mass flow controllers (MKS 1259, 200 ml min^{-1}; MKS instruments, Methuen, MA, United States) at a flow rate of 200 ml min^{-1}. CO_2 release rates (MCO_2 in nmol g^{-1} min^{-1}) were measured with a differential infrared gas analyser (DIRGA, URAS 4, 0–100 ppm, Hartmann & Braun, Frankfurt, Germany). Tracheal pressure was measured via a cannulated spiracle. A modified piece of PE 10 tubing was connected to the tracheal system via one spiracle (usually the second or third thoracic spiracle on the right side of the animal). The tubing was connected to a pressure sensor (SenSym, SDXL 010D4, Sensortechnics, Puchheim/Germany) via thin steel tubes (inner diameter 0.25 mm). An automatic microliter syringe (Hamilton micro lab p, Hamilton, Switzerland; V=10 µl) was connected to the steel tubes via a T-piece. This allowed to remove small samples of air necessary to calibrate volume changes against pressure changes. The voltage output of the pressure sensor was amplified with a custom made amplifier 400-fold to obtain a resolution in the order of 1 Pa. Calibration of the pressure sensor was checked using a custom made pressure calibration system that uses a water or mercury column to generate a certain differential pressure. Movements of the animals' abdomens were controlled by a reflex light barrier (SFH900, Siemens, Germany) linearised by means of a resistor network. The device sends infrared light to the tip of the abdomen and measures the intensity of the light reflected back from the abdomen. In a subset of the experiments, the PO_2 within the tracheal system was also measured through a second spiracle using the method described in Hetz et al. [11]. Data acquisition of all sensors was done via a 16-channel A to D converter board (Data Translation, DT 2821) to a personal computer using custom made scripts of the TurboLab® data acquisition software package for DOS-Computers (MDZ Bührer & Partner GbR, Stockdorf, Germany). Recording rates were 1 or 10 s^{-1} for high-speed recordings, respectively.

In order to determine the volume changes in the tracheal system, we set up a plethysmometer that allowed us to calibrate the volume decrease of the tracheal system during the F-period (Fig. 1B) against the pressure decrease within the tracheal system (Fig. 1A). Thus, we were able to characterise the intratracheal pressure decrease simultaneously with the tracheal volume decrease. This had to be done experimentally since the tracheal system was expected to be highly compliant as has been shown in diapausing silkworm pupae [12]. To characterise the compliance (volume changes divided by pressure changes) of the tracheal system, we used the computer-driven syringe to withdraw small volumes of air (3 to 10 µl) from the tracheal system repeatedly. We calibrated pressure changes against volume changes (Fig. 1C) and plotted it against the average tracheal pressure (highest pressure+lowest pressure divided by 2). Compliance was measured over the whole sub-atmospheric pressure range while the pupa was in the C-period (Fig. 1A). The pressure differences (highest pressure−lowest pressure) in the F-period together with the compliance values of a certain pressure range were used to calculated the volumes taken

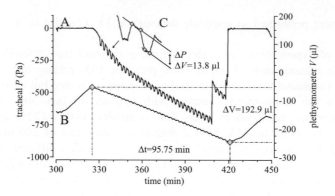

Fig. 1. Original data from a plethysmometry experiment. Tracheal pressure (A, left axis) is measured simultaneously with chamber volume (B, right axis). Compliance of the tracheal system is determined by repeatedly removing small volumes of air from the tracheal system and determining the corresponding pressure changes (C).

up in the F-period. From the fractional concentration fO_2 in the ambient air, the amount of O_2 taken up was calculated (Fig. 3B).

3. Results

The intratracheal pressure did not decrease linearly as expected but showed a biphasic course. From 0 Pa to about −300 Pa, the pressure fell almost exponentially with time whereas the pressure decrease rate below −300 Pa showed a almost linear decrease (Figs. 1A and 4C). Tracheal volume, however, decreased linearly indicating a constant oxygen uptake rate of the animal from the tracheal system (Fig. 1B). As a result, the compliance of the tracheal system was not constant too. In all pupae compliance increased about 3-fold in the range of 0 to −300 Pa from about 20 to 60 nl Pa^{-1} and then slowly decreased between −400 and −1000 Pa to about 40 nl Pa^{-1}. Pressure increase occurred very fast ($N=10$, $n=200$), lasting only 0.3 to 0.9 s within the first part of the F-period (Fig. 2, left side). The

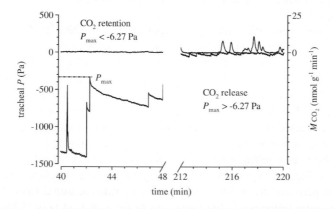

Fig. 2. Tracheal pressure (left axis) and CO_2 release (right axis) of a *Attacus* pupa. Total CO_2 retention occurs in the F-period when the maximum tracheal pressure (P_{max}) is low (left part), whereas CO_2 release may occur when the pressure difference between tracheal system and atmosphere is near zero (right part).

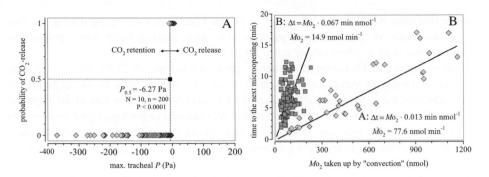

Fig. 3. (A) Probability plot of CO_2 release in 200 pressure increase events. Maximum pressure is plotted against a CO_2 release peak (probability 1) or total CO_2 retention (probability 0). At a maximum tracheal pressure of -6.27 Pa, the probability of CO_2 retention is 0.5. (B) Time to the next microopening from the same experiments. (A) Group of data where total retention of CO_2 occurred. (B) Group of data when small releases of CO_2 were detectable. Note the shorter time differences in the B-group indicating a higher opening frequency.

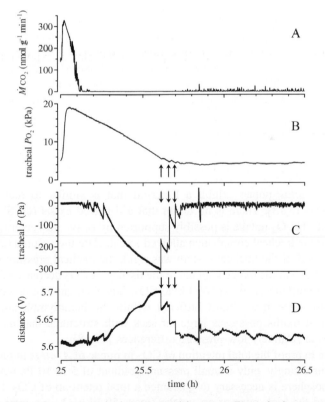

Fig. 4. Synopsis of CO_2 release (A), tracheal oxygen partial pressure (B), tracheal pressure (C) and abdomen length (D), in an *Attacus* pupa. The arrows indicate the effect of air uptake on tracheal PO_2 and pupal volume.

pressure rise rates were 20 to 2200 Pa s^{-1} with the fasted rates occurring during the first part of the F-period when tracheal pressure was low. During these parts, convective volume uptake rates reached values up to 50 µl s^{-1}.

Total retention of CO_2 occurred at tracheal pressures below -6.27 Pa (Fig. 2, left side; Fig. 3A). A probit fit yielded a pressure of -6.27 Pa where 50% of the experiments statistically resulted in total CO_2 retention (Fig. 3A) mainly in the first part of the F-period ($N=10$, $n=200$, $p<0.0001$). We therefore divided the data into two subgroups depending on the maximum tracheal pressure. If the maximum pressure was below -6.27 Pa, the data were assigned to the A-group, if the pressure was above -6.27 Pa, the data were assigned to the B-group (Fig. 3B).

A plot of the time to next microopening against the amount of oxygen taken up by convection (calculated from the pressure difference, the compliance and fractional concentration fO_2 of the inspired air), yielded a linear relation. The time to the next microopening was 0.013 min/nmol of oxygen taken up for the A-group and 0.067 min/nmol for the B-group (Fig. 3B). The records also show an increase in spiracle opening frequency.

Oxygen uptake mainly by convection could be detected within large inspirations at the beginning of the F-period (see the arrows in Fig. 4B, C and D). The amount of air sucked into the tracheal system in this example (10.5, 14.1 and 8.2 µl; in terms of oxygen: 91.9, 122.9 and 71.4 nmol of O_2) leads to a noticeable increase in tracheal oxygen partial pressure (Fig. 4B) that in turn allows the animal to close its spiracles for some minutes. Later, in the F-period, the tracheal PO_2 is maintained around 4.5 kPa mainly by diffusion of O_2 into the tracheal system (Fig. 4B). The mainly diffusive O_2 uptake can be derived from the low-pressure differences between atmosphere and tracheal system (Fig. 4C) and the small output of CO_2 from the tracheal system (Fig. 4A). The time between two small CO_2 release peaks is shorter than the time between two pressure increase events indicating an increase in the frequency of microopenings too.

4. Discussion

Diapausing *A. atlas* pupae exhibit a F-period that is similar to that described for *Hyalophora* pupae [6,13]. There is no doubt that a F-period exists (cf. Slama [14]) and there are no hints that O_2 uptake is possibly supported by active movements [14–16]. The determination of the tracheal compliance allowed to calculate the volume (and O_2) uptake rates in the F-period. If the tracheal system was rigid, the tracheal pressure decreased to a much lower level due to the oxygen uptake of the tissues. A PO_2 decrease of 15 kPa would lead to a pressure difference of $-15\,000$ kPa. CO_2, however, can not compensate for the pressure decrease since it is almost buffered within the hemolymph and tissues. The tracheal system of moths possesses large air sacs with structures that may allow these volume changes at relatively low-pressure differences [17,18].

We were able to proof the total retention of CO_2 in pupae of *A. atlas* in the beginning of the F-period. Surprisingly, only a small pressure gradient of 5 to 10 Pa between tracheal system and atmosphere is necessary to guarantee a total retention of CO_2. From the swift pressure rise and the high rates of air uptake (max. 50 µl s^{-1}), one may argue that the spiracles have to be widely opened in a single flutter event. However, morphological data from Schmitz and Wasserthal [19] show that a single spiracle in *Attacus* pupae consists of an oval shaped valve, a maximum of 80 μm wide and about 600 μm long. Adjacent to the valve lies the atrium that may form a tube of the same area and a height of about 800 μm. In a first approximation, we can simplify one open spiracle as a tube with a mean diameter R of 0.08 mm, an opening area A of 0.02 mm^2 and a length L of 0.8 mm. Applying the law of Hagen-Poiseuille (with $\eta=0.0182$ mPa s) to calculate the laminar flow rate of air through the spiracle, we yield a steady state air flow rate of 267 μl s^{-1} for a pressure difference of 250 Pa. This flow rate is five times higher than our measured values and thus high enough to guarantee the high-pressure rise rates of up to 2200 Pa s^{-1} measured in our experiments. However, the dense filter apparatus in *Attacus* pupae [19] will certainly contribute some resistance to flow. If our morphological assumptions were right, the maximum velocity of air through one spiracle is about 4 m s^{-1} and should explain the total retention of CO_2 and maybe H_2O.

The problem of oxygen uptake persists in the later F-period. From unpublished data, we know the single spiracle conductance G for CO_2 of 70 nmol kPa^{-1} min^{-1}. The conductance for oxygen should be slightly higher due to the smaller molecule. The huge PO_2 difference of 15 kPa between trachea and atmosphere (Fig. 4B) should result in an oxygen uptake rate of 18.8 nmol s^{-1} by diffusion. At a mean CO_2 release rate of 60 nmol min^{-1}, and a respiration ratio of 0.7 for pupae, the O_2 uptake (85.7 nmol min^{-1}) within 5 s should supply sufficient O_2 for 1 min. If we take the morphometric data of A (0.02 mm^2), L (0.8 mm) and a ΔPO_2 of 15 kPa together with Krogh's coefficient of diffusion (494.4 nmol mm^{-1} min^{-1} kPa^{-1} after Dejours [20]) to calculate the O_2 uptake rate by pure diffusion, we get 3.1 nmol s^{-1}, about 20% of the rate determined in our experiments. Since morphometric data cannot be simply converted between convection and diffusion, some more experiments have to be performed to get a final result. The time to the next microopening in the B-group (Fig. 3B) may therefore show the deviation from the data of the A-group, when no CO_2 release occurred. From the time between two microopenings in the A-group, a mean O_2 uptake rate of 77.6 nmol min^{-1} could be determined, which is in the range of the uptake rates measured in the plethysmometer (84.6 nmol min^{-1} from $\Delta V=192.9$ μl and $\Delta t=95.75$ min in Fig. 1) or calculated from CO_2 release although the tracheal PCO_2 increase was not taken into account. However, the O_2 uptake rate by convection in the B-group (14.9 nmol min^{-1}) can only explain 20% of the time to the next microopening (14.9 nmol min^{-1} divided by 77.6 nmol min^{-1}). We therefore strongly assume that the other 80% are taken up by diffusion (when CO_2 release was detectable). Looking at the original data in Fig. 4A, B and C, we can see that despite a negligible pressure gradient, the tracheal PO_2 can be precisely regulated. The regulation in *A. atlas* obviously occurs by means of adapting the conductance of the spiracles within the F-period by changing the opening duration from only one second when "passive suction ventilation" is possible to some seconds when mainly diffusion serves for O_2 uptake. Low respiratory water loss rates are then not the primary stimulus but the effect of these low duty cycles of spiracle opening but should be carefully discussed as long as no experimental data exist [21]. Although our morphometric calculations of spiracle conductance were mainly depending on very coarse estimations, we assume that oxygen uptake during F-period may easily occur through one single spiracle.

References

[1] J.R.B. Lighton, D. Garrigan, Ant breathing: testing regulation and mechanism hypotheses with hypoxia, J. Exp. Biol. 198 (1995) 1613–1620.

[2] B.N. Burkett, H.A. Schneiderman, Roles of oxygen and carbon dioxide in the control of spiracular function in cecropia pupae, Biol. Bull. 147 (1974) 274–293.

[3] H.A. Schneiderman, C.M. Williams, Discontinuous carbon dioxide output by diapausing pupae of the giant silkworm, *Platysamia cecropia*, Biol. Bull. 105 (2) (1953) 382.

[4] H.A. Schneiderman, C.M. Williams, An experimental analysis of the discontinuous respiration of the cecropia silkworm, Biol. Bull. 109 (1) (1955) 123–143.

[5] S.K. Hetz, Untersuchungen zu Atmung, Kreislauf und Säure-Basen-Regulation an Puppen der tropischen Schmetterlingsgattungen *Ornithoptera, Troides* und *Attacus*. Doctoral thesis. Zoologie I, Erlangen (1994) 1–216.

[6] R.I. Levy, H.A. Schneiderman, Discontinuous respiration in insects: 2. Direct measurement and significance of changes in tracheal gas composition during respiratory cycle of silkworm pupae, J. Insect Physiol. 12 (1966) 83–104.

[7] J.B. Buck, S. Friedman, Cyclic CO_2 release in diapausing pupae: III. CO_2 capacity of the blood: carbonic anhydrase, J. Insect Physiol. 2 (1958) 52–60.

[8] H.A. Schneiderman, Discontinuous respiration in insects—role of the Spiracles, Biol. Bull. 119 (3) (1960) 494–528.

[9] P. Kestler, Respiration and respiratory water loss, in: K.H. Hoffmann (Ed.), Environmental Physiology and Biochemistry of Insects, Springer Verlag, Berlin, Heidelberg, 1984, pp. 137–183.

[10] P. Kestler, Saugventilation verhindert bei Insekten die Wasserabgabe aus dem Tracheensystem, Verh. Dtsch. Zool. Ges. (1980) 306.

[11] S.K. Hetz, et al., Direct oxygen measurements in the tracheal system of lepidopterous pupae using miniaturized amperometric sensors, Bioelectrochem. Bioenerg. 33 (2) (1994) 165–170.

[12] A.P. Brockway, H.A. Schneiderman, Strain gauge transducer studies on intratracheal pressure and pupal length during discontinuous respiration in diapausing silkworm pupae, J. Insect Physiol. 13 (1967) 1413–1451.

[13] R.I. Levy, H.A. Schneiderman, Discontinuous respiration in insects: 4. Changes in intratracheal pressures during the respiratory cycle of silkworm pupae, J. Insect Physiol. 12 (1966) 465–492.

[14] K. Slama, Active regulation of insect respiration, Ann. Entomol. Soc. Am. 92 (6) (1999) 916–929.

[15] K. Slama, A new look at insect respiration, Biol. Bull. 175 (2) (1988) 289–300.

[16] K. Slama, L. Neven, Active regulation of respiration and circulation in pupae of the codling moth (*Cydia pomonella*), J. Insect Physiol. 47 (11) (2001) 1321–1336.

[17] L.T. Wasserthal, Oscillating haemolymph circulation and discontinuous tracheal ventilation in the giant silk moth *Attacus atlas* L., J. Comp. Physiol. 145 (1981) 1–15.

[18] L.T. Wasserthal, The open haemolymph system of holometabola and its relation to the tracheal space, in: F. Harrison, M. Locke (Eds.), Microscopic Anatomy of Invertebrates, Wiley-Liss, New York, 1997.

[19] A. Schmitz, L.T. Wasserthal, Comparative morphology of the spiracles of the Papilionidae, Sphingidae, and Saturniidae (Insecta: Lepidoptera), Int. J. Insect Morphol. Embryol. 28 (1–2) (1999) 13–26.

[20] P. Dejours, Principles of Comparative Respiratory Physiology, 1st ed., North Holland Publishing, Amsterdam, Oxford, 1975.

[21] S.L. Chown, Respiratory water loss in insects, Comp. Biochem. Physiol., A 133 (3) (2002) 791–804.

ELSEVIER

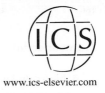

www.ics-elsevier.com

Multiple sets of arsenic resistance genes are present within highly arsenic-resistant industrial strains of the biomining bacterium, *Acidithiobacillus caldus*

Marla Tuffin, Peter de Groot,
Shelly M. Deane, Douglas E. Rawlings*

*Department of Microbiology, University of Stellenbosch, Room 306, JC Smuts Building Block A de Beer,
Private Bag X1, Stellenbosch, Western Cape, Matieland, 7602, South Africa*

Abstract. The moderately thermophilic, sulfur-oxidizing bacterium *Acidithiobacillus caldus* is an important role player in continuous-flow biooxidation processes associated with the biooxidation of arsenopyrite concentrates. Certain isolates of these bacteria have been exposed to high concentrations of arsenic for many years and have become highly arsenic-resistant. We investigated the arsenic resistance genes of the highly resistant strains of *At. caldus* and compared these with those of less arsenic-resistant isolates. Up to three sets of arsenic resistance genes were found in the most resistant strains. One set of genes was located on a 12-kb Tn*21*-like transposon flanked by Tn*21*-like 40-bp inverted repeats (IR) and the transposon was active in the bacterium, *Escherichia coli*. This transposon was present only in highly arsenic-resistant strains and contained an unusual *ars* operon with *arsR*, *arsC*, two *arsD*-like, two *arsA*-like and *arsB* genes. Situated between the *arsA* and *arsB* genes are two open reading frames encoding for NADH oxidase-like enzyme and a protein with a CBS domain that is also present in IMP dehydrogenases. Deletion of one copy of the *arsDA* genes occurred readily but there were no marked differences in arsenic resistance in the deleted clones. The second set of arsenic resistance genes appeared to be related to the first set although some of the genes were missing. The third set was distantly related and appeared to be present on the chromosomes of all *At. caldus* strains irrespective of whether they had been exposed to elevated levels of arsenic. © 2004 Elsevier B.V. All rights reserved.

Keywords: Biomining bacteria; Arsenopyrite biooxidation; Tn*21*-like transposon; Arsenic resistance

* Corresponding author. Tel.: +27 21 808 5848; fax: +27 21 808 5846.
E-mail address: der@sun.ac.za (D.E. Rawlings).

0531-5131/ © 2004 Elsevier B.V. All rights reserved.
doi:10.1016/j.ics.2004.07.026

1. Introduction

A biooxidation process in which a consortium of bacteria is used to decompose gold-bearing arsenopyrite concentrates prior to extraction of the gold by cyanide was developed in the 1980s [1–3]. Mineral concentrate biooxidation takes place at 40 °C and pH 1.6 in a series of highly aerated continuous-flow tanks that is dominated by the iron-oxidizing bacterium *Leptospirillum ferriphilum* and the sulfur-oxidizing bacterium *Acidithiobacillus caldus*. During the early laboratory stages of development of the biooxidation process, oxidation of the arsenopyrite concentrate was slow and inefficient because the bacteria were sensitive to the high concentrations of arsenic that were released. Arsenic inhibition was so severe that after a period of aeration, the mineral suspension was transferred to an unaerated tank where the pH was adjusted to 3.5 and the precipitated arsenic removed by settling. The mineral suspension was transferred to a fresh tank where aeration was continued. Initially more than one arsenic precipitation step was required. Separation of arsenic from the insufficiently oxidized arsenopyrite was complicated and the process was uneconomic. However, over a period of about 2 years, the bacterial consortium became sufficiently resistant to arsenic so that no arsenic precipitation steps were required. The residence time of the mineral concentrate in the series of aeration tanks was reduced from about 12 to less than 7 days. In 1986, the first commercial arsenopyrite biooxidation plant was built at the Fairview gold mine near the town of Barberton in South Africa [4]. After 3 years of operation, not only had the total residence time of the mineral in the biooxidation tanks been reduced to a little over 3 days, but also the quantity of mineral concentrate in suspension had been increased from 10% to 19% w/v.

We wished to investigate what genetic changes were required to permit a consortium of bacteria to increase their tolerance to total arsenic in solution from less than 1 to 13 g/l. Unfortunately, no samples of the early biooxidation bacterial consortium were maintained and, therefore, it is not possible to compare the bacteria in the arsenic-sensitive and arsenic-tolerant consortia. However, isolates of the same species of bacteria as found in the biooxidation tanks that are unlikely to have been exposed to high levels of arsenic can be compared with the highly arsenic tolerant bacteria. Here we report on our investigation of the arsenic resistance genes in the bacterium *At. caldus*.

In biological systems arsenic typically exists in two oxidation states, arsenite (AsIII) and arsenate (AsV). Arsenic resistance mechanisms have been reviewed extensively [5–8]. The minimal set of genes that confer resistance to both arsenite and arsenate are known as the *arsR*, *arsB* and *arsC* genes. The gene product, ArsR, is an arsenic-responsive gene regulator, ArsB, a membrane-located arsenite efflux pump and ArsC an arsenate reductase required to reduce arsenate to arsenite prior to its export from the cell by ArsB. Other frequently encountered arsenic resistance-associated genes are *arsA* and *arsD*. ArsA is an ATPase that forms a complex with ArsB and assists in the export of arsenite, while ArsD is a second regulator that controls the upper level of *ars* gene expression. More recently, another gene, *arsH* [9 10], has been found in several bacteria although its function is not yet clear and *arsM*, a putative As(III)-methyltransferase gene, has been found in the archaeon, *Halobacterium* [11].

2. Isolation of arsenic resistance genes from *At. caldus* strain #6

The construction of a gene bank from a strain of *At. caldus* that was isolated from arsenopyrite biooxidation tanks at the Fairview mine will be described elsewhere. The gene bank was transformed into the arsenic sensitive *Escherichia coli* strain ACSH50I^q [10] and the transformants screened for arsenate and arsenite resistance. Three families of genes that conferred resistance to either 1.0 mM arsenate, 0.5 mM arsenite or both were identified. Representatives of two of these families were fully sequenced and the third partly sequenced. These sequences were analysed and the genes that they contained identified by comparing the amino acid sequences of the translated open reading frames with proteins that had been deposited in the GenBank database. The genes present on the two fully sequenced clones that conferred arsenic-resistance to *E. coli* are indicated in Fig. 1.

The arsenic resistance genes in clone family A were contained within a 12.2-kb transposon that has Tn*21*-like inverted repeat (IR) sequences and a Tn*21* family-like resolvase and transposase. Between the transposase genes, arsenic resistance genes with high amino acid sequence homology to *arsR*, *arsC*, duplicate copies of *arsD* and *arsA* as well as an *arsB* were found. Between the second copy of *arsA* and the single copy of *arsB*, two open reading frames called orf7 and orf8 were found. The 470-aa-long predicted product of orf7 had clear homology to the 447-aa NADH-dependent dehydrogenase (36% identity/52% similarity) from the bacterium *Thermoanaerobacter tencongensis*. The product of orf8 (158 aa) had highest homology (39% identity/62% similarity) over approximately its entire length to what is known as the cystathione-β-synthase (CBS) [12] domain of a membrane protein from *Desulfitobacterium hafiense*. This domain is also present in IMP dehydrogenases. Arsenic-sensitive cells of *E. coli* transformed with clone

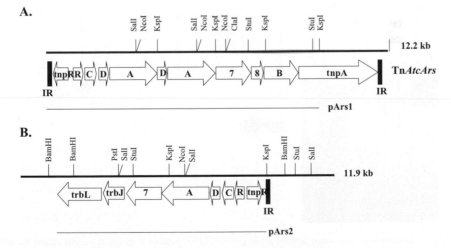

Fig. 1. Two of the sets of genes that conferred arsenic resistance to *E. coli*. IR, inverted repeats; *tnpR* and *tnpA* are genes for resolvase and transposase, respectively; R, C, D, A and B are *ars* genes; 7 is orf7; 8 is orf8; *trpL* and *trbJ* are homologous to conjugation genes from the Ti plasmid of *A. tumefaciens*.

I26 (Fig. 1) were resistant to arsenate and arsenite. These results and a more detailed analysis of the sequence will be reported elsewhere.

Clone family B contained a Tn21-like IR sequence followed by a series of genes that was similar to those found on pArs1, except that there was only a single copy of arsD and arsA and there was no orf8, arsB, tnpA or a second IR present. The genes that were present had an identical sequence to their counterparts in clone family A. E. coli cells when transformed with clone pArs2 were resistant to low levels of arsenate but not arsenite. The arsenate resistance conferred by clone pArs2 is puzzling because no arsB gene was present and in current models, a functional ArsB is required to enable the arsenate that is reduced to arsenite by ArsC to be pumped out of a cell.

The third family of clones has not been fully sequenced as yet, but appears to contain arsR, arsC and arsB genes that are different from those on the Tn21-like transposon.

3. Only the highly arsenic-resistant strains of At. caldus have extra arsenic resistance genes

We obtained six strains of At. caldus [13]. Of the three strains that had been previously exposed to arsenic, two strains (#6 and MNG) were isolated from arsenopyrite concentrate biooxidation tanks and one ('f') from a nickel ore biooxidation tank, the inoculum which had originated from an arsenopyrite biooxidation tank some years previously. Three strains which were unlikely to have been exposed to high levels of arsenic originated from Birch Coppice (BC13) and a coal spoil (KU) in the United Kingdom and from a bioreactor in Brisbane, Australia (C-SH12). Total DNA was isolated from each strain, digested with the restriction enzyme BamHI and the fragments separated on an agarose gel (Fig. 2A).

This DNA was transferred to a nylon membrane and probed with a labelled arsC gene from a related bacterium, Acidithiobacillus ferrooxidans, or the arsDA genes from At.

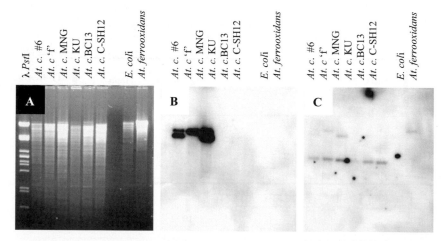

Fig. 2. (A) Ethidium-bromide-stained agarose gel of genomic DNA isolated from six At. caldus strains including genomic DNA from E. coli and A. ferrooxidans (strain ATCC33020). (B) Southern hybridisation analysis of the gel shown in A using the arsDA genes from At. caldus strain #6 as a probe. (C) As for B but using the arsC gene from At. ferrooxidans as probe.

caldus strain #6. When the six isolates of *At. caldus* were probed with the *At. caldus arsDA* genes, only the three isolates that had been previously exposed to arsenic gave a positive hybridisation signal. A similar result was obtained when the *At caldus arsB* genes was used as a probe (not shown). When the six *At. caldus* isolates were probed with a heterologous *At. ferrooxidans arsC* (Fig. 2C) or *arsB* probe (not shown), a positive hybridisation signal was obtained for all six *At. caldus* strains, suggesting that all *At. caldus* strains had the third set of *ars* genes but that only the highly arsenic-resistant strains had the transposon-located *ars* genes.

4. Arsenic resistance is conferred by *At. caldus ars* genes expressed in *E. coli*

Cloned Tn*AtcArs* genes present on construct pArs1 were transformed into an *E. coli* chromosomal *ars* deletion strain (ACSH50I^q) [10] and assayed for the ability to grow in the presence of arsenite and arsenate. Resistance was compared with *E. coli* (pUM3), which contained the *E. coli* R773 *arsR*, *arsB* and *arsC* genes cloned into vector pBR322 [14]. *E. coli* ACSH50I^q cells containing pArs1 were considerably more resistant to both arsenite and arsenate than untransformed cells, but slightly less resistant than cells containing the *arsRBC* genes present on pUM3 (Fig. 3).

To investigate the effect of the *arsDA* duplication, plasmid pArs1ΔDA from which one of the duplicate *arsDA* copies was removed (a 2.2-kb *Ksp*I deletion of pArs1) was assayed for arsenic resistance. The arsenite and arsenate resistance of cells containing pArs1ΔDA or pArs1 was not markedly different. Growth of *E. coli* ACSH50I^q cells containing pArs1Δ78, from which orfs 7 and 8 had been deleted (pArs1 with a 1.9 kb *Ksp*I deletion, Fig. 1), was examined in both arsenite and arsenate. Although pArs1Δ78 constructs were slightly less resistant to arsenite or arsenate than pArs1, the decrease in resistance was small (Fig. 3). A similar result was obtained with plasmid pArs1orf7* that had a frame-shift mutation introduced at the *Cla*I site in orf7 (not shown). A problem experienced in all constructs containing an *arsDA* duplication was that spontaneous *arsDA* deletions occurred in a varying proportion of such plasmids. The occurrence of these spontaneous deletions indicated that these arsenic resistance results should not be over interpreted. Nevertheless, the deliberate deletion of either *arsDA* or orfs 7 and 8 did not appear to have a marked effect on arsenic resistance in *E. coli*.

The low level of arsenate resistance conferred to *E. coli* ACSH50I^q cells by plasmid pArs2 is not shown.

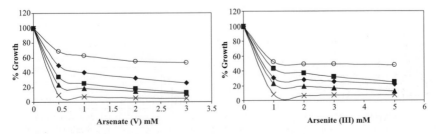

Fig 3. Growth of *E. coli* ACSHI^q transformants in LB plus arsenite or arsenate containing the following: (O–O) pUM3; (■–■) pArs1; (♦–♦) pArs1ΔDA; (▲–▲) pArs1Δ78; (×–×) vector control.

5. Origin of the *ars* genes on the Tn*21*-like transposon

As the bacteria that have been subjected to high concentrations of arsenic appeared to have acquired the Tn*AtcArs* transposon, we were interested in discovering from where the transposon or arsenic resistance genes might have originated. Mineral biooxidation takes place in open tanks and is not a sterile process. It is possible that the **ars**-gene containing transposon could have been introduced from bacteria that were present on the ore, concentrate, soil, water, low-grade fertilizer or the air that was introduced into the biooxidation tanks. We therefore used the amino acid sequences for each of the arsenic resistance proteins to search for proteins with related sequences using the BLASTP program, and used alignments of the sequences to construct phylogenetic trees for four of the *ars* gene products. These are shown in Fig. 4.

Comparison of the sequences of the Ars proteins with those of other bacteria (including ArsA not shown) indicated that, with the exception of ArsR, the Ars proteins present on the Tn*21*-like transposon form a deep branch within the Gram-negative

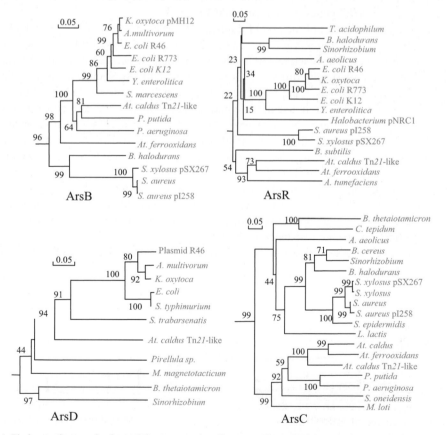

Fig. 4. Phylogenetic trees for four of the Ars proteins. Sequence alignments were made using CLUSTALX and the trees drawn using DNAMAN. Bootstrap values are indicated at the branch points.

Proteobacteria. The Tn*21*-like ArsR together with the ArsR of *At. ferrooxidans* and *Agrobacterium tumefaciens* forms a cluster that groups closer to the ArsR of Gram-positive bacteria than other Gram-negative bacteria. As the Tn*21*-like transposon-located Ars proteins occur on deep branches, it is not possible to discern their origin by sequence comparison.

6. Discussion

Southern blotting experiments (only some of which have been shown) indicated that the three strains of *At. caldus* that had been exposed to high levels of arsenic during their history had additional *ars* genes that were not present in strains of *At. caldus* that were not known to have been previously exposed to high levels of arsenic. These *ars* genes were present on a Tn*21*-like transposon. At least two of the arsenic resistance strains (#6 and MNG) had the second, truncated copy of the Tn*AtcArs* transposon. The second partial Tn*AtcArs* was not completely sequenced, but genes found downstream had products that were related to a group of conjugation proteins, TrbL (24/38%; identity/similarity) and TrbJ (31/55%; identity/similarity), to which the conjugation proteins of the *A. tumefaciens* Ti plasmids also belong. The means by which the truncated Tn*21*-like *ars* genes were acquired by some *At. caldus* strains is not certain, but the presence of the *trbL*-and *trbJ*-like genes suggested that they may be located on a plasmid or have been integrated into the chromosome via a plasmid.

The third set of presumably chromosomal *ars* genes are clearly different and, based on the signals obtained from Southern hybridisation experiments, they appear to be more closely related to those of *At. ferrooxidans* than to those of the Tn*21*-like transposon. Interestingly, the signals obtained with the *arsC* probe all occurred on the same size *Bam*HI fragment irrespective of the strain from which the DNA was isolated (Fig. 2). Dopson et al. [15] carried out hybridisation experiments with *At. caldus* strain KU and obtained a homology signal using the *E. coli* R773 *arsB* gene on pUM3 as a probe although they did not succeed in isolating the *ars* genes.

The arrangement of *ars* genes on the Tn*AtcArs* is unusual in that, in two of the *At. caldus* strains, there was a duplication of the *arsDA* genes. The effect of this duplication is unclear. Not only was the duplication rather unstable in *E. coli*, but when the second copy of *arsDA* genes was deleted, there was no consistent difference in the levels of resistance to either arsenite or arsenate. There may possibly be differences in *ars* gene regulation but this has not yet been tested. A second unusual feature was the presence of orf7 that codes for an NADH-dependent oxidoreductase-like enzyme and orf8 that appears to encode a protein with a CBS-like domain. Deletion of these genes also had no marked effect on arsenic resistance in *E. coli*. We tested whether the gene products of orfs 7 and 8 might play a role in the reduction of arsenate by testing for arsenate resistance in an *E. coli trxA* (thioredoxin) *gshA* (responsible for the synthesis of glutathione) double mutant (not shown). However, arsenate resistance was greatly reduced in the *E. coli* double mutant and the products of orfs 7 and 8 did not appear to encode for an NADH-dependent arsenate reduction mechanism that alleviated the requirement for thioredoxin or glutathione in *E. coli*.

Acknowledgements

We wish to thank BHP-Billiton, the National Research Foundation (Pretoria) and Stellenbosch University for financial support.

References

[1] P.C. Van Aswegen, et al., Developments and innovations in bacterial oxidation of refractory ores, Miner. Metall. Process. 8 (1991) 188–192.

[2] D.E. Rawlings, Heavy metal mining using microbes, Annu. Rev. Microbiol. 56 (2002) 65–91.

[3] D.E. Rawlings, D. Dew, C. du Plessis, Biomineralization of metal-containing ores and concentrates, Trends Biotech. 21 (2003) 38–44.

[4] D.E. Rawlings, S. Silver, Mining with microbes, Bio/Technology 13 (1995) 773–779.

[5] C. Cervantes, et al., Resistance to arsenic compounds in microorganisms, FEMS Microbiol. Rev. 15 (1994) 355–367.

[6] S. Silver, L.T. Phung, Bacterial heavy metal resistance: new surprises, Annu. Rev. Microbiol. 50 (1996) 753–789.

[7] B.P. Rosen, Families of arsenic transporters, Trends Microbiol. 7 (1999) 207–212.

[8] R. Mukhopadhyay, et al., Microbial arsenic: from geocycles to genes and enzymes, FEMS Microbiol. Rev. 26 (2002) 311–325.

[9] C. Neyt, et al., Virulence and arsenic resistance in Yersiniae, J. Bacteriol. 179 (1997) 612–619.

[10] B.G. Butcher, S.M. Deane, D.E. Rawlings, The chromosomal arsenic resistance genes of *Thiobacillus ferrooxidans* have an unusual arrangement and confer increased arsenic and antimony resistance to *Escherichia coli*, Appl. Environ. Microbiol. 66 (2000) 1826–1833.

[11] G. Wang, et al., Arsenic resistance in *Halobacterium* strain NRC-1 examined by using an improved gene knockout system, J. Bacteriol. 186 (2004) 3187–3194.

[12] A. Bateman, The structure of a domain common to archaebacteria and the homocystinuria disease protein, Trends Biochem. 22 (1997) 12–13.

[13] P. deGroot, S.M. Deane, D.E. Rawlings, A transposon-located arsenic resistance mechanism from a strain of *Acidithiobacillus caldus* isolated from commercial, arsenopyrite biooxidation tanks, Hydrometallurgy 71 (2003) 115–123.

[14] M.L.T. Mobley, et al., Cloning and expression of R-factor mediated arsenate resistance in *Escherichia coli*, Mol. Gen. Genet. 191 (1983) 421–426.

[15] M. Dopson, E.B. Lindström, K.B. Hallberg, Chromosomally encoded arsenical resistance of the moderately thermophilic acidophile *Acidithiobacillus caldus*, Extremeophiles 5 (2001) 247–255.

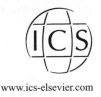

www.ics-elsevier.com

Selenium prevents spontaneous and arsenite-induced mutagenesis

Toby G. Rossman*, Ahmed N. Uddin

The Nelson Institute of Environmental Medicine, New York University School of Medicine, United States

Abstract. Selenium (Se) and arsenic are next-door neighbors on the periodic table and have similar chemical properties as metalloids. Arsenic antagonizes selenium toxicity in a number of organisms. Inorganic arsenic in drinking water is a human carcinogen while selenium compounds are anticarcinogenic in animals and humans. Our previous work showed that arsenite enhanced solar UV-induced skin cancer in the hairless mouse and caused delayed mutagenesis in human HOS cells. Here, we assess the abilities of three selenium compounds to antagonize arsenite. Sodium selenite is far more toxic to HOS cells than selenomethionine and Se-(methyl)selenocysteine in a 10-day clonality assay. When concentrations subtoxic in the clonality assay were assessed for long-term effects on growth, selenite, but not the organic compounds, caused a delayed inhibitory effect after 3 weeks. None of the Se compounds effectively blocked arsenite toxicity. Both organoselenium compounds blocked spontaneous and arsenite-induced delayed mutagenesis. The mechanism of delayed mutagenesis by arsenite is not known, but reactive oxygen species may play a role. We suggest that the antimutagenic action of organoselenium might result from up-regulation of the selenoproteins GSH peroxidase and thioredoxin reductase, which would protect against spontaneous and arsenite-induced oxidative DNA damage. © 2004 Elsevier B.V. All rights reserved.

Keywords: Arsenic; Selenium; Cell culture; Toxicity; Mutagenicity

1. Introduction

The problem of trace element imbalance in the diet is of global concern. Selenium (Se) is an essential trace element. Due to soil variations, crops and forage in some areas can be Se deficient or cause Se toxicity. Severe Se deficiency (<10 μg/day) is limited to China where it causes Keshan's and Kaschin-Beck disease. Suboptimal dietary intakes of selenium that

---

    * Corresponding author. Tel.: +1 845 731 3616; fax: +1 845 351 3489.
    E-mail address: rossman@env.med.nyu.edu (T.G. Rossman).

0531-5131/ © 2004 Elsevier B.V. All rights reserved.
doi:10.1016/j.ics.2004.09.038

are not sufficient to cause disease may predispose to various cancers [1]. Although inorganic Se is sometimes found in dietary supplements, Se is found predominantly as L-selenocysteine, selenomethionine (Se-met) and Se-methylseleno-L-cysteine (SMSC) in foods. Its nutritional role is mediated through selenoproteins in which Se is covalently bound as selenocysteine. There are at least 23 selenoproteins, most of whose functions are unknown (reviewed in Ref. [2]). Se is viewed as a trace element needed for antioxidant defense or redox regulation mainly because of its essential role in glutathione peroxidase (GPX) and thioredoxin reductase (TR) (reviewed in Ref. [3]).

Very large numbers of people worldwide are exposed to high levels of arsenic in drinking water. As a result of this exposure, these populations are at increased risk for a number of cancers and other diseases [4,5]. Selenium and arsenic are next-door neighbors on the periodic table and have similar chemical properties as metalloids. As early as the1930s, it became clear that arsenic could antagonize selenium toxicity in livestock and fowl [6,7]. Since arsenite antagonized Se, the ability of Se to antagonize arsenic compounds was examined. Selenite protected against some aspects of arsenite toxicity in vivo [8] and may have played a protective role in arsenic-induced lung cancers in smelter workers [9]. It also blocked arsenite-induced chromosome aberrations in lymphocytes in vitro [10] and in vivo [11]. Selenite reduced the toxicity of As_2O_3, a trivalent arsenic compound used in chemotherapy of some leukemias [12]. Selenized yeast containing mainly Se-met, given to arsenic-exposed individuals in Inner Mongolia for 14 months, caused significantly greater decreases in clinical signs and symptoms and a greater decrease in the arsenic content of blood, urine and hair, compared with controls [13].

Although there is no doubt that arsenite is a human carcinogen, unlike many carcinogens it is only weakly mutagenic, and usually only at highly toxic concentrations. Until recently, arsenite carcinogenesis had no animal model. This laboratory demonstrated that arsenite in drinking water enhances skin cancer induction by solar UV light in mice, but is not a complete carcinogen [14,15]. Thus, arsenite may be able to partner with a variety of genotoxic insults to cause cancers in humans. Se deficiency may be one such insult. It has been suggested that in some parts of the world with high arsenic in the drinking water, the low Se levels in soil may exacerbate the arsenic toxicity and carcinogenicity [16].

Based on a previously developed assay to measure spontaneous mutagenesis [17], we showed that human osteosarcoma cells (HOS) could be mutagenized by exposure to low concentrations of arsenic, but only after many generations of exposure [18]. This enabled us to address the question whether Se compounds affect spontaneous or arsenite-induced "delayed" mutagenesis, and might therefore counteract arsenite-induced carcinogenesis in humans.

2. Materials and methods

2.1. Cell culture and clonal survival

Human Osteosarcoma TE85 (HOS) cells, obtained from American Type Culture Collection (Rockville, MD), were cultured in α-MEM containing 10% heat-inactivated fetal bovine serum (Gemini Bio Products, Calabasas, CA) at 37 °C in 5% CO_2. For clonal survival, 500 cells were seeded in 60-mm dishes (in triplicate) in 5 ml medium. Stock solutions of 1 mM sodium arsenite, 10 mM sodium selenite, 10 mM Se-met and 10 mM SMSC (Sigma, St. Louis, MO) were prepared in sterile distilled water and stored at −20 °C. An aliquot of stock solution was thawed, diluted, and added after attachment (~4 h) and the cultures were incubated until colonies were visible (7–10 days). Colonies were fixed in methanol, stained with 0.5% crystal violet in 50% methanol and counted.

2.2. Mutagenesis assay

This assay is based on that of Rossman et al. [17]. To cleanse pre-existing *HPRT* mutants, cells were grown in HAT medium (medium with 100 µM hypoxanthine, 0.4 µM aminopterin and 16 µM thymidine) for 14 days. Cells (10^6) were seeded in medium containing sodium arsenite and/or selenium compounds. Mutants were allowed to accumulate during 6 weeks of growth, subculturing every week. The final cell count and plating efficiency were assessed at each subculture. 10^6cells were then distributed into 10 100-mm dishes in medium containing 0.1 µg/ml 6-thioguanine (6-TG). The plating efficiency in nonselective medium was also determined. After 12–14 days, mutant colonies were stained with 0.5% crystal violet in 50% methanol and scored. The mutant fraction (F) was calculated by dividing the number of mutant colonies (M) by the number of cells seeded, corrected for the plating efficiency. The generations (g) were approximated as the base 2 logarithm of the ratio of the total cell population size to the size of the initial population, corrected for plating efficiency.

2.3. Neutral Red assay

For the Neutral Red assay, 5×10^3 cells are seeded in wells of Microtitre plates. Test agents are added after cell attachment, and cells are incubated for 48 h, after which time Neutral Red (50 µg/ml) is added to the medium and the cells are incubated for 3 h. The medium is removed carefully from the culture and cells washed with a 1% formaldehyde−1% $CaCl_2$ solution, and the dye is extracted by addition of 0.2 ml of 1% acetic acid+50% ethanol for at least 10 min. The absorbance is read at 540 nm on a microtitre plate reader.

3. Results

3.1. Effects of inorganic and organic selenium compounds on clonal survival and growth rate of HOS cells

The toxicities of sodium selenite, Se-met, and SMSC were determined in a clonal survival assay. Selenite is more toxic to HOS cells than is either organoselenium compound (Fig. 1A). SMSC becomes toxic at concentrations >15 µM. Se-met was the least toxic of the three compounds. Long-term growth is necessary for determining spontaneous mutation rates. When concentrations of these compounds that did not reduce clonal survival were used to study long-term growth, it was noted that 4 µM selenite reduced the growth rate starting after 1 week (Fig. 1B). There was no effect on growth of either organoselenium compound at 10 µM (data not shown).

3.2. Effects of selenium compounds on arsenite toxicity in HOS cells

The abilities of non-toxic concentrations of the three Se compounds to reduce the toxicity of arsenite, as measured in the Neutral Red assay, were analyzed (Fig. 2). At 1.25

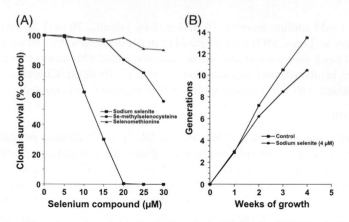

Fig. 1. (A) Effects of three Se compounds on clonal of survival of HOS cells. (B) Delayed effect of selenite on growth rate of HOS cells.

μM arsenite (~36% growth inhibition), all three compounds had a very slight protective effect, even though all were at molar excess. Only selenite and (to a lesser degree) Se-met were somewhat protective against 2.5 μM arsenite (~64% inhibition), and none of the compounds protected against 5 μM arsenite (~69% inhibition).

3.3. Effects of organic selenium compounds on spontaneous and arsenite-induced mutagenesis

Because selenite had a delayed inhibitory effect on the growth rate (Fig. 1B), which would affect the mutation rate, only the two organoselenium compounds were assayed for their abilities to block the accumulation of mutants in cultures growing for 6 weeks. Spontaneous mutagenesis was drastically reduced by both compounds (Fig. 3). Both

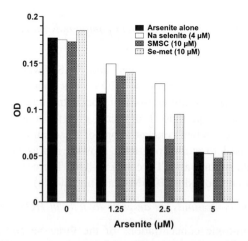

Fig. 2. Effect of selenium compounds on toxicity of arsenite as measured in the Neutral Red assay.

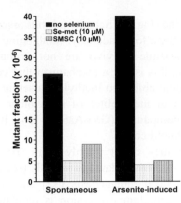

Fig. 3. Effect of organoselenium compounds on accumulation of mutants over a 6-week period.

compounds were also able to block the increased mutagenesis caused by arsenite in these cells.

4. Discussion

We confirmed previous reports [19,20] that selenite is more toxic to cells than organoselenium compounds. Selenite is toxic because it reacts with glutathione (GSH) to form selenodiglutathione (see Fig. 4). This can be converted to the anion GS-Se$^-$, which then redox cycles, producing oxidant stress [3,16,19] and apoptosis [21].

Selenium is reported to counteract some of the effects of arsenic in vivo [8,11] and in vitro [6,22]. In this study, none of the Se compounds were strongly protective against the arsenite toxicity, but the organoselenium compounds did protect against both spontaneous and (low-dose) arsenite-induced delayed mutagenesis, suggesting different mechanisms for these events.

In vivo, arsenite undergoes a series of methylations and reductions to the less toxic dimethyl arsenic acid (DMA^V), which is excreted in the urine [23]. Selenium is also

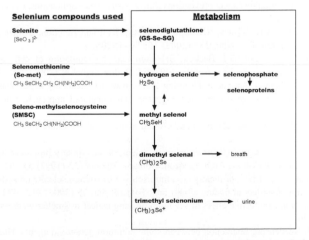

Fig. 4. In vivo metabolism of the selenium compounds used (based on Ref. [4]).

methylated and excreted in urine (Fig. 4). Selenite inhibits arsenic methylation [24,25] and selenite and arsenite may compete for S-adenosyl-methionine or GSH [26,27]. However, the effects of selenite on arsenite in vivo are not primarily through inhibition of methylation [28]. In any case, this is not a mechanism that could not be operative here, since HOS cells show very little ability to methylate arsenite [18]. Arsenite and selenite enhance the biliary excretion of metabolites of each other [6,29], possibly through a formation of a diglutathione compound [(GS)$_2$AsSe]$^-$ [30]. It is not known whether this compound forms in these cultured cells.

Spontaneous mutagenesis may result mainly from oxidative DNA damage [31]. Arsenite also increases oxidative DNA damage in cells (reviewed in Ref. [5]). Selenite blocks hydrogen peroxide-induced mutagenesis [32] and oxidative damage to DNA, proteins and lipids [33]. Selenoprotein expression is regulated by Se supply and cells growing in high selenite have increased activities of these enzymes [34,35]. Taken together, this suggests that Se-containing GPX and TR may be responsible for its antimutagenic effects. However, selenite, but not Se-met, was able to block arsenite-induced heme oxygenase expression, a marker of oxidant stress [36] so it is possible that Se-met blocks arsenite-induced mutagenesis by a different mechanism or else arsenite-induced mutagenesis occurs by a non-oxidative pathway.

Acknowledgements

This work was supported by United States Public Health Service Grants R01 CA73610 and P42 ES10344, and is part of NYU's Nelson Institute of Environmental Medicine Center programs supported by Grants ES00260 from NIEHS and CA16087 from NCI. ANU was supported by a Post-doctoral fellowship from the Cancer Research and Prevention Foundation, USA.

References

[1] P.C. Raich, et al., Selenium in cancer prevention: clinical issues and implications, Cancer Investig. 19 (2001) 540–553.
[2] R.F. Burk, K.E. Hill, A.K. Motley, Selenoprotein metabolism and function: evidence for more than one function for selenoprotein P, J. Nutr. 133 (2003) 1517S–1520S.
[3] R.C. McKenzie, J.R. Arthur, G.J. Beckett, Selenium and the regulation of cell signaling, growth and survival: molecular and mechanistic aspects, Antioxid. Redox Signal. 4 (2002) 339–351.
[4] National Research Council, Arsenic in Drinking Water, National Academy Press, Washington, DC, 2000.
[5] T.G. Rossman, Mechanism of arsenic carcinogenesis: an integrated approach, Mutat. Res. 533 (2003) 37–66.
[6] O.A. Levander, Metabolic interrelationships between arsenic and selenium, Environ. Health Perspect. 19 (1977) 159–164.
[7] D.J. Hoffman, et al., Interactive effects of arsenate, selenium, and dietary protein on survival, growth, and physiology in mallard ducklings, Arch. Environ. Contam. Toxicol. 22 (1992) 55–62.
[8] S. Chattopadhyay, et al., Effect of dietary co-administration of sodium selenite on sodium arsenite-induced ovarian and uterine disorders in mature albino rats, Toxicol. Sci. 75 (2003) 412–422.
[9] L. Gerhardsson, et al., Protective effect of selenium on lung cancer in smelter workers, Br. J. Ind. Med. 42 (1985) 617–626.
[10] L. Beckman, I. Nordenson, Interaction between some common genotoxic agents, Hum. Hered. 36 (1986) 397–401.

[11] S. Biswas, G. Talukder, A. Gharma, Prevention of cytotoxic effects of arsenic by short-term dietary supplementation with selenium in mice in vivo, Mutat. Res. 441 (1999) 155–160.

[12] J.Y. Yeh, et al., Modulation of the arsenic effects on cytotoxicity, viability, and cell cycle in porcine endothelial cells by selenium, Endothelium 10 (2003) 127–139.

[13] W. Wang, et al., Effects of selenium supplementation on arsenism: an intervention trial in Inner Mongolia, Environ. Geochem. Health 24 (2002) 359–374.

[14] T.G. Rossman, et al., Arsenite is a cocarcinogen with solar ultraviolet radiation for mouse skin: an animal model for arsenic carcinogenesis, Toxicol. Appl. Pharm. 176 (2001) 64–71.

[15] F.J. Burns, et al., Arsenic-induced enhancement of UVR carcinogenesis in mouse skin: a dose–response, Environ. Health Perspect. 112 (2001) 599–603.

[16] J.E. Spallholtz, L.M. Boylan, M.M. Rhaman, Environmental hypothesis: is poor dietary selenium intake an underlying factor for arsenososis and cancer in Bangladesh and West Bengal, India? Sci. Total Environ. 323 (2004) 21–32.

[17] T.G. Rossman, E.I. Goncharova, A. Nádas, Modeling and measurement of the spontaneous mutation rate in mammalian cells, Mutat. Res. 328 (1995) 21–30.

[18] K. Mure, et al., Arsenite induces delayed mutagenesis and transformation in Human Osteosarcoma cells at extremely low concentrations, Environ. Mol. Mutagen. 41 (2003) 322–331.

[19] M.S. Stewart, et al., Selenium compounds have disparate abilities to impose oxidative stress and induce apoptosis, Free Radic. Biol. Med. 26 (1999) 42–48.

[20] C.L. Shen, W. Song, B.C. Pence, Interactions of selenium compounds with other antioxidants in DNA damage and apoptosis in human normal keratinocytes, Cancer Epidemiol. Biomark. Prev. 10 (2001) 385–390.

[21] J. Lu, et al., Selenite induction of DNA strand breaks and apoptosis in mouse leukemic L1210 cells, Biochem. Pharmacol. 47 (1994) 1531–1535.

[22] A. Sweins, Protective effect of selenium against arsenic-induced chromosomal damage in cultured human lymphocytes, Hereditas 98 (1983) 249–282.

[23] D.J. Thomas, M. Styblo, S. Lln, The cellular metabolism and systemic toxicity of arsenic, Toxicol. Appl. Pharmacol. 176 (2001) 127–144.

[24] J.P. Buchet, R. Lauwerys, Study of inorganic arsenic methylation by rat liver in vitro: relevance for the interpretation of observations in man, Arch. Toxicol. 57 (1985) 125–129.

[25] M. Styblo, D.J. Thomas, Selenium modifies the metabolism and toxicity of arsenic in primary rat hepatocytes, Toxicol. Appl. Pharmacol. 172 (2001) 56–61.

[26] E.M. Kenyon, M.F. Hughes, O.A. Levander, Influence of dietary selenium on the disposition of arsenate in the female B6C3F1 mouse, J. Toxicol. Environ. Health 51 (1997) 279–299.

[27] Z. Gregus, A. Gyurasics, I. Csanaky, Effects of arsenic-, platinum-, and gold-containing drugs on the disposition of exogenous selenium in rats, Toxicol. Appl. Pharmacol. 57 (2000) 22–31.

[28] I. Csansky, Z. Gregus, Effect of selenite on the deposition of arsenate and arsenite in rats, Toxicology 186 (2003) 33–50.

[29] Z. Gregus, A. Gyurasics, L. Koszorus, Interactions between selenium and group Va-metalloids (arsenic, antimony, bismuth) in the biliary excretion, Environ. Toxicol. Pharmacol. 5 (1998) 89–99.

[30] J. Gailer, et al., A metabolic link between arsenite and selenite: the seleno-bis(S-glutathionyl) arsinium ion, J. Am. Chem. Soc. 122 (2000) 4637–4639.

[31] K. Mure, T.G. Rossman, Reduction of spontaneous mutagenesis in mismatch repair deficient and proficient cells by dietary antioxidants, Mutat. Res. 480–481 (2001) 85–95.

[32] G. Bronzetti, et al., Antimutagenicity of sodium selenite in Chinese hamster V79 cells exposed to azoxymethane, methylmethanesulfonate and hydrogen peroxide, Mutat. Res. 523–524 (2003) 21–31.

[33] K. El-Bayoumy, The protective role of selenium on genetic damage and on cancer, Mutat. Res. 475 (2001) 123–139.

[34] S.W. Lewin, et al., Selenium supplementation acting through the induction of thioredoxin reductase and glutathione peroxidase protects the human endothelial cell, Biochim. Biophys. Acta 1593 (2002) 85–92.

[35] C. Ip, Y. Dong, H.E. Ganther, New concepts in selenium chemoprevention, Cancer Metastasis Rev. 21 (2002) 281–289.

[36] S. Taketani, et al., Selenium antagonizes the induction of human heme oxygenase by arsenite and cadmium ions, Biochem. Int. 23 (1991) 625–632.

International Congress Series 1275 (2004) 180–188

ELSEVIER

www.ics-elsevier.com

Zn and Cd accumulation in *Potamonautes warreni* from sites in the North–West Province of South Africa

S. Thawley[a,*], S. Morris[a], A. Vosloo[b]

[a]*School of Biological Sciences, University of Bristol, Woodland Road, Bristol BS8 1UG, UK*
[b]*North–West University, Potchefstroom, South Africa*

Abstract. The freshwater crab, *Potamonautes warreni*, is endemic to rivers of the North–West Province, South Africa. Parts of this province are heavily mined for gold, diamonds and platinum. The rivers inhabited by *P. warreni* are therefore vulnerable to metal pollution from industry, as well as from other anthropogenic activities. Measurements of Zn and Cd in crab tissues (gill, midgut gland, muscle and carapace), sediments and water from sites on three tributaries of the Limpopo River near the town of Rustenburg were made. Ambient and accumulated Zn and Cd concentrations and water Na and Ca concentrations were used to investigate factors affecting metal accumulation. Zn and Cd concentrations in *P. warreni* varied between sites and tissues and a negative relationship was found at some sites between water Na and Ca concentrations and metal burdens of crabs. Sediment and water metal concentrations were not representative of metal accumulation in the crab tissues, indicating the importance of including biota in monitoring programs. © 2004 Elsevier B.V. All rights reserved.

Keywords: Zn; Cd; Accumulation; Freshwater crab; South Africa

1. Introduction

Cd and Zn are transition metals with similar chemistries. An important difference between them is that Zn is essential, being found in every body cell as a constituent of

---

* Corresponding author. Tel.: +44 117 9287478; fax: +44 117 9257374.
E-mail address: s.thawley@bristol.ac.uk (S. Thawley).

0531-5131/ © 2004 Elsevier B.V. All rights reserved.
doi:10.1016/j.ics.2004.09.036

proteins [1], while Cd is thought to have no biological function. Cd and Zn have a strong affinity for sulphydryl-containing ligands such as the amino acids cysteine and histidine [2] and have toxic effects on proteins and ion channels (for a review, see Ref. [3]). In humans, Cd produces toxic effects on the human kidney and was thought to cause Japanese Itai-itai disease [4].

Cd and Zn find their way into the environment by natural (e.g., volcanic eruptions and erosion of rocks) and anthropogenic means. Cd is recovered for many uses as a by-product during smelting of Zn, Pb, Zn–Cu and complex ores as it is found concentrated in sulphide minerals, along with Zn, Cu, Pb and Hg [5]. About 60% of all anthropogenic Cd emissions into the atmosphere occur through Zn and Cu production [6].

Zn is used in alloys (e.g., brass), in galvanising (especially of iron) and in pharmaceuticals. Cd has many uses; for example, it is used in electroplating, in pigments, in plastic stabilizers and in batteries [5]. However, only 5% of Cd which is put to these uses is recovered [5], resulting in an inevitable increase in environmental Cd. Air, water and soil Cd concentrations in areas unaffected by human activities are usually very low, in contrast to concentrations in polluted areas [7].

Heavy metals can have effects on different aspects of the physiology of aquatic animals, for example, oxygen consumption [8], water permeability [9] and osmoregulation [10] (for a review, see Ref. [11]). Considering the toxicity of these metals, Cd in particular, it is important to be able to monitor their levels in the environment in an accurate and representative way.

Concentrations of metals can be analysed in water samples, sediment samples and biota taken from study sites. Using water samples to assess water quality in terms of metal contamination, and also to identify pollution sources, can be inconclusive due to fluctuations in dissolved constituents within short time intervals [12]. These fluctuations are due to daily and seasonal changes in water flow, changing pH and redox conditions, salinity, temperature and detergent concentrations in the water. Metal concentrations found in water are usually very low, and so, there are also analytical problems associated with this [13]. Sediment analysis may be more useful to detect pollution problems and sources, especially for contaminants which are rapidly adsorbed by particulate matter and consequently would not remain in water samples for long [12]. When river flow is low, particulate matter suspended in the water settles to the river bed and is incorporated into the sediment. When sediments are used to monitor metal pollution in rivers, factors such as water flow (after high water discharge, a lower degree of contamination would be measured due to erosion of the river bed sediments) and particle size of sediments need to be taken into account [12].

Biomonitoring, where accumulated metal concentrations in biota are measured, offers an alternative to sediment and water sampling for the purposes of identifying areas at risk from metal pollution. Biomonitors provide "time-integrated measures of those portions of the total ambient metal load that are of direct ecotoxicological relevance" [13]. When sediments and water samples are analysed for metals, it is the total metal concentration that is measured. However, the total metal concentration may not be a definitive way of analyzing whether metal uptake and toxicity are causing a problem at a site. Zn uptake occurs in proportion to ambient total Zn concentrations, for example, in *Palaemon elegans*, [14], but it is generally considered that the free metal ion is the form of Cd and Zn that is available to aquatic organisms (in crustaceans [15,16]; in rainbow trout [17]). Factors other than total metal concentration alter the free metal ion concentration of freshwater, for example, pH and salinity [18] and concentration of humic materials [19]. To examine whether factors controlling metal speciation and uptake at a site (e.g., metal concentration, salinity, temperature, pH) are combining to produce toxic effects or metal accumulation in biota, it is necessary to measure aspects of the biota themselves, as well as metal concentrations in the sediment.

Potamonautes warreni (Calman) is a true freshwater crab found in parts of the North–West Province, South Africa. Its potential use as an indicator organism has been investigated in studies of tissue accumulation of Cu [20] and Cd and Zn [21].

The present study was aimed at quantifying concentrations of Zn and Cd in sediment, water and tissues of *P. warreni* from six river sites in the heavily mined Rustenburg area of the North–West Province of South Africa. Ca and Na concentrations in the water at each site were also measured to provide measures of salinity and water hardness in order to investigate whether high salinity and/or water hardness could provide protection against metal accumulation.

2. Materials and methods

2.1. Study location

Six sites were chosen near the city of Rustenburg in the North–West Province of South Africa (Fig. 1). A preliminary study where eight sites were sampled for crabs, sediment and water in both January and February 2002 enabled identification of sites to study in greater detail the following year. There are two sites on each of the three rivers Elands, Leragane and Hex. They are all tributaries of the Limpopo.

2.2. Sample collection and preparation

Crabs, water and sediment were collected from six sites near the town of Rustenburg, North–West Province, South Africa in February 2003 (Fig. 1). At each site, crabs were caught either by hand as they set out on terrestrial excursions beside the rivers, or by baited line from the bottom of the rivers. Between 6 and 11 crabs were caught at each site. Haemolymph and urine samples were taken on site and were subsequently acidified 1:1 with 0.1 mmol l^{-1} HNO$_3$. At each site, six water samples (250 ml) were taken from the areas where crabs had been caught. Water samples were later acidified (12 ml water + 980 μl concentrated HNO$_3$) and stored until analysis. Sediment samples were taken by placing a corer 80 mm into the substrate at six different areas within the vicinity of the river site. Sediment samples were later dried and sieved.

Crabs were weighed, sexed and dissected by removing chelae muscle, midgut gland, gills and a section of dorsal carapace from above the pericardium. Tissue samples were frozen, and all water, sediment and tissues were transported to Bristol for preparation and metal analyses.

Tissue and sediment samples were weighed and wet-ashed in 10 ml of a 5:1 nitric acid/ perchloric acid mixture heated to approximately 100 °C for 3 h using reflux condensation to prevent sample loss. Sediment digests were filtered prior to metal analyses.

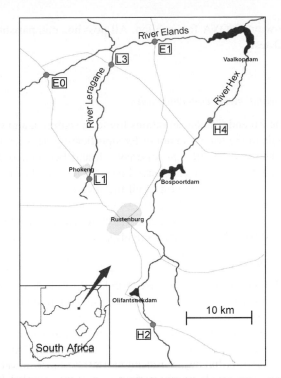

Fig. 1. The geographical position of Rustenburg field sites (E0, E1, L1, L3, H2 and H4) within South Africa showing roads and major towns.

2.3. Zn and Cd analysis

All digests were analysed for Cd and Zn content using graphite furnace atomic absorption spectrophotometry (GFAAS) (GBC 960A, GBC Melbourne). Standards were prepared daily from 1 mg l^{-1} Cd and Zn stock solutions. All glassware and polyethylene autosampler cups were acid washed using the following procedure: soaking in 30% V/V HCl overnight, soaking in 30% V/V HNO_3 overnight and rinsed copiously with double-distilled water before use.

2.4. Na and Ca analysis

Water samples were analysed for Na and Ca concentrations by atomic absorption spectrophotometry (AAS; GBC 906). Samples were diluted with 5.9 mmol l^{-1} $CsCl_2$ (for Na analysis) or 7.2 mmol l^{-1} $LaCl_3$ (for Ca analysis) to suppress chemical interference.

2.5. Statistical analysis

Tissue data were log-transformed to produce equal variances, and nested ANOVA was carried out for each metal. Cd carapace concentrations were analysed separately by one-way ANOVA due to heterogeneous variances when compared with other tissues. Sediment Cd data were log-transformed to normalise the data. Sediment and water data were analysed using one-way ANOVA for each metal. Water Na and Ca concentrations were analysed using one-way ANOVA for each ion. All post hoc comparisons were carried out using Tukey's HSD test.

3. Results

3.1. Sediment and water metal concentrations

Table 1 shows the Zn and Cd concentrations found in sediment and water samples from the six sites. Zn levels in the water did not differ significantly between the sites ($P=0.214$, $F=1.52$, $df=5,29$). The only significant difference found between sediment Zn concentrations was between the highest (E0) and lowest levels (H4) ($P=0.032$). Cd water concentrations in site E1 were the lowest of all the sites ($P=0.01$). Cd in the water of L1 was significantly higher than that at H4 ($P=0.01$). Cd in the sediment was highest in L3 ($P=0.036$). Cd in the sediment from L1 was lower than that from L3 ($P<0.0001$) and both of the Hex sites ($P=0.043$, $P=0.003$, respectively).

3.2. Tissue Zn concentrations

In crabs from H4, highest Zn burdens were found in the muscle compared with all other tissues ($P<0.001$) (Table 2). More Zn was present in both the midgut gland ($P=0.001$) and the gill ($P=0.007$) than in the carapace of H4 crabs. Crabs from H2 ($P=0.023$) and E1 ($P=0.003$) showed higher Zn burdens in muscle than in carapace; crabs from E0 showed higher Zn burdens in midgut gland than in the muscle ($P=0.007$). Crabs from L3 contained more Zn in carapace ($P=0.0008$), midgut gland ($P=0.0276$) and muscle ($P=0.0071$) than H2. Crabs from L3 also contained more Zn in carapace than E1 ($P=0.03$) and H4 ($P=0.0001$) and more Zn in midgut gland than H4 ($P=0.013$). Crabs from E0 contained more Zn in their carapace ($P=0.0001$) and midgut gland ($P=0.0033$) than those from H4. Crabs from E0 also contained more Zn in their midgut gland than crabs from H2 ($P=0.0073$). Crabs from E1 had more Zn in their gill ($P=0.0211$) and midgut gland

Table 1

Mean Cd and Zn concentrations measured in sediment ($\mu g \ g^{-1}$) and water ($\mu g \ ml^{-1}$) collected from Rustenburg field sites in February 2003

Site	E0	L1	L3	E1	H2	H4
Cd						
Sediment	0.0497a	0.0196bdf	0.1671abc eg	0.0523c	0.0467de	0.0678fg
	(0.012)	(0.004)	(0.029)	(0.018)	(0.005)	(0.015)
Water	0.00016a	0.00018bc	0.00017d	0.00009abdef	0.00016e	0.00014cf
	(0.00001)	(0.00001)	(0.00002)	(0.00000)	(0.00001)	(0.00001)
Zn						
Sediment	24.26a	16.42	20.58	23.40	16.91	11.07a
	(2.02)	(1.76)	(5.78)	(1.72)	(1.73)	(1.99)
Water	0.135	0.0622	0.135	0.145	0.117	0.163
	(0.019)	(0.004)	(0.042)	(0.044)	(0.012)	(0.042)

S.E.M. in brackets. $N=6$ for sediment and water data except L1 Zn water ($N=5$). For tissues, Cd sediment and Zn water data were also log transformed. Matching letters indicate significant differences ($p<0.05$): lower case letters indicate differences between sites of the same sediment/water.

Table 2
Mean Cd and Zn concentrations measured in *P. warreni* tissues ($\mu g \ g^{-1}$) collected from Rustenburg field sites in February 2003

Site	E0	L1	L3	E1	H2	H4
Cd						
Carapace	7.751ab	6.815	5.057ac	5.183bd	7.522cd	5.995
	(0.445)	(0.578)	(0.495)	(0.598)	(0.434)	(0.596)
Gill	0.109A	0.172aAB	0.085	0.119	0.046aA	0.056A
	(0.034)	(0.020)	(0.014)	(0.019)	(0.006)	(0.024)
Midgut gland	0.255aAB	0.084aA	0.128	0.234A	0.134AB	0.161AB
	(0.031)	(0.009)	(0.032)	(0.036)	(0.031)	(0.024)
Muscle	0.066B	0.064B	0.100	0.113A	0.058B	0.072B
	(0.018)	(0.010)	(0.032)	(0.026)	(0.008)	(0.010)
Zn						
Carapace	104.58a	42.89	246.14bcd	34.84bA	22.52cA	8.86adABC
	(28.17)	(13.80)	(89.78)	(8.08)	(4.76)	(2.56)
Gill	133.93	177.42	89.36	214.35a	39.04	31.41aAD
	(30.33)	(92.05)	(33.43)	(69.24)	(9.70)	(11.67)
Midgut gland	214.95abA	47.74	235.72cd	184.85e	32.90ac	29.46bdeBE
	(41.56)	(13.00)	(91.62)	(50.50)	(4.95)	(4.74)
Muscle	64.62A	153.29	374.96a	391.01bA	51.29abA	121.14CDE
	(9.03)	(68.87)	(114.48)	(130.92)	(7.78)	(42.34)

S.E.M. indicated in brackets. N=6 (E0), 7 (L1), 7 (L3), 11 (E1), 10 (H2) and 10 (H4). All tissue data except Cd carapace were log transformed. Matching letters indicate significant differences (p<0.05): lower case letters indicate differences between sites of the same tissue; upper case letters indicate differences between tissues at the same site.

(P=0.0394) than crabs from H4 and those from E1 had more Zn in their muscle than crabs from H2 (P=0.0232).

3.3. Tissue Cd concentrations

At all sites, Cd accumulated most in the carapace (Table 2). Crabs from E0 (P=0.02, P=0.001, respectively), H2 (P=0.001, P=0.016, respectively) and H4 (P=0.0001, P=0.001) all contained more Cd in midgut gland than in either the gill or the muscle. Crabs from L1 contained more Cd in their gill than in either their midgut gland (P=0.014) or muscle (P<0.0001). Crabs from E1 contained more Cd in their midgut gland than in their muscle (P=0.017). There was no significant difference between tissue Cd concentrations from L3 (P=0.395, F=0.985, df=2,16).

Table 3
Mean Ca and Na concentrations (mmol l^{-1}) of water from six sites near Rustenburg, South Africa

Site	E0	L1	L3	E1	H2	H4
Na	0.974	1.421	0.597	1.635	2.171	1.921
	(0.021)	(0.013)	(0.002)	(0.003)	(0.0037)	(0.013)
Ca	0.641a	2.106	0.876	0.633a	1.540	1.454
	(0.0040)	(0.005)	(0.005)	(0.001)	(0.0048)	(0.005)

S.E.M. shown in brackets. Matching letter indicates no significant difference. N=(Na,Ca) E0 (6,6), L1 (6,5), L3 (5,5), E1 (5,5), H2 (6,6), H4 (5,5).

Carapace from H2 contained more Cd than carapace from either L3 ($P=0.027$) or E1 ($P=0.025$). Carapace from E0 contained more Cd than carapace from either L3 ($P=0.039$) or E1 ($P=0.039$). Gill from L1 contained more Cd than gill from H2 ($p=0.0003$). Midgut gland from E0 contained more Cd than midgut gland from L1 ($p=0.0369$).

3.4. Na and Ca water concentrations

Table 3 shows Na and Ca concentrations of water samples from the six sites (note that no significant differences are denoted by matching letters which is different from the other tables in this study). Na water concentrations were all significantly different from one another ($P<0.0001$). Na concentrations were in the following order: L3< E0<L1<E1<H4<H2. Ca water concentrations were all significantly different from each other ($P<0.0001$), except for between sites E0 and E1 ($P=0.779$). Ca concentrations were in the following order: E0/E1<L3<H4<H2<L1. Site H2 had the most Ca and Na in combination, of all the sites.

4. Discussion

Na concentrations can provide a measure of the salinity of the water. A high Na concentration (compared to other freshwater sites) indicates a high Cl concentration since the major mineral source of Na is NaCl [1]. Both sites on the Hex river had high Na and Ca water concentrations when compared to the other sites. It is likely that there would be a constant low free metal ion concentration in comparison with other sites, due to increased complexation of Cd and Zn with Cl ions, and therefore, low metal uptake and accumulation resulted in these crabs.

The free ion as the bioavailable form of the metal has been used to explain the negative relationship between metal uptake/toxicity with salinity (e.g., Refs. [22–24]; for a review, see Ref. [25]). In saline or alkaline water, there are higher concentrations of OH^- and Cl^- present which chelate Cd and Zn resulting in less metal available to the aquatic biota.

Ca water concentrations have been shown to have an inverse relationship with Cd accumulation in the shore crab Carcinus maenas [26]. Wright [26] suggests that this is due to an activation of Ca uptake mechanisms in low Ca conditions, and that subsequent increased accumulation of Cd is due to 'accidental' uptake via Ca uptake routes. Cd uptake is likely to be via routes of Ca uptake in crustacean gill [27], and Zn and Ca are thought to share common uptake routes in freshwater fish gill [28].

There are three factors brought about by low Na and Ca water conditions which interplay to affect metal uptake rates and accumulation. The first is the bioavailable metal concentration (in high salinity, the free metal ion concentration is low due to the formation of metal chlorides) [25]. Secondly, stimulation of Na and Ca uptake mechanisms in low salinity may allow incidental uptake of Zn and Cd ions, as suggested by Wright [26]. Finally, competition between the major ions (Na and Ca) and heavy metal ions (Cd and Zn) for uptake sites (for example, Ref. [29]) can occur.

If Na and Ca water concentrations are examined and used to predict which sites should contain crabs with high metal burdens using these three factors, L3 should be the site with highest metal burdens in crabs, while the Hex sites should have 'cleaner' animals. This prediction can be confirmed from our data, especially for Zn tissue concentrations. Site L1 had the highest water Ca concentration and had low Zn concentrations in crab tissues; however, it had one of the highest gill Cd concentrations of all the sites.

Factors other than salinity are likely to be controlling metal accumulation in the crab tissues, for example, pH and temperature. These factors have been shown experimentally to produce altered metal uptake by aquatic animals [22,30]. It is likely that differences in metal uptake and accumulation rates produced by variables such as pH are due to changes in both metal speciation and physiology of the animal [13].

Concentrations of accumulated metals in crabs from E0, E1 and L3 were not reflected in the ambient metal concentrations in terms of comparing metal concentrations between sites. The river Leragane flows through mining areas before reaching L3 just before the confluence with the Elands. If only water and sediment samples were taken and analysed from these sites, the actual effect of the metals on the biota would have gone unnoticed.

Cd and Zn concentrations in the six study sites of such a small area (approximately 30×40 km) varied when measured in sediments, water and crab tissues. Factors such as Na and Ca concentration also varied, and it is likely that they have some control over metal accumulation and toxicity. Therefore, in order to maximise the relevance of monitoring programs, it is necessary to examine accumulation in the biota themselves, as well as in sediment and water. This is especially important when such a wide range of factors control the toxicity of metals.

Although field identification placed the crab species caught in this study as *P. warreni*, studies have shown that *P. unispinus* inhabits tributaries of the Limpopo [31]. The species used remains to be ascertained by analysing a variable other than morphological characteristics.

Acknowledgements

Thanks are due to Daléne van Heerden, Arno de la Rey, Andre Laas and Andrew Glendinning for their field assistance. The project was funded by NERC. The attendance of S. Thawley at the 3rd ICCPB was supported by an SEB/COB travel grant.

References

[1] R.J.P. Williams, J.J.R. da Silva, The Natural Selection of the Chemical Elements, Bath Press, Bath, 1996.
[2] B.L. Vallee, D.D. Ulmer, Biochemical effects of mercury, cadmium and lead, Annu. Rev. Biochem. 41 (1972) 91–129.
[3] T. Kiss, O.N. Osipenko, Toxic effects of heavy metals on ionic channels, Pharmacol. Rev. 46 (1994) 245–267.
[4] S. Satarug, M.R. Moore, Adverse health effects of chronic exposure to low-level cadmium in foodstuffs and cigarette smoke, Environ. Health Perspect. 112 (2004) 1099–1103.
[5] J.O. Nriagu, Production, uses, and properties of cadmium, in: J.O. Nriagu (Ed.), Cadmium in the Environment Part 1: Ecological Cycling, Wiley, Chichester, 1980, pp. 35–70.
[6] J.O. Nriagu, Cadmium in the atmosphere and in precipitation, in: J.O. Nriagu (Ed.), Cadmium in the Environment Part 1: Ecological Cycling, Wiley, Chichester, 1980, pp. 71–114.
[7] B. Raspor, Distribution and speciation of cadmium in natural waters, in: J.O. Nriagu (Ed.), Cadmium in the Environment Part 1: Ecological Cycling, Wiley, Chichester, 1980, pp. 147–236.
[8] M.D. Ahern, S. Morris, Respiratory, acid–base and metabolic responses of the freshwater crayfish *Cherax destructor* to lead contamination, Comp. Biochem. Physiol. A 124 (1999) 105–111.

[9] A.D. Rasmussen, et al., The effects of trace metals on the apparent water permeability of the shore crab *Carcinus maenas* (L.) and the brown shrimp *Crangon crangon* (L.), Mar. Pollut. Bull. 31 (1995) 60–62.

[10] M.D. Ahern, S. Morris, Accumulation of lead and its effects on Na balance in the freshwater crayfish *Cherax destructor*, J. Exp. Zool. 281 (1998) 270–279.

[11] J.M. Bouquegneau, R. Gilles, Osmoregulation and pollution of the aquatic medium, in: R. Gilles (Ed.), Mechanisms of Osmoregulation in Animals, Wiley, Chichester, 1979, pp. 563–580.

[12] U. Forstner, Cadmium in polluted sediments, in: J.O. Nriagu (Ed.), Cadmium in the Environment Part 1: Ecological Cycling, Wiley, Chichester, 1980, pp. 305–364.

[13] P.S. Rainbow, Biomonitoring of heavy metal availability in the marine environment, Mar. Pollut. Bul. 31 (1995) 183–192.

[14] S.L. White, P.S. Rainbow, Regulation of zinc concentration by *Palaemon elegans* (Crustacea:Decapoda): zinc flux and effects of temperature, zinc concentration and moulting, Mar. Ecol. Prog. Ser. 16 (1984) 135–147.

[15] D. Nugegoda, P.S. Rainbow, Effect of a chelating agent (EDTA) on zinc uptake and regulation by *Palaemon elegans* (Crustacea: Decapoda), J. Mar. Biol. Ass. U.K. 68 (1988) 25–40.

[16] D. Nugegoda, P.S. Rainbow, Salinity, osmolality, and zinc uptake in *Palaemon elegans* (Crustacea: Decapoda), Mar. Ecol. Prog. Ser. 55 (1989) 149–157.

[17] P. Part, O. Svanberg, A. Kiessling, The availability of cadmium to perfused rainbow trout gilld in different water qualities, Water Res. 19 (1985) 427–434.

[18] D.R. Turner, M. Whitfield, A.G. Dickson, The equilibrium speciation of dissolved components in freshwater and seawater at 25 °C and 1 atm pressure, Geochim. Cosmochim. Acta 45 (1981) 855–881.

[19] R.F.C. Mantoura, A. Dickson, J.P. Riley, The complexation of metal with humic materials in natural waters, Estuar. Coast. Mar. Sci. 6 (1978) 387–408.

[20] V.E. Steenkamp, H.H. du Preez, H.J. Schoonbee, Bioaccumulation of copper in the tissues of *Potamonautes warreni* (Calman) (Crustacea, Decapoda, Branchiura), from industrial, mine and sewage-polluted freshwater ecosystems, South Afr. Tydskr Dierk 29 (1994) 152–161.

[21] M.J. Sanders, H.H. du Preez, J.H.J. van Vuren, Monitoring cadmium and zinc contamination in freshwater systems with the use of the freshwater river crab, *Potamonautes warreni*, Water SA 25 (1999) 91–98.

[22] J. O'Hara, The influence of temperature and salinity on the toxicity of cadmium to the fiddler crab, *Uca pugilator*, Fish. Bull. 71 (1973) 149–153.

[23] D.A. Wright, The effect of salinity on cadmium uptake by the tissues of the shore crab *Carcinus maenas*, J. Exp. Biol. 67 (1977) 137–146.

[24] I.P. Zanders, W.E. Rojas, Salinity effects on cadmium accumulation in various tissues of the tropical fiddler crab, *Uca rapax*, Environ. Pollut. 94 (1996) 293–299.

[25] D.A. Wright, Trace metal and major ion interactions in aquatic animals, Mar. Pollut. Bull. 31 (1995) 8–18.

[26] D.A. Wright, The effect of calcium on cadmium uptake by the shore crab *Carcinus maenas*, J. Exp. Biol. 67 (1977) 163–173.

[27] C. Lucu, V. Obersnel, Cadmium influx across isolated *Carcinus* gill epithelium, J. Comp. Physiol. B 166 (1996) 184–189.

[28] C. Hogstrand, et al., Mechanisms of zinc uptake in gills of freshwater rainbow trout: interplay with calcium transport, Am. J. Physiol. 270 (1996) R1141–R1147.

[29] D.J. Spry, C.M. Wood, A kinetic method for the measurement of zinc influx in vivo in the rainbow trout and the effects of waterborne calcium on flux rates, J. Exp. Biol. 142 (1989) 425–446.

[30] J.M. Laporte, et al., Combined effects of water pH and salinity on the bioaccumulation of inorganic mercury and methylmercury in the shore crab, *Carcinus maenas*, Mar. Pollut. Bull. 34 (1997) 880–893.

[31] S.R. Daniels, et al., Carapace dentition patterns, morphometrics and allozyme differentiation amongst two toothed freshwater crab species (*Potamonautes warreni* and *P. unispinus*) (Decapoda:Brachyura:Potamonautidae) from river systems in South Africa, J. Zool. Lond. 255 (2001) 389–404.

International Congress Series 1275 (2004) 189–194

ELSEVIER

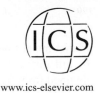

www.ics-elsevier.com

Mechanism of acute copper toxicity in euryhaline crustaceans: implications for the Biotic Ligand Model

A. Bianchini[a,*], S.E.G. Martins[b], I.F. Barcarolli[b]

[a]Departamento de Ciências Fisiológicas, Fundação Universidade Federal do Rio Grande (FURG),
Av. Itália km 8, Campus Carreiros, 96201-900, Rio Grande, RS, Brazil
[b]Programa de Pós-Graduação em Oceanografia Biológica, FURG, Brazil

Abstract. The Biotic Ligand Model (BLM) for copper is largely based on data obtained from freshwater fish and is currently calibrated to protect freshwater invertebrates. The extrapolation from fish to invertebrates must rely on the general assumption that the mechanisms of toxicity induced by copper in the sensitive invertebrates are the same as those observed in the less sensitive teleost fish. Therefore, the need for more invertebrate data is a critical area for the improvement of the BLM for freshwater and for its extension to brackish and marine waters. Results from our recent studies have shown that in low salinities the mechanism of acute toxicity in euryhaline crustaceans sensitive to copper is similar to that observed in freshwater fish and crustaceans, i.e., iono- and osmoregulatory imbalance induced by Na^+,K^+-ATPase inhibition. However, other results clearly indicate that the same mechanism of toxicity is not evident in euryhaline crustaceans more tolerant to copper. They also indicate that in sea water the mechanism of acute copper toxicity either in sensitive or more tolerant species is definitely not associated with an iono- and osmoregulatory imbalance, as opposed to marine teleost fish. © 2004 Elsevier B.V. All rights reserved.

Keywords: Acute toxicity; Biotic Ligand Model; Copper; Euryhaline crustaceans

1. Introduction

The Biotic Ligand Model (BLM) is a computational model developed to perform risk assessment involving several metals, including copper [1,2]. This model attempts to

* Corresponding author. Tel.: +55 53 233 6853; fax: +55 53 233 6850.
E-mail address: adalto@octopus.furg.br (A. Bianchini).

0531-5131/ © 2004 Elsevier B.V. All rights reserved.
doi:10.1016/j.ics.2004.08.074

predict metal toxicity to aquatic organisms on the basis of metal speciation and effects at the gill surface, i.e., the biotic ligand [3–6]. The BLM for copper is largely based on data obtained from freshwater fish and is currently calibrated to protect freshwater invertebrates [5,6]. However, the extrapolation from fish to invertebrates must rely on the general assumption that the mechanism of toxicity induced by copper in invertebrates are the same as those observed in teleost fish. Therefore, the need for more invertebrate data is a critical area for the improvement of the BLM for freshwater and for its extension to brackish and marine waters. Thus, the aim of the present paper is to highlight this need and briefly describe the findings on the mechanisms of acute copper toxicity in aquatic animals, especially fish and crustaceans.

This paper is divided into two main sections: a brief background on the BLM for copper, and a summary on the mechanism of acute copper toxicity in aquatic animals, including our recent findings in euryhaline crustaceans. Conclusions based on the findings reported and their implications for the BLM are also considered in the last section of this paper.

2. Copper and the BLM

Copper is an essential nutrient to aquatic organisms. However, it causes toxicity when present in elevated concentrations in the water. Consequently, the emission of this metal into the environment is currently under regulation. This regulation is largely based on the total concentration of metal in effluents or/and in the environment although the United States Environmental Protection Agency's current water quality criteria corrects for water hardness. In addition to hardness, which offers some protection against acute copper exposure [7,8], other water chemistry parameters ameliorate the effects of acute exposure to this metal. The effects of acute exposure to copper are influenced by pH [7–10] and dissolved organic matter [8,10,11].

The protective effects of various water chemistry parameters have been modelled in the Biotic Ligand Model (BLM) for copper [5,6]. The BLM simultaneously accounts for the speciation and complexation of dissolved metal and competitive binding of metal and other cations at the site of action, the gill. The premise behind the model is that there is a strong correlation between the metal concentration in/on the target and the subsequent acute toxicity [12,13].

In light of the above, it is clear that water chemistry and the presence of food (organic matter) in the experimental medium profoundly modify copper toxicity to aquatic animals. Unfortunately, most of the information and knowledge on copper toxicity is available only for freshwater environments after acute exposure, a situation that normally does not involve the presence of food in water. Despite the important differences in the amount of possible copper ligands (Cl^-, SO_4^{2-}, NOM, $S_2O_3^{2-}$, sulfide, Br^-, and $B(OH)_4^-$) or competitors (Na^+, Mg^{2+}, Ca^{2+}, K^+, and Sr^{2+}) in freshwater, brackish, and seawater, copper toxicity studies and attempts to validate the BLM in estuarine and marine animals are scarce. However, it is known that the relative acute toxicity of copper to invertebrates varies in freshwater and salt water. Toxicity is greater in freshwater than in marine waters. LC50 values are generally less than 0.5 mg L^{-1} and range from 0.006 to >225 mg L^{-1}. These differences could be mainly attributed to the water chemistry, as discussed above, and routes of copper accumulation.

Since the primary site of toxic action for waterborne copper in freshwater fish is the gill [14, for review], this organ is the correct "target" for the BLM for freshwater. However, the situation is different in salt water because ionic Cu^+ is much less prevalent and cationic competition from Na^+, Ca^{2+}, Mg^{2+}, K^+, and Sr^{2+} at Cu-gill binding sites will also be stronger in saltwater. Furthermore, the situation is complicated for fish in saltwater because they drink to replace water lost by osmosis across the gills [15]. This water is absorbed in the gut, so this tissue could be an important "target" for Cu^+ interactions in brackish and marine fish. It is important to note here that information regarding the routes of copper accumulation and the mechanism of copper toxicity in brackish and marine invertebrates is scarce. In this case, the situation is quite different from saltwater fish, since marine invertebrates in general are osmoconformers, but are still ionoregulators [15]. This condition strongly suggests that the gill may become the main site of toxicity for copper in marine invertebrates as opposed to fish, where both gills and gut seems to be involved in copper accumulation and toxicity.

In summary, the BLM was originally developed for freshwater environments. It is largely based on data obtained from fish and is currently calibrated to protect invertebrates that are much more sensitive to copper based on toxicity data for *Daphnia* sp. [5,6]. However, the extrapolation from fish to invertebrates must rely on the general assumption that the mechanisms of toxicity induced by copper in the sensitive invertebrates are the same as those in the less sensitive teleost fish. So, a better understanding of the routes of accumulation and mechanisms of acute copper toxicity in brackish and marine invertebrates is imperative for future extension of the BLM to saltwater environments.

3. Mechanisms of acute copper toxicity in euryhaline crustaceans

Parallel to the development of the BLM, evidence elucidating the physiological mechanism of acute copper toxicity in freshwater fish and crustaceans has been accumulating.

Copper is considered as an osmoregulatory toxicant to freshwater animals. In fact, several authors have demonstrated that acute exposure to waterborne copper significantly reduced plasma sodium and chloride concentration in different freshwater fish species. This effect is associated with a reduced ion uptake at the gills level, which is believed to be due to an inhibition of the Na^+,K^+-ATPase located at the basolateral membrane of the gill epithelium [14, for review].

Regarding freshwater crustaceans, information about the mechanism of acute copper toxicity is scarce. In *Daphnia magna*, a reduced whole body sodium concentration was reported after few hours of exposure to high concentrations of copper [16]. Recently, it was demonstrated that waterborne copper exposure ($100~\mu g~L^{-1}$) induced 77% reduction of the sodium uptake in the amphipod *Gammarus pulex*. In this case, an inhibition of the Na^+,K^+-ATPase was also reported [17].

It is well known that the gills are the main site of active transport of Na^+ and Cl^- from the water into the extracellular fluid of the animal, and that branchial Na^+,K^+-ATPase activity is directly related to the Na^+ and Cl^- uptake across the gills. Furthermore, it is well demonstrated that this uptake is essential to counteract the diffusive ion loss through the gills and excretory organs in freshwater fish and crustaceans [18–21]. Thus, the Na^+,K^+-

ATPase inhibition induced by waterborne copper exposure seems to be the key site of acute copper toxicity for both freshwater fish and crustaceans. Despite that, other recent findings reported in the literature suggest that the impact of copper on other mechanisms involved in Na^+ and Cl^- uptake at the gills level should be considered [14, for review]. As suggested by Grosell et al. [14], a possible competition between Cu^+ and Na^+ by the Na^+ channels at the gill apical membrane, as well as an inhibition of the carbonic anhydrase activity after copper exposure also should be investigated.

As discussed above, the mechanism of acute copper toxicity in freshwater fish and crustaceans is relatively well known. However, information on the mechanisms of acute copper toxicity in euryhaline or marine animals is scarce. In *Opsanus beta*, a marine teleost fish, osmoregulatory disturbances have been reported to occur after copper exposure [22]. According to these authors, marine fish gills accumulate copper when the metal concentration in the water is high. However, it is discussed at what extension the degree of accumulation reflects the physiological effects observed after acute or chronic exposure to copper. The Na^+,K^+-ATPase from *O. beta* seems to be insensitive to copper, since its activity in both gill and intestine was not inhibited after exposure for 30 days [22]. In fact, a recent study has demonstrated that different Na^+,K^+-ATPase isoforms are expressed according to salinity in teleost fish. Thus, it is possible that these different isoforms could show different sensitivities to copper [23].

Regarding estuarine or marine crustaceans, there are no reports in the literature about the mechanism of copper toxicity. Recent studies developed in our laboratory aimed to determine the mechanisms of acute copper toxicity in two euryhaline crustaceans, the isopod *Excirolana armata* and the crab *Chasmagnathus granulata*, in a wide range of salinity. Up to date, results obtained show that in low salinities and in either the presence or the absence of food the mechanism of acute toxicity in the isopod, a copper sensitive species, is similar to that observed in freshwater fish and crustaceans [24], i.e., an iono- and osmoregulatory imbalance induced by Na^+,K^+-ATPase inhibition. However, results clearly indicate that in the crab, a copper tolerant species, the same mechanism of acute toxicity is not evident [25]. As recently reported for silver [26], a metal showing a similar mechanism of acute toxicity to that observed for copper in freshwater fish and crustaceans [14, for review], our data indicate that in sea water this mechanism is definitely not associated with an iono- and osmoregulatory imbalance at the hemolymph or whole body level. However, as reported for silver [26], ionoregulatory impairments at the cellular level cannot be ruled out.

4. Conclusions

The BLM was already validated and calibrated for copper using data from freshwater organisms. However, this model is largely based on data obtained from freshwater fish and is currently calibrated to protect freshwater invertebrates [5,6]. The extrapolation from fish to invertebrates must rely on the general assumption that the mechanism of toxicity induced by copper in the sensitive invertebrates is the same as those observed in the less sensitive teleost fish. According to the findings reported in the present paper, the key mechanism of acute copper toxicity in freshwater fish and crustaceans [14, for review], as well as in euryaline crustaceans exposed to copper in low salinities [24,25], is based on an iono- and osmoregulatory imbalance associated with an inhibition of the gill Na^+,K^+-ATPase. Thus, these findings clearly support the extrapolation done in the current version of the BLM for copper. However, further studies are needed for a better understanding of the key mechanism of acute toxicity in estuarine and marine fish and crustaceans exposed to copper in seawater. Despite the fact that there are strong evidences that copper is also an osmoregulatory toxicant in marine fish, our recent findings clearly indicate that the key mechanism of toxicity in euryhaline crustaceans exposed to copper in seawater is definitely not associated with an ionoregulatory imbalance at the hemolymph or whole body level.

Acknowledgements

This work was financially supported by the International Copper Association. A. Bianchini is a research fellow from the Brazilian CNPq (Proc. #302734/2003-1). S.E.G. Martins and I.F. Barcarolli are graduate fellows from the Brazilian CNPq (CT-Hidro).

References

[1] HydroQual, Biotic Ligand Model (BLM)-User's Guide for Version a008, HydroQual, New Jersey, 1999.

[2] P.R. Paquin, J.W. Gorsuch, S. Apte, et al., The biotic ligand model: a historical overview, Comp. Biochem. Physiol., C 133 (2002) 3–35.

[3] P.R. Paquin, D.M. DiToro, R.S. Santore, et al., A biotic ligand model of the acute toxicity of metals: III. Application to fish and Daphnia exposure to Ag. 822-E-99-001. Technical report, Washington: Environmental Protection Agency, Office of Water Regulations and Standards, 1999.

[4] J.C. McGeer, et al., A physiologically based biotic ligand model for predicting the acute toxicity of waterborne silver to rainbow trout in freshwaters, Environ. Sci. Technol. 34 (2000) 4199–4207.

[5] R.C. Santore, DiToro, DM, P.R. Paquin, A biotic ligand model of the acute toxicity of metals: II. Application to acute copper toxicity in freshwater fish and daphnia. Technical report, Washington: Environmental Protection Agency, Office of Water Regulations and Standards, 1999.

[6] R.C. Santore, D.M. Di Toro, P.R. Paquin, et al., Biotic Ligand Model of the acute toxicity of metals: 2. Application to acute copper toxicity in freshwater fish and Daphnia, Environ. Toxicol. Chem. 20 (10) (2001) 2397–2402.

[7] G.K. Pagenkopf, Gill surface interaction model for trace-metal toxicity to fishes: role of complexation, pH, and water hardness, Environ. Sci. Technol. 17 (1983) 342–347.

[8] R.J. Erickson, D.A. Benoit, V.R. Mattson, et al., The effects of water chemistry on the toxicity of copper to fathead minnows, Environ. Toxicol. Chem. 15 (1996) 181–193.

[9] R.F. Cusimano, D.F. Brakke, G.A. Chapman, Effects of pH on the toxicities of cadmium, copper, and zinc to steelhead trout (Salmo gairdneri), Can. J. Fish Aquat. Sci. 43 (1986) 1497–1503.

[10] P.G. Welsh, J.F. Skidmore, D.J. Spry, et al., Effects of pH and dissolved organic carbon on the toxicity of copper to larval fathead minnow (Pimephales promelas) in natural waters of low alkalinity, Can. J. Fish Aquat. Sci. 50 (1993) 1356–1362.

[11] V.M. Brown, T.L. Shaw, D.G. Shurben, Aspects of water quality and the toxicity of copper to rainbow trout, Water Res. 8 (1974) 797–803.

[12] R.K. MacRae, D.E. Smith, N. Swoboda-Colberg, et al., Copper binding affinity of rainbow trout (Oncorhynchus mykiss) and brook trout (Salvelinus fontinalis) gills, Environ. Toxicol. Chem. 18 (1999) 1180–1189.

[13] D.M. Di Toro, H.E. Allen, H.L. Bergman, et al., Biotic Ligand Model of the acute toxicity of metals: 1. Technical basis, Environ. Toxicol. Chem. 20 (10) (2001) 2383–2396.

[14] M. Grosell, C. Nielsen, A. Bianchini, Sodium turnover rate determines sensitivity to acute copper and silver exposure in freshwater animals, Comp. Biochem. Physiol., C 133 (2002) 287–303.

[15] K. Schmidt-Nielsen, Fisiologia Animal: Adaptação e Meio Ambiente, Santos Editora, São Paulo, 1996.
[16] I. Holm-Jensen, Osmotic regulation in *Daphnia magna* under physiological conditions and in the presence of heavy metals, K. Dan. Vidensk. Selsk., Biol. Medd. 20 (11) (1948) 4–64.
[17] S.J. Brooks, C.L. Mills, The effect of copper on osmoregulation in the freshwater amphipod *Gammarus pulex*, Comp. Biochem. Physiol. 135 (2003) 527–537.
[18] P.C. Castilho, I.A. Martins, A. Bianchini, Gill Na+,K+-ATPase and osmoregulation in the estuarine crab, *Chasmagnathus granulata* Dana, 1851 (Decapoda, Grapsidae), J. Exp. Mar. Biol. Ecol. 256 (2001) 215–227.
[19] G. Flik, T. Kaneko, A.M. Greco, et al., Sodium dependent transport, Fish Physiol. Biochem. 17 (1997) 385–396.
[20] A. Péqueux, Osmotic regulation in crustaceans, J. Crustac. Biol. 15 (1995) 1–60.
[21] S.F. Perry, The chloride cell: structure and function in the gills of freshwater fishes, Annu. Rev. Physiol. 59 (1997) 325–347.
[22] M. Grosell, et al., Effects of prolonged copper exposure in the marine gulf toadfish (*Opsanus beta*) II: copper accumulation, drinking rate and Na$^+$,K$^+$-ATPase activity in osmoregulatory tissues, Aquat. Toxicol. 68 (2004) 263–275.
[23] J.G. Richards, J.W. Semple, P.M. Schulte, Pattern of Na+,K+-ATPase isoform expression in rainbow trout (*Oncorhynchus mykiss*) following abrupt salinity transfer, Integr. Comp. Biol. 42 (2003) 1300.
[24] S.E.G. Martins. Mecanismos e limiares de toxicidade aguda do cobre no caranguejo eurialino *Chasmagnathus granulata* Dana, 1851 (Decapoda, Brachyura, Grapsidae): implicações para o modelo do ligante biológico. MSc thesis. Fundação Universidade Federal do Rio Grande. Rio Grande, RS, Brazil, 2004.
[25] Mecanismos e limiares de toxicidade aguda do cobre no isópodo eurialino *Excirolana armata* Dana, 1852 (Isopoda-Cirolanidade): implicações para o modelo do ligante biológico. MSc thesis. Fundação Universidade Federal do Rio Grande. Rio Grande, RS, Brazil, 2004.
[26] A. Bianchini, R.C. Playle, C.M. Wood, et al., Mechanism of acute silver toxicity in marine invertebrates, Aquat. Toxicol. (2004) (submitted for publication).

International Congress Series 1275 (2004) 195–200

ELSEVIER

www.ics-elsevier.com

Gill damage in *Oreochromis mossambicus* and *Tilapia sparrmanii* after short-term copper exposure

Daléne van Heerden[a,*], Louwrens R. Tiedt[b], André Vosloo[a]

[a]*School for Environmental Sciences and Development, North-West University, Potchefstroom Campus, Private Bag X6001, Potchefstroom 2520, South Africa*
[b]*Laboratory for Electron Microscopy, North-West University, Potchefstroom Campus, Potchefstroom, South Africa*

Abstract. *Oreochromis mossambicus* and *Tilapia sparrmanii* were exposed to 600 μg L^{-1} and 4.4 mg L^{-1}, respectively, of waterborne copper for 24 h. The arithmetic mean thickness of gill epithelium (H_{ar}), using a morphometric technique, was measured after 4 and 24 h of exposure for both fish species. Copper exposure caused the arithmetic thickness of gill epithelium in *O. mossambicus* to increase to 4.92±0.210 μm, after 24 h of exposure, which was significantly higher than the corresponding control value of 2.97±0.131 μm and that of the 4 h exposure value (3.08±0.142 μm), while the 4 h exposure value did not differ from the control values. The gill epithelial thickness of 6.07±0.156 μm for *T. sparrmanni* exposed to copper was already significantly higher than the control value of 4.96±0.205 μm after only 4 h of exposure. The increase in epithelial thickness remained during the entire 24 h of exposure, with the value for the exposed fish after 24 h (5.56±0.190 μm) being significantly higher than that of the control fish (4.99±0.137 μm). © 2004 Published by Elsevier B.V.

Keywords: Tilapia; *Oreochromis mossambicus*; *Tilapia sparrmanii*; Gill damage; Copper; Gas exchange

1. Introduction

Although an essential element for numerous enzymatic systems in fish, copper is extremely toxic in high concentrations [1]. Amongst others, high copper levels can cause fast generation of reactive oxygen species [2]. It also binds histidine-, cystein- and methionine-containing proteins, resulting in dysfunction [3].

* Corresponding author. Tel.: +27 18 299 2512; fax: +27 18 299 2503.
E-mail address: drkdvh@puk.ac.za (D. van Heerden).

0531-5131/ © 2004 Published by Elsevier B.V.
doi:10.1016/j.ics.2004.08.071

Fish gills are, due to their large surface area, the prime target for copper in water. In low-sodium water (typically ion-poor soft water) copper will be taken up through the apical sodium pathway in gills, inhibiting sodium uptake via gills. This is associated with the inhibition of Na^+/K^+ATP-ase [3,4]. The disruption of branchial ion regulation, due to high copper levels in water, can cause mortality in fish [5].

Copper was reported to also cause severe gill damage in *Prochilodus scrofa*, which included epithelial lifting, cell swelling and chloride and mucus cell proliferation. The damage from a 96-h copper exposure recovered only after 7 days [6]. Copper exposure for 24 h caused a significant increase in epithelial thickness in *Oncorhynchus mykiss* gills. Recovery of the increase epithelial thickness occurred within 48 h after exposure was terminated [7]. This increase in epithelial thickness was largely due to hypertrophy of epithelial cells, which was found to be most characteristic of heavy metal exposure (for review see Ref. [8]). Gill damage can be linked to impaired physiological function in fish [9].

Lease et al. [10] found gill histopathology to be useful as an early-warning tool to monitor fish health in the environment.

The present study compares changes in epithelial thickness in both *Tilapia sparrmanii* and *Oreochromis mossambicus* during a 24-h exposure to copper with control values at the same sampling times taken from fish where no copper was added to holding tanks.

2. Materials and methods

Mozambique tilapia (*O. mossambicus*) were obtained from the Aquaculture study group of the Stellenbosch University, Stellenbosch, South Africa. Banded tilapia (*T. sparrmanii*) were caught in Boskop Dam, Potchefstroom, South Africa. Fish were kept in dechlorinated tap water in the laboratory for at least 1 week prior to the experiments. Feeding was stopped 2 days before the experiments. Fish were divided into four groups (two exposure and two experimental groups of nine fish each) and transferred to four aerated tanks at least 12 h before the onset of experiments. Copper, in the form of copper sulphate ($CuSO_4 \cdot 5H_2O$) was added to the exposure tanks for a final calculated copper concentration of 600 µg L^{-1} for Mozambique Tilapia and 4.4 mg L^{-1} for Banded Tilapia. Abovementioned concentration for exposing *O. mossambicus* was based on concentrations used by Nussey et al. [11] for 96 h copper exposure but, due to the unavailability of data, the exposure concentration for Banded Tilapia was estimated from concentrations where physiological changes were detected (Van Aardt, unpublished results).

After 4 and 24 h of exposure, six copper-exposed fish and six control fish were stunned with a blow to the head and the second left gill arch was exposed and clamped both dorsally and ventrally with tongue forceps to stop blood flow. The arch was cut outside the forceps and immersed in ice-cold Todd's fixative [12]. Forceps were removed and fixing continued for at least 24 h at +20 °C.

Gill samples were treated at the Laboratory of Electron Microscopy, Potchefstroom University, South Africa. After fixing with Todd's fixative, gill filaments were cut from gill arch, post-fixed in 2% osmium tetroxide, stained with 2% uranile acetate and dehydrated in acetone. Filaments were then embedded in Spurr resin [13].

Semithin (1 μm) saggital sections were cut from gill filaments and stained with 0.5% toluidine blue. Digital images were taken at 100 times magnification and pictures were analyzed using a cycloidal grid [14] (Grid C) as described in Refs. [7,15], where the grid constant was 16.5 μm.

Data sets were tested for normal distribution by using a modified Kolmogorov–Smirnov (KS) test [16]. Two-way analysis of variance (ANOVA), using Tukey HSD post-hoc test (Statistica Version 6.1, STATSOFT) was used to determine statistical significance of data. All results were given in mean±standard error of the mean (S.E.M).

3. Results

Since water chemistry affects the bioavailability of copper, we cannot compare the concentrations of copper, as used in the experiments, to available copper LC_{50} values for *O. mossambicus* and *T. sparrmanii*. We ascertained that all fish survived the 24-h exposure period.

The two fish species reacted differently to copper exposure, as indicated by the changes in epithelial thickness (Figs. 1 and 2). Exposure to copper caused an increase in the epithelial thickness in the gills of *O. mossambicus* only after 24 h of exposure, where the epithelial thickness of 4.92±0.210 μm showed significant increase compared to both the control value of 2.97±0.131 μm and the 4 h exposure value of 3.08±0.142 μm. The 4 h exposure value was not significantly higher than the corresponding control value of 3.09±0.085 μm (Fig. 1).

Unlike *O. mossambicus*, significant increase in epithelial thickness in gills of *T. sparrmanii* occurred already after 4 h of copper exposure, where the value of exposed fish was 6.07±0.156 μm compared to the control value of 4.96±0.205 μm. The increased epithelial thickness of copper-exposed fish compared to that of control fish remained

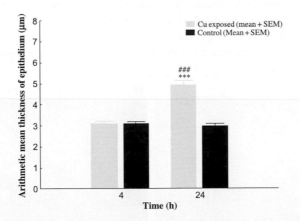

Fig. 1. Arithmetic mean thickness of gill epithelium of *O. mossambicus* exposed to 600 μg L^{-1} copper for 4 and 24 h as well as in gills of control fish sampled at these same time points as exposed fish. Means±S.E.M are given. Asterisks indicate statistically significant differences ($P<0.001$) between copper-exposed and control fish sampled at the same time point. Significant differences ($P<0.001$) between fish exposed for 4 and 24 h, respectively, are indicated with #'s ($N=23$ for 4 h exposed fish and $N=25$ for the others).

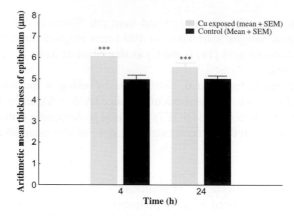

Fig. 2. Arithmetic mean thickness of gill epithelium of *T. sparrmanii* exposed to 4.4 mg L^{-1} copper for 4 and 24 h as well as in gills of control fish sampled at these same time points as exposed fish. Means±S.E.M is given. Asterisks indicate statistically significant differences ($P<0.001$) between copper-exposed and control fish sampled at the same time point. Significant differences ($P< 0.001$) between fish exposed for 4 and 24 h, respectively, are indicated with #'s ($N=25$).

constant for the rest of the experiment, with the value after 24 h exposure being 5.56±0.190 µm and that of the control 4.99±0.137 µm (Figs. 2 and 3).

4. Discussion

There are differences between basal H_{ar} values of different fish species. *O. mossambicus* has a mean basal H_{ar} value of 3.03 µm while *T. sparrmanni* has a mean basal H_{ar} value of 4.98 µm (this study). Studies done in Refs. [7,17] showed basal H_{ar} values for *O. mykiss* of 3.73 and 4.2 µm, respectively. In another study on the effects of copper on gill structure of *O. mykiss*, the mean basal H_{ar} value was found to be 3.9 µm (Van Heerden and Vosloo, unpublished results). Since there was no significant difference between the basal H_{ar} in three separate studies on *O. mykiss*, measuring mean arithmetic epithelial thickness indicates that this technique could be used to compare the changes in

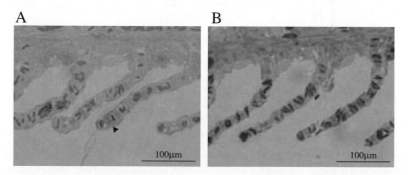

Fig. 3. Light micrographs of saggital sections through secondary lamellae of *T. sparrmanii* gills. Micrograph A shows gills exposed to copper for 4 h, where thickening of epithelium because of hypertrophy (▶) can clearly be seen as opposed to gills from control fish (B).

epithelial thickness within species from different experiments or collected from different locations during field based studies.

Although sublethal, the concentrations of copper used during these experiments were enough to cause severe gill damage in both *O. mossambicus* and *T. sparrmanii* as indicated by the highly significant increase in gill epithelial thickness during the 24 h copper exposure. An increase in gill epithelial thickness can lead to a decrease in the relative diffusion capacity of gills epithelium [17], which in turn could cause tissue hypoxia, as indicated in rainbow trout by an accumulation of HIF-1α proteins [7].

The thickening of epithelium in gills of fish exposed to copper was caused by hypertrophy in both pavement cells as well as lamellar telangiectasis as found during previous studies [6,7]. This is believed to be a compensatory response to keep metals from entering gill cells. Although it is indicated that the effects of copper exposure on gills could be reversed to a certain extent [6,7], permanent damage, for instance an increase in the number of necrotic and apoptotic cells, due to hypertrophy could occur [18].

Since we have found downstream physiological effects associated with the thickening of gill epithelium due to copper exposure in rainbow trout, further studies are now undertaken to determine whether or not H_{ar} can successfully be used as a general biomarker of environmental stress from metal impacted field sites. Downstream physiological effects measured in rainbow trout included an accumulation of hypoxia inducible factor-1α (HIF-1α) [7], as well as decrease in both pH_a and P_aO_2 (Van Heerden and Vosloo, unpublished results) after 4 h exposure to copper.

5. Conclusion

The results of this study supports the results from a similar study done on rainbow trout, proving that morphometric measurements on gills of fish could be an easy and effective indicator of toxic exposure. Since the gill damage occurred early during copper exposure, toxic effect could be detected before irreversible damage occurs.

References

[1] A.G. Heath, Water Pollution and Fish Physiology, CRC Press, Florida, 1995.
[2] Z.L. Harris, J.D. Githlin, Genetic and molecular basis for copper toxicity, Am. J. Clin. Nutr. 63 (1996) 836S–841S.
[3] M. Grosell, C.M. Wood, Copper uptake across rainbow trout gills: mechanisms of apical entry, J. Exp. Biol. 205 (2002) 1179–1188.
[4] C.M. Wood, Toxic responses of the gill, in: W.H. Benson, D.W. Schleuh (Eds.), Target Organ Toxicity in Marine and Freshwater Teleosts, Taylor and Francis, Washington, DC, 2001, pp. 1–87.
[5] D.J. Laurén, D.G. McDonald, Acclimation to copper by rainbow trout, *Salmo gairdneri*: physiology, Can. J. Fish. Aquat. Sci. 44 (1987) 99–104.
[6] C.C.C. Cerqureira, M.N. Fernandes, Gill tissue recovery after copper exposure and blood parameter responses in the tropical fish *Prochilodus scrofa*, Ecotox. Environ. Saf. 52 (2002) 83–91.
[7] D. Van Heerden, A. Vosloo, M. Nikinmaa, Effects of short-term copper exposure on gill structure, metallothionein and Hypoxia Inducible Factor-1α (HIF-1α) levels in Rainbow trout (*Oncorhynchus mykiss*), Aquat. Toxicol. 69 (2004) 271–280.
[8] J. Mallat, Fish gill structural changes induced by toxicants and other irritants: a statistical review, Can. J. Fish Aquat. Sci. 42 (1985) 630–648.
[9] D.F. Woodward, R.G. Riley, C.E. Smith, Accumulation, sublethal effects, and safe concentration of a refined oil as evaluated with cutthroat trout, Arch. Environ. Contam. Toxicol. 12 (1983) 455–464.

[10] H.M. Lease, et al., Structural changes in gills of Lost River suckers exposed to elevated pH and ammonia concentrations, Comp. Biochem. Physiol. C, Comp. Pharmacol. Toxicol. 134 (2003) 491–500.

[11] G. Nussey, J.H.J. Van Vuuren, H.H. Du Preez, Effect of copper on the haematology and osmoregulation of the Mozambique tilapia, *Oreochromis mossambicus*, Comp. Biochem. Physiol. C, Comp. Pharmacol. Toxicol. 111 (1995) 369–380.

[12] W.J. Todd, Effects of specimen preparation on the apparent ultrastructure of micro-organisms, in: H.C. Aldrich, W.J. Todd (Eds.), Ultrastructure Techniques for Micro-Organisms, Plenum, New York, 1986, p. 87.

[13] A.R. Spurr, A low-viscosity epoxy resin embedding medium for electron microscopy, J. Ultrastruct. Res. 26 (1969) 31–43.

[14] C.V. Howard, M.G. Reed, Unbiased Steriology: Three-Dimensional Measurement in Microscopy, BIOS Scientific Publishers, Oxford, 1998.

[15] H. Tuurala, Relationships between secondary lamellar structure and dorsal aortic oxygen tension in *Salmo gairdneri* with gills damaged by zinc, Ann. Zool. Fenn. 20 (1983) 235–238.

[16] G.E. Dallal, L. Wilkinson, An analytic approximation to the distribution of Liliefors's test statistic for normality, Am. Stat. 40 (1986) 294–296.

[17] J. Lappivaara, M. Nikinmaa, H. Tuurala, Arterial oxygen tension and the structure of the secondary lamellae of the gills in rainbow trout (*Oncorhynchus mykiss*) after acute exposure to zinc and during recovery, Aquat. Toxicol. 32 (1995) 321–331.

[18] Z. Dang, et al., Cortisol increases Na^+/K^+-ATPase density in plasma membranes of gill chloride cells in the freshwater Tilapia *Oreochromis mossambicus*, J. Exp. Biol. 203 (2002) 2349–2355.

International Congress Series 1275 (2004) 201–208

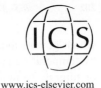

www.ics-elsevier.com

Combining studies of comparative physiology and behavioural ecology to test the adaptive benefits of thermal acclimation

Robbie S. Wilson[a],*, Ian A. Johnston[b]

[a]School of Life Sciences, The University of Queensland, St. Lucia, Brisbane, QLD 4072, Australia
[b]Gatty Marine Laboratory, University of St. Andrews, St. Andrews, Fife KY16 8LB, United Kingdom

Abstract. The effects of temperature on the reproductive behaviour of male eastern mosquito fish (*Gambusia holbrooki*) offer a novel system for examining the adaptive significance of thermal acclimation and developmental plasticity. The mating system of mosquito fish is dominated by male sexual coercion, which means that males rarely display to females, females almost never cooperate during copulations, and all matings are achieved by sneaky copulations. Throughout their native range, *G. holbrooki* also experience a wide seasonal range of temperatures and males display reproductive behaviours across different seasons between 18 and 34 °C. Preliminary experiments have revealed that temperature markedly influences both the propensity of males to follow females and their ability to obtain sneaky copulations. In addition, traits that are integral to obtaining sneaky copulations, such as swimming performance, are modified by acclimation temperature. Future studies will address the potential benefits and costs of temperature acclimation and the relative importance of altered locomotory performance and postcopulatory factors in determining reproductive success. © 2004 Elsevier B.V. All rights reserved.

Keywords: Sneaky mating; Beneficial acclimation hypothesis; Temperature

1. Introduction

Temperature affects the performance of all physiological traits in ectotherms [1]. Whole animal traits such as metabolic rate, and burst and sustained locomotor performance,

* Corresponding author. Tel.: +61 7 3365 1390; fax: +61 7 3365 1655.
E-mail address: rwilson@zen.uq.edu.au (R.S. Wilson).

0531-5131/ © 2004 Elsevier B.V. All rights reserved.
doi:10.1016/j.ics.2004.08.078

which govern much of the behavioural activities of organisms, are also highly influenced by temperature [1,2]. In aquatic ectotherms, the ability to select favourable microclimates or migrate to new habitats in response to daily or seasonal temperature change is often very limited. Many species can respond to long-term changes in temperature (usually seasonal changes) by changing their underlying physiology, often resulting in major changes in protein expression and tissue ultrastructure [3], a process known as thermal acclimation. Comparative physiologists have been relatively successful at documenting the mechanisms underlying these acclimation responses [1,4] and the responses to seasonal temperature change show wide variation between species [3].

For almost a century, comparative physiologists have assumed that all acclimation responses of organisms are beneficial. However, critics of the adaptationist program have highlighted that there are many alternatives to adaptive scenarios [5,6], including genetic drift, past selection, genetic correlations, and historical attributes [7]. Thus, to understand the evolutionary significance of a physiological response, it must be experimentally examined, not just assumed to be beneficial. During the last decade, physiologists have been adopting a more hypothesis-driven approach to examining evolutionary questions. A wide range of studies has utilized the strengths of this evolutionary approach in comparative physiology to create a deeper understanding of the evolution of physiological systems [8–10]. At the forefront of this approach are the recent studies of the adaptive significance of acclimation. The beneficial acclimation hypothesis (BAH) was proposed to describe the assumption that all acclimation responses enhance the fitness of an individual organism [11]. Using strict hypothesis-driven experimental designs, several studies have very successfully examined the benefits of temperature-induced phenotypic changes, in both the bacterium *Escherichia coli* and the fruit fly *Drosophila*. In contrast with predictions, most experimental tests of the BAH have rejected the generality of the assumption that all acclimation changes are beneficial [4,11–14]. Given that these studies used rigorous experimental designs to test and reject a long-held assumption within comparative physiology, they have been widely used as model examples for the necessity to test adaptive scenarios rather than simply assuming them.

Much of the rigorous nature of these experimental studies was afforded by the careful selection of model study organisms. The huge number of replicates, short generation times, and comparatively simple laboratory maintenance are all important advantages of utilizing these study species. However, there are also several important limitations with using either bacteria or *Drosophila* for testing the benefits of acclimation responses. In the majority of these studies, organisms have been reared at different temperatures over one or more generations at constant or fluctuating temperatures. A consequence of this experimental design is that temperature-induced developmental plasticity and 'reversible' temperature acclimation responses are confounded [15]. Temperature is known to interact with development in ectotherms, in some cases, to affect developmental outcome and the adult phenotype. In the case of fish, development temperature can affect vertebrae number, pigmentation patterns, sex ratios, ultimate body size [3], and the number of myotomal muscle fibres [16]. The reaction norms for developmental plasticity can be complex and have several components and be distinct from those observed for temperature acclimation responses in the same physiological system (Johnston and Wilson, in press). As comparative physiologists, most of our understanding of acclimation responses is based on the plethora of studies illuminating the particular reversible responses of organisms (mostly vertebrates), and their underlying mechanisms, to seasonal changes in the environment [1]. Whilst previous tests of the BAH have elegantly demonstrated the fitness consequences of developmental acclimation responses in organisms with short generation times, the adaptive benefits of more seasonal-type (or reversible) acclimation responses still remain to be investigated [15].

In many cases, the physiological traits under investigation in temperature acclimation studies were proxies of fitness, making analyses of only gross estimations or correlations of fitness possible. It was this difficulty with obtaining good estimates of fitness for physiological traits (in this case acclimation) that led to previous empirical tests of the BAH using analyses of growth and survival of *E. coli* over many generations, where good estimates or even direct measures of fitness could be obtained. However, a new experimental system needs to be established to allow the adaptive benefits and costs of temperature-induced developmental acclimation and seasonal-type temperature acclimation responses to be independently assessed. The purpose of this paper is to summarise some of our current research aimed at developing a new protocol for testing the adaptive benefits of thermal acclimation. In addition, we argue that many of the techniques that are routinely utilized in behavioural ecology could be effectively used to address novel questions related to and temperature adaptation and acclimation of physiological traits.

2. Using mating behaviour to study thermal acclimation in male mosquitofish

The effect of temperature on the reproductive behaviour of male eastern mosquito fish (*Gambusia holbrooki*) offers a novel system for examining questions about the adaptive significance of thermal acclimation and developmental plasticity. A long and successful history exists within behavioural ecology of studying the effects of variation in behaviour and morphology on the reproductive success of individual organisms. By utilizing the effects of temperature on the ability of male mosquito fish to obtain matings and subsequently sire offspring, it would be possible to test the benefits of thermal acclimation and developmental plasticity on their reproductive success.

The eastern mosquito fish is a small live-bearing poeciliid fish native to the southeastern waterways of the United States. Introduced as a combatant against mosquito populations, *G. holbrooki* is now distributed across most states of the United States (including Alaska) and most of the world's continents. Their broad temperature tolerance has led to their successful colonization of a wide range of thermal environments, from tropical to subarctic waterways [17]. Throughout their native range, *G. holbrooki* experience a wide seasonal range of temperatures, with males displaying reproductive behaviours and females giving birth over the range of temperatures of at least 18–34 °C (Ref. [17]; Wilson, unpublished data).

The mating system of *G. holbrooki* is dominated by male sexual coercion. This means that males almost never display to females, males have drab colours, females never cooperate during copulations, and all matings are achieved by thrusting of the almost intromittent organ toward the female genital pore. Thus, males almost solely rely on a sneaky strategy to obtain matings and often use extended bouts of male–male combat to obtain territories around uncooperative females to allow a greater number of coercive mating attempts [18–22].

An important requirement for utilizing the mating behaviour of male *G. holbrooki* to test hypotheses concerning temperature acclimation and adaptation is that the performance of sneaky mating is influenced by acute changes in temperature. Preliminary experiments reveal that male *G. holbrooki* attempt sneaky copulations across the temperature range of at least 14–34 °C (Fig. 1), representing one of the widest reproductively active temperature ranges for any ectotherm. To examine the effect of temperature on mating behaviour, male *G. holbrooki* were observed when introduced into an aquarium with a small group of mature females (Wilson, in preparation). Mating behaviour was found to be highly dependent on environmental temperature, and the total time males spent following females in pursuit of sneaky copulations varied from approximately 50% of their time at 14 °C to almost 95% of their time at 26 °C (Wilson, in preparation). The number of mating attempts performed by male *G. holbrooki* was also found to significantly vary across this temperature range (Fig. 1), suggesting that the thermal dependence of sneaky mating could be used as a measure of performance for analyses of thermal acclimation and adaptation.

Whole animal traits that most likely underlie the performance of sneaky mating behaviours, such as activity metabolism and burst and sustained locomotor performance, are highly influenced by acute changes in temperature (Ref. [23]; Wilson, unpublished data). In a study of thermal acclimation of aerobic performance, Hammill et al. [23] found that male *G. holbrooki* possessed the capacity to acclimate their maximum sustainable swimming performance following exposure to 18 or 30 °C for 2 months [23] (Fig. 2). The maximum sustainable swimming speeds of male *G. holbrooki* were 20% greater at 18 °C for the 18 °C-acclimated fish, and 15% greater at 30 °C for 30 °C-acclimated fish [23], indicating a classical tradeoff in performance following acclimation to a new temperature regime. Thus, the thermal acclimation of an aerobic measure of swimming performance suggests that the ability of male *G. holbrooki* to obtain matings and defend territories may also be influenced by acclimation.

Some of the possible physiological mechanisms associated with the acclimation responses observed in the swimming performance of male *G. holbrooki* were also investigated by Hammill et al. [23]. Cold acclimation was associated with a 40% increase

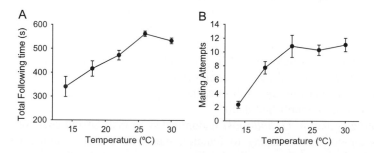

Fig. 1. Influence of temperature on (A) the time spent following females, and (B) the total number of mating attempts, by male eastern mosquitofish (*G. holbrooki*) during a 10-min observation period. Data represent mean±S.E. (*n*=10 for each test temperature) (Wilson, in preparation).

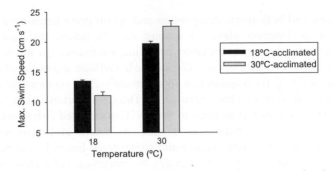

Fig. 2. Effect of temperature on the maximum sustained swimming performance of male mosquitofish, *G. holbrooki*, acclimated to either 18 or 30 °C for 2 months. Swimming performance at each test temperature was significantly different between acclimation groups ($n=15$ for each acclimation group tested at each temperature). Data represent mean±S.E. (data sourced from Ref. [23]).

in the total cross-sectional area of slow twitch and intermediate muscle in male *G. holbrooki*, reflecting an increase in average fibre diameter [23]. An S58 antibody raised against chicken slow skeletal muscle myosin stained a subset of the slow fibres identified by myosin ATPase staining. The number of S58-positive muscle fibres was 50% greater in 30 °C-acclimated than 18 °C-acclimated male *G. holbrooki*, implying that different MyHCs are being expressed in cold- and warm-acclimated individuals [23].

The effect of temperature on the sneaky-mating behaviour of male *G. holbrooki* was examined after exposure of fish to either 18 or 30 °C for 6 weeks (Fig. 3) (Wilson et al., in preparation). The total time each male spent in pursuit of females for sneaky copulations was determined at both experimental temperatures. Male *G. holbrooki* acclimated to 18 °C spent a greater amount of time following females at 18 °C than the 30 °C group, whilst there was no difference between the groups when tested at 30 °C (Fig. 3). Future studies will investigate the ability of male *G. holbrooki* from different acclimation temperatures to obtain sneaky copulations and sire offspring.

Various reproductive and postcopulatory processes could also have marked effects on the benefits of thermal acclimation for male *G. holbrooki*. Factors such as the motility and

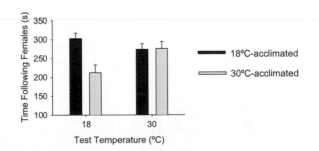

Fig. 3. Effect of thermal acclimation on the total time male *G. holbrooki* spent following females in pursuit of copulations at 18 and 30 °C during a 5-min period when introduced into an aquarium with two mature females. Significant differences were detected between acclimation groups at both test temperatures ($n=20$ for each acclimation group). Data represent mean±S.E. (data sourced from Wilson et al., in preparation).

viability of sperm and both sperm competition and sperm precedence could all influence the role thermal acclimation plays for mating success across different temperatures [24,25]. For example, thermal acclimation has a huge influence on the total number of sperm available in the ejaculate of male *G. holbrooki* (Wilson, unpublished data) (Fig. 4). Fish maintained at 32 °C for 6 weeks had approximately three times as many sperm cells in a single ejaculate than fish acclimated to 18 °C. Thus, fish acclimated to 32 °C may only require one third the number of matings of the 18 °C-acclimated fish to release the same number of sperm into the female genital tract. As many of the techniques for the assessment of postcopulatory mate choice and competition have already been developed for *G. holbrooki* and other poeciliid fish [26,27], the importance of thermal acclimation on postcopulatory performance of male *G. holbrooki* would also be an interesting area for future discussion and research. Studies could also utilize modern genetic microsatellite analyses of paternity to examine the relative reproductive success of male *G. holbrooki* from different acclimation and developmental temperature environments [28].

Other potential study systems already exist for combining analyses of behavioural ecology and comparative physiology for examining questions related to temperature adaptation in ectotherms. For example, body temperature has been reported to influence the call structure of many species of frogs [29,30]. Calling in male frogs represents one of the most energetically demanding sustainable activities for any ectotherm [31]. The implications of temperature-mediated variation in call structure on their ability to attract mates remain to be explored. Most of our current knowledge of selection and divergence of thermal performance traits is based on physiological systems that are not directly related to either the ability to attract or acquire matings. Measures of whole animal performance that have a direct connection with the ability to acquire mates and reproduce are likely to be under strong directional selection. Predictions that thermal performance traits related to mating performance would demonstrate greater or more rapid divergence between populations or species from different thermal environments could be tested. Incorporating analyses of behavioural ecology into studies of comparative physiology could also address the importance of sexual selection on the evolution of thermal dependence curves, both through phenotypic acclimation and, over several generations, via genetic adaptation.

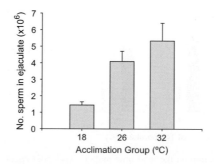

Fig. 4. Influence of acclimation temperature on the total number of sperm cells present in a stripped ejaculate from male eastern mosquitofish (*G. holbrooki*). Data represent mean±S.E. (n=10 for each acclimation group) (Wilson, unpublished data).

3. Conclusions

Although this research is still at an early stage of development, we suggest that the mating performance of male eastern mosquitofish is an interesting system for examining questions related to both temperature adaptation and acclimation. The mosquitofish has been introduced throughout most of the world's continents and now inhabits a wide diversity of thermal environments, from localities that experience highly variable daily fluctuations in temperature to daily stable but seasonally shifting conditions. Future research will address the benefits and costs of thermal acclimation to the reproductive success of male *G. holbrooki* as well as the detailed physiological mechanisms involved.

Acknowledgments

We thank the Royal Society of Engineering and Science UK and the Australian Research Council for funding. R.S.W. is currently an ARC Postdoctoral Fellow at UQ. We also thank a UQ Startup Fund that allowed the principal author to attend this symposium.

References

[1] C.L. Prosser, Comparative Animal Physiology, John Wiley and Sons, New York, 1979.

[2] I.A. Johnston, A.F. Bennett, Animals and Temperature: Phenotypic and Evolutionary Adaptation. Society for Experimental Biology Seminar Series, Cambridge University Press, Cambridge, 1996.

[3] I.A. Johnston, G.K. Temple, Thermal plasticity of skeletal muscle phenotype in ectothermic vertebrates and its significance for locomotory behaviour, J. Exp. Biol. 205 (2002) 2305–2322.

[4] R.B. Huey, D.A. Berrigan, Testing evolutionary hypotheses of acclimation, in: I.A. Johnston, A.F. Bennett (Eds.), Animals and Temperature: Phenotypic and Evolutionary Adaptation. Society for Experimental Biology Seminar Series, Cambridge University Press, Cambridge, 1996, pp. 205–237.

[5] T. Garland Jr., P.A. Carter, Evolutionary physiology, Ann. Rev. Ecolog. Syst. 56 (1994) 579–621.

[6] M.E. Feder, A.F. Bennett, R.B. Huey, Evolutionary physiology, Ann. Rev. Ecolog. Syst. 31 (2000) 315–341.

[7] S.J. Gould, R.C. Lewontin, The spandrels of San Marco and the Panglossian Paradigm: a critique of the adaptationist programme, Proc. R. Soc. Lond. 205 (1979) 581–598.

[8] J.G. Kingsolver, R.B. Huey, Evolutionary analyses of morphological and physiological plasticity in thermally variable environments, Am. Zool. 38 (1998) 545–560.

[9] A.F. Bennett, R.E. Lenski, Experimental evolution and its role in evolutionary physiology, Am. Zool. 39 (1999) 346–362.

[10] T.J. Bradley, A.E. Williams, M.R. Rose, Physiological responses to selection for desiccation resistance in *Drosophila*, Am. Zool. 39 (1999) 337–341.

[11] A.M. Leroi, et al., Temperature acclimation and competitive fitness: an experimental test of the beneficial acclimation assumption, Proc. Natl. Acad. Sci. U. S. A. 91 (1994) 1917–1921.

[12] A.F. Bennett, R.E. Lenski, Evolutionary adaptation to temperature: VI. Phenotypic acclimation and its evolution in *Escherichia coli*, Evolution 51 (1997) 36–44.

[13] R.B. Huey, et al., Testing the adaptive significance of acclimation: a strong inference approach, Am. Zool. 39 (1999) 323–336.

[14] P. Gibert, R.B. Huey, G.W. Gilchrist, Locomotor performance of *Drosophila melanogaster*: interactions among developmental and adult temperatures, age, and geography, Evolution 55 (2001) 205–209.

[15] R.S. Wilson, C.E. Franklin, Testing the beneficial acclimation hypothesis, Trends Ecol. Evol. 17 (2002) 66–70.

[16] I.A. Johnston, et al., Embryonic temperature modulates muscle growth characteristics in larval and juvenile herring, J. Exp. Biol. 201 (1998) 623–646.

[17] A.H. Arthington, L.N. Lloyd, Introduced poeciliids in Australia and New Zealand, in: G.K. Meffe, F.F. Snelson Jr. (Eds.), Ecology and Evolution of Livebearing Fishes (Poeciliidae), Prentice Hall, New Jersey, 1989.

[18] A. Bisazza, G. Marin, Male size and female mate choice in the eastern mosquitofish (*Gambusia holbrooki*, Poeciliidae), Copeia 1991 (1991) 730–735.

[19] M.A. McPeek, Mechanisms of sexual selection operating on body size in the mosquito fish (*Gambusia holbrooki*), Behav. Ecol. 3 (1992) 1–12.

[20] A. Bisazza, G. Marin, Sexual selection and sexual size dimorphism in the eastern mosquitofish *Gambusia holbrooki* (Pisces Poeciliidae), Ethol. Ecol. Evol. 7 (1995) 169–183.

[21] A. Pilastro, E. Giacomello, A. Bisazza, Sexual selection for small size in male mosquitofish (*Gambusia holbrooki*), Proc. R. Soc. Lond., B 264 (1997) 1125–1129.

[22] J.L. Gould, et al., Female preferences in a fish genus without female mate choice, Curr. Biol. 9 (1999) 497–500.

[23] E. Hammill, R.S. Wilson, I.A. Johnston, Sustained swimming performance and muscle structure are altered by thermal acclimation in male mosquitofish, J. Therm. Biol. 29 (2004) 251–257.

[24] M. Andersson, Sexual Selection, Princeton University Press, Princeton, NY, 1994.

[25] C.W. Petersen, R.R. Warner, Sperm competition in fishes, in: T.R. Birkhead, A.P. Moller (Eds.), Sperm Competition and Sexual Selection, Academic Press, London, 1998.

[26] J.P. Evans, M. Pierotti, A. Pilastro, Male mating behaviour and ejaculate expenditure under sperm competition risk in the eastern mosquitofish, Behav. Ecol. 14 (2002) 268–273.

[27] J.P. Evans, et al., Directional postcopulatory sexual selection revealed by artificial insemination, Nature 421 (2003) 360–363.

[28] L. Zane, et al., Microsatellite assessment of multiple paternity in natural populations of a live-bearing fish, *Gambusia holbrooki*, J. Evol. Biol. 12 (1999) 61–69.

[29] H.C. Gerhardt, Temperature coupling in the vocal communication system of the gray tree frog, *Hyla versicolor*, Science 199 (1978) 992–994.

[30] D.C. Gayou, Effects of temperature on the mating call of *Hyla versicolor*, Copeia 1984 (1984) 733–738.

[31] T.U. Grafe, J. Thein, Energetics of calling and metabolic substrate use during prolonged exercise in the European treefrog *Hyla arborea*, J. Comp. Physiol., B 171 (2001) 69–76.

International Congress Series 1275 (2004) 209–217

ELSEVIER

www.ics-elsevier.com

Ontogenetic patterns in thermal adaptation of fish vs. long-term temperature trends in large rivers

F. Schiemer[a,*], H. Keckeis[a], H. Nemeschkal[b], E. Schludermann[a], G. Winkler[a], I. Zweimüller[a]

[a]*Department of Limnology, Institute of Ecology and Conservation Biology, University of Vienna, Althanstrasse 14, A-1090 Vienna, Austria*
[b]*Department of Systematic Zoology and Developmental History, Institute of Zoology, University of Vienna, Althanstrasse 14, A-1090 Vienna, Austria*

Abstract. Rheophilic fish species characteristic of large river systems are finely tuned during early ontogenetic development to the seasonal temperature regime of their main nursery habitats in the inshore zones of rivers. River regulation and the construction of hydropower dams have disrupted the balance between requirements and the field conditions. Frequently, temperatures fall below the optimal range in regulated rivers due to faster runoff and reduced inshore retention capacity. Under such conditions, growth through the "critical period" during the life history is retarded resulting in high mortality rates. This is a main reason for the decline of stocks and a critical state of recruitment of many riverine species. The trends caused by long-term climatic changes have to be similarly addressed from the point of view of match or mismatch between requirements and the predicted changes in environmental conditions. Long-term trends in the temperature development have been analyzed for the Austrian Danube. The potential effect of such trends is tested against the temperature dependence of embryogenesis and a growth model developed for one of our target species, the cyprinid *Chondrostoma nasus*. Field data on individual daily growth rates of larval fish, based on otolith analysis, show that the present conditions are critical. The consequences of global change for rheophilic fish species in large river systems are discussed. © 2004 Elsevier B.V. All rights reserved.

Keywords: Fish larvae; Critical stage; Ontogenetic niche; Differentiation; Energetics; Efficiencies; Ecophysiology; Growth model; Global change; Match–mismatch

* Corresponding author. Tel.: +43 1 4277 54340; fax: +43 1 4277 9542.
E-mail address: friedrich.schiemer@univie.ac.at (F. Schiemer).

0531-5131/ © 2004 Elsevier B.V. All rights reserved.
doi:10.1016/j.ics.2004.09.039

1. Introduction

Along the river course, characteristic fish associations are adapted to prevailing temperature regimes. The longitudinal thermal profile of rivers resembles to some extent the latitudinal geographical pattern. Local success of species is dependent on the match or mismatch between requirements and field conditions during the early life history, which is the critical phase, the bottleneck, deciding on success or failure of a species. The fine tuning between requirements and environmental conditions has been considerably disrupted by river engineering (dams, reduction of inshore retention [1]). Global warming is a further factor which has to be taken into account.

The study analyzes (a) the thermal ranges and ontogenetic niche shifts of characteristic species during the early life history, (b) its optima and constraints with regard to temperature, (c) identifies long-term trends in the temperature development of the Danube river and (d) analyzes the potential effects of such trends on characteristic fish species.

2. The thermal niche of riverine fish species

Three fish species are representative for the longitudinal distribution of fish in European rivers. Brown trout (*Salmo trutta*) is characteristic for the upper rithral zone. The nase (*Chondrostoma nasus*) is a cyprinid, typical for large and structured river systems and a representative of the barbel-zone [2,3]. The roach (*Rutilus rutilus*), again a cyprinid, is a eurytopic species occurring in the upper and lower potamal stretches and different types of stagnant water bodies [4]. A comparison of the thermal niche dimensions of the three species with respect to the position in the thermal gradient, the optimum and tolerance range during embryogenesis (until hatching) and the early larval (nase and roach) or juvenile phase (brown trout) shows that the viable range for embryogenesis is similar in all three species (in the order of 9–10 °C) and widens with

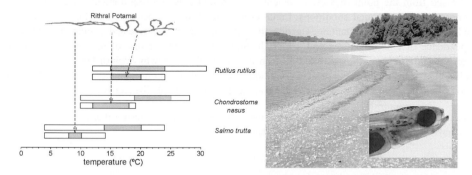

Fig. 1. The viable (white) and the optimal temperature range (grey) of embryogenesis (lower bar) and larval development (upper bar) of three species characteristic for different fish regions along the longitudinal range of rivers. The upper insert presents a sketch on the hydromorphological and biocoentic zonation, rithral and potamal of rivers as physiographically determined by a.o. current velocity pattern, substrate. Data on thermal ranges according to: *S. trutta*, embryogenesis [5]; early juvenile period [6]. *C. nasus*, embryogenesis [7]; larval period [8]. *R. rutilus*, embryogenesis [9], larval period [10]. The photo shows a characteristic nursery zone for rheophilic fish in the Danube and a larval nase.

stage and size. There is a distinct shift in optimal temperatures from egg development to the later stages which is more expressed in the two riverine species trout and nase than in roach and which apparently reflects the rise of temperature after the spawning periods in rivers (Fig. 1).

3. Microhabitat requirements and thermal niche shifts in the nase, *C. nasus*

C. nasus has become a flagship species for the ecology and conservation of large European rivers. The thermal requirements of the species are closely linked to conditions of larger and structurally rich river sections. A clear habitat shift in the course of the life cycle is apparent: rithral gravel bars are required for spawning. The spawning period occurs characteristically in April at river temperatures between 8 and 12 °C [11]. As larval microhabitats richly structured inshore zones of rivers are required which offer a combination of low current velocity, high production of zooplankton as larval food and refuge possibilities in the case of floods. With increasing size, the preferred microhabitats shift towards more lotic conditions.

Detailed experimental studies have been carried out on the early life history stages recognizing that they are critical for recruitment. Fig. 2 provides information on the temperature dependence of egg development [7]. Embryogenesis under constant conditions takes place over a range between 10 and 19 °C. Mortality increases strikingly below and above this range. It is of significance to note that temperature not only determines duration but also changes the pattern of development: at higher values the hatching of the embryos, the up-swimming of larvae and the onset of exogenous feeding occur at a distinctly smaller body size (tissue weight), at a less advanced stage of lower morphological differentiation but with a higher remaining yolk reserve (Fig. 2b). This strategic shift indicating trade-offs between size, duration and the conservation of energy reserves is schematically outlined in Fig. 2c.

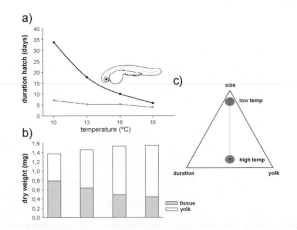

Fig. 2. Temperature dependence of (a) duration of embryogenesis, full line: fertilization until hatching, broken line: hatching until onset of feeding; (b) size of larvae at hatching (grey) and the remaining yolk reserve (white) and (c) temperature induced shifts between size, duration and yolk reserve at hatching.

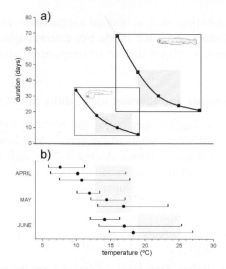

Fig. 3. (a) Temperature dependence of duration of embryogenesis from fertilization until hatch and from hatch to the end of the larval period. The rectangles delineate the temperature window (range of viable temperatures, range of low mortality), the shaded zone indicates the optimal ranges (see text). (b) Monthly mean temperature (black point) and range for April, May and June in a cold year (upper line), respectively a warm year (middle line) from the series of 1951–1995. The lower line represents the prognosis for 2050 based on the trend analysis. Inserted is the optimal temperature range for embryogenesis (April, May) and the larval period (June).

Fig. 3a illustrates the temperature dependence of stage duration of embryogenesis and the larval period. It clearly shows the shift in the viable and the optimum range in the consecutive stages, which occurs within a short period of time and developmental phase. A distinct succession of thermal adaptations is evident. This shift is very pronounced—in the order of 8–10 °C in the first phase of ontogeny—and occurs over a short period of time (duration) in the order of days.

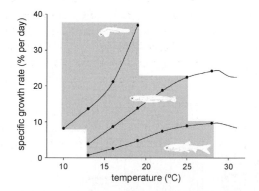

Fig. 4. Growth rates of three ontogenetic phases of *C. nasus* grown during larval phase over a wide range from 10 to 28 °C under constant temperatures and ad libitum food supply (for methodological details, see Refs. [7,8]). Since embryogenesis is limited to a temperature range between 10 and 19 °C, larval growth at higher temperatures were studied from larvae hatched at 16 °C.

Table 1
Size dependent growth rates in dependence of temperature, calculated as the allometric function $G=aW^b$

	A	B
15 °C	0.0997	0.298
20 °C	0.1994	0.249
25 °C	0.3003	0.236

Temperature dependence of larval growth rates has been experimentally studied over a wide experimental range from 10 to 28 °C. A Gompertz type model of the form:

$$F_{(T,D)} = A_c \exp\left[e^{\alpha T} D^\gamma\right] = A_c \exp\left[e^{\alpha T} D^{\gamma \ln D}\right]$$

could be fitted over the whole temperature range applied to the experimental data for the larval and juvenile period in terms of body length and dry weight (dwt) by polynomial regression with temperature and age (duration) as the independent variables.

Fig. 4 compares specific growth rates during embryogenesis, the larval and the early juvenile period. Growth rates are particularly high during the egg development phase (i.e. the conversion from yolk into tissue, data from Kamler et al. [7]) and decrease with size and stage. The size dependence between the onset of exogenous feeding (1–5 mg dwt) to the juvenile stage (over 100 mg dwt) at different temperatures are given in Table 1. The figure also illustrates both the shift and an expansion of the thermal niche from the larval to the early juvenile period by an increase of Q_{10}-values for growth with size (Table 2).

It is well established that within the early life history the period from onset of feeding until full yolk resorption of larvae (mixed feeding period) and the larval period of entirely exogenous feeding is the most critical [12–14]. The morphological differentiation related to the sensory, feeding, swimming and respiratory functions has to occur fast. Considering the low metabolic scope and the high and competitive requirements for growth, differentiation and maintenance, the temperature range providing for optimal fitness has to be defined by a combination of characteristics:

- energetics, both power and efficiencies, determine the scope for growth and development,
- the attained body size of characteristic stages are significant with regard to the swimming, escape and feeding performances and determine the "point of no return",
- duration, the time required to reach a certain stage relates to the cumulative risks larval fish are exposed to in a stochastic nursery microhabitat.

There is indication that within the viable temperature range the various functions are accelerated with temperature at different speeds [15] leading to a set of different solutions.

Table 2
Q_{10}-values of growth over the range of linear increase (13–25 °C)

Size class (mg dry weight)	1–5	5–30	30–50	50–80	80–200
Q_{10}	3.34	3.30	3.68	3.84	4.41

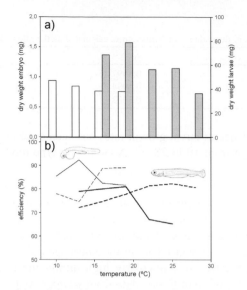

Fig. 5. (a) Temperature dependence of size of larvae at the onset of exogenous feeding (white) and at the end of the larval phase. Note that for hatching larvae and finite larval size different scales are used. (b) Assimilation efficiency (*A/C* in percent): solid lines; production efficiency (*P/A*): broken lines. Embryogenesis (data from Refs. [1,7]): thin lines; exogenously feeding larvae [1,8]: thick lines.

At present, we cannot answer the question if they are the result of trade-offs and constraints or represent an adaptive strategy in the sense that different solutions provide an array of chances under stochastic environmental conditions with frequently occurring suboptimal conditions (temperature, food, oxygen supply, water velocity), which will have cumulative effects.

In order to define the "optimum range", Fig. 5 compares two major fitness qualities during early ontogeny and its dependence from temperature. The upper panel compares body size at hatching (white) and the finite larval size (grey; note the different scale). At higher temperatures, both of these endpoints are attained at smaller body mass. The lower panel compares bioenergetic efficiencies: it is interesting to note that temperature dependence of assimilation efficiency ($A/C \times 100$) decreases in the upper viable range during both phases while production efficiency ($P/C \times 100$) increases. This comparison illustrates that optimality cannot be narrowly defined.

4. Merging field ecology, global trends, bioenergetics and conservation

How do these requirements match with conditions larval fish encounter in the field?

In order to answer this question, we have to assess the relevant environmental conditions and their spatiotemporal variability in the larval microhabitats in the inshore zones of rivers [3]. Richly structured inshore zones are the main nurseries of riverine fish. They are characterized by higher temperatures and a higher plankton (=food) production compared to the main stem of the river, depending on the water retention ("Inshore Retention Concept": [16]).

Fig. 6 provides an example of a detailed study on early larval growth in an inshore location with high water retention of the free-flowing Danube downstream of Vienna in Austria with comparatively good growth conditions. The individual growth pattern can be traced-back from daily ring formations using the otolith microstructure. The growth trajectories of two larvae show that the growth rates are not synchronized. The grey band represents the growth variability encountered within a group of larvae analyzed from a particular catch. The overall slope of the growth band of the cohort can be compared with continuous temperature recordings in the nursery microhabitat. Inserted are the continuous temperature recordings in the nursery microhabitat.

The overall slope of the growth band can be compared with the temperature dependent growth rates in terms of larval length found in the experimental cultures. It becomes apparent that suboptimal conditions are decisive for low growth rates in the field leading to prolonged risks in a stochastic environment.

How critical are the present temperature conditions and what are the long-term trends?

The trends illustrated in Fig. 7 are analyzed for the conditions in high retention inshore zones. It has to be emphasized that the observed trends not only represent global climatic changes but that they are additionally influenced by other impacts on the river system (hydropower dams, connectivity of the river–floodplain system).

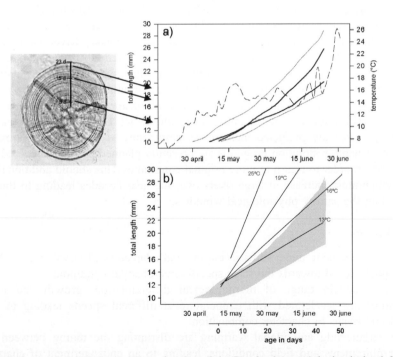

Fig. 6. (a) Early larval growth in an inshore location of the Danube (see text) back-calculated from daily increments of the otoliths of larvae collected at a specific date. Two individual growth trajectories (solid line) and the width of the "growth band" (shaded). Broken line: continuous temperature recordings in the nursery habitat. (b) Experimental growth data compared to field growth.

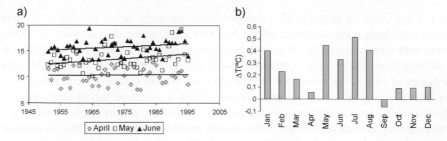

Fig. 7. (a) Long-term trends (1951–1996) of inshore temperature regime calculated from the daily readings and the divergence pattern of inshore temperatures at highly structured inshore locations in the free-flowing Austrian Danube downstream of Vienna. The trends (linear regressions) are given for the April, May and June when most spawning activities and early fish development takes place. (b) Seasonal pattern of temperature changes in fish nursery habitats calculated for a 10-year period.

In order to outline the match–mismatch between the physiological requirements and the field situation in a high quality nursery situation, the temperature dependence of stage duration are set in comparison to the conditions for April, May and June, when early life history takes place in the field. Monthly means and the range of daily values have been selected for a year with low and high temperatures from the series from 1951 to 1995. The third line represents the prognosis for 2050 based on the trend analysis. The graph clearly demonstrates that present temperature conditions are suboptimal and embryonic development is retarded. The same holds good for the larval phase. River engineering, the straightening of the river course and the loss of inshore retention zones have reduced the overall spring temperatures and a disruption in the synchronization between the physiological program of riverine species and the environmental temperature regime. At a first glance, it would mean that over a time scale of approximately 100 years global warming could improve the situation and counteract the deficiencies caused by engineering. Even the predicted increase in temperature is outside the optimal range. On the other hand, restoration programs are presently planned and implemented (e.g. for the Danube) in order to return to more original conditions. This should additionally speed up the temperature increase in large rivers over the next decades leading to the risks of overshooting the narrow physiological windows.

5. Conclusions

Distinct ontogenetic niche shifts in the thermal adaptation of larval stages of riverine fish are finely tuned towards the stage-specific microhabitat conditions.

Within a certain range of morphological differentiation, growth and metabolic expenditures are accelerated with temperature at different speeds leading to a set of different end-points in character combination.

River engineering and global warming are disrupting the tuning between physiological requirements and field conditions, leading to an endangerment of characteristic species.

Programs defined to analyze their ecophysiological requirements are essential for guiding management, restoration and conservation.

References

[1] F. Schiemer, H. Keckeis, E. Kamler, The early life history stages of riverine fish: ecophysiological and environmental bottlenecks, CBP, A 133 (2003) 439–449.

[2] M. Penaz, *Chondrostoma nasus*—its reproduction strategy and possible reasons for a widely observed population decline—a review, in: A. Kirchhofer, D. Hefti (Eds.), Conservation of Endangered Freshwater Fish in Europe, Birkhäuser Verlag, Bern, 1996, pp. 279–285.

[3] F. Schiemer, Fish as indicators for the assessment of the ecological integrity of large rivers. Proceedings on a workshop on ecological integrity in Vienna, Hydrobiologia 422/423 (2000) 271–278.

[4] F. Schiemer, W. Wieser, Epilogue: food and feeding, ecomorphology, energy assimilation and conversion ion cyprinids, Environ. Biol. Fishes 33 (1992) 223–227.

[5] A.F. Ojanguren, F. Brana, Thermal dependence of embryonic growth and development in brown trout, J. Fish Biol. 62 (2003) 580–590.

[6] A.F. Ojanguren, F.G. Reyes-Gavilan, F. Brana, Thermal sensitivity of growth, food intake and activity of juvenile brown trout, J. Therm. Biol. 26 (2001) 165–170.

[7] E. Kamler, H. Keckeis, E. Bauer-Nemeschkal, Temperature-induced changes of survival, development and yolk-partitioning in *Chondrostoma nasus*, J. Fish Biol. 53 (1998) 658–682.

[8] H. Keckeis, et al., Survival, development and food energy partitioning of nase larvae and early juveniles at different temperatures, J. Fish Biol. 59 (2001) 45–61.

[9] W. Wieser, et al., Growth rates and growth efficiencies in larvae and juveniles of *Rutilus rutilus* and other cyprinid species: effects of temperature and food in the laboratory and in the field, Can. J. Fish. Aquat. Sci. 45 (1988) 943–950.

[10] W.M. Mooij, O.F.R. Van Tongeren, Growth of 0+ roach (*Rutilus rutilus*) in relation to temperature and size in a shallow eutrophic lake: comparison of field and laboratory observations, Can. J. Fish. Aquat. Sci. 47 (1990) 960–967.

[11] H. Keckeis, Influence of river morphology and current velocity conditions on spawning site selection of *Chondrostoma nasus* (L.), Arch. Hydrobiol., Suppl. 113 Large Rivers 10 (2001) 51–64.

[12] J.H.S. Blaxter, The effect of temperature on larval fishes, Neth. J. Zool. 42 (1992) 336–357.

[13] E. Kamler, Early Life History of Fish. An Energetics Approach, Chapman & Hall, 1992, 267 pp.

[14] W. Wieser, Energetics of fish larvae, the smallest vertebrates, Acta Physiol. Scand. 154 (1995) 279–290.

[15] C.C. Lindsay, A.N. Arnason, A model for responses of vertebral numbers in fish to environmental influences during development, Can. J. Fish. Aquat. Sci. 42 (1981) 31–38.

[16] F. Schiemer, et al., The "inshore retention concept" and its significance for large rivers, Arch. Hydrobiol., Suppl. 135 (2001) 509–516.

International Congress Series 1275 (2004) 218–225

ELSEVIER

www.ics-elsevier.com

Placental function in lizards

Michael B. Thompson[a,*], Susan M. Adams[a], Jacquie F. Herbert[a],
Joanna M. Biazik[b], Christopher R. Murphy[b]

[a]*Integrative Physiology Research Group, School of Biological Sciences, The University of Sydney, Australia*
[b]*Anatomy & Histology and Institute for Biomedical Research, The University of Sydney, Australia*

Abstract. Frequent evolution of viviparity in squamate reptiles provides excellent models for study of the transition from oviparity to viviparity, and the evolution of complex placentae. Embryonic reptiles have a chorioallantoic placenta at the embryonic pole of the egg, and an omphaloplacenta at the abembryonic pole. The uterus of viviparous reptiles and mammals exhibits common plasma membrane transformation including uterodome formation associated with pregnancy. The transition from oviparity to viviparity requires few changes: (1) reduction in an eggshell, (2) delay of expulsion of oviposition/birth, (3) increased vascularisation of the uterus for gas exchange. We used immunohistochemistry to address the question of eggshell thinning in a range of species, and SEM and TEM to infer the functions of different placental regions in one species with a complex placenta. We conclude that: (1) changes in the calcium channels among species accompany the evolution of viviparity; (2) the omphaloplacenta has a role in nutrient transport via apocrine secretion and histotrophy; (3) the placentome has a role in nutrient transport, but not via apocrine secretion; (4) the paraplacentome of the chorioallantoic placenta has a major role in gas exchange. © 2004 Elsevier B.V. All rights reserved.

Keywords: Viviparity; Evolution; Calcium; Omphaloplacenta; Placentotrophy

1. Introduction

Live-bearing, or viviparity, has evolved many times in animals, resulting in many mechanisms of nutrient transport to embryos growing within the mother's body [1]. Mechanisms of nutrient transport within the Amniota are constrained, however, by the highly conserved nature of the extraembryonic membranes that form the embryonic

---

* Corresponding author. Tel.: +61 2 9351 3989; fax: +61 2 9351 4119.
E-mail address: thommo@bio.usyd.edu.au (M.B. Thompson).

0531-5131/ © 2004 Elsevier B.V. All rights reserved.
doi:10.1016/j.ics.2004.08.055

placental structures [2]. Nevertheless, viviparity has evolved approximately 100 times within one major amniote clade, the squamate reptiles (lizards and snakes) [1], and the occurrence of a plasma membrane transformation seems widespread, if not universal, in lizards [3,4]. The occurrence of such a large number of independent origins of viviparity within one clade suggests that few molecular changes are required for viviparity to evolve, providing an excellent model system in which to investigate the evolution of viviparity. Within the Squamata, the lizard family Scincidae exhibits the largest number of independent origins of viviparity [5] and displays the greatest range of placental complexities [6]. Consequently, we have used the Scincidae as our model to address questions of the evolution of viviparity.

Given that eggs of oviparous lizards contain all the nutrients required for embryonic development except oxygen and water [2], the retention of eggs in the uterus during the early stages of the evolution of viviparity requires only: (1) reduction in an eggshell to facilitate gas and water exchange, (2) delay of expulsion of the conceptus, and (3) increased vascularisation of the uterus for gas exchange. Consequently, there is no need for the appearance of any novel anatomical features to facilitate viviparity in its simplest form.

The extraembryonic membranes of viviparous species develop into two structurally and spatially separated placentae, one at the embryonic pole (the chorioallantoic placenta) and one at the abembryonic pole (the omphaloplacenta) [2]. The maternal placental contribution to each of these placentae also becomes anatomically differentiated (e.g., Biazik [7]). Despite the differentiation of the placentae, their functions have never been demonstrated, although there have been a number of suggestions as to their functions [8,2].

In this paper, we draw on our recent work on Australian skinks to review the changes in the three parameters required in the transformation from oviparity to viviparity, particularly the reduction in the eggshell, and we review available data to interpret the functions of the omphaloplacenta and chorioallantoic placenta.

2. Reduction in eggshell

All oviparous squamates produce an eggshell composed of organic and, in most, a calcareous component, although the details vary among taxa [9,10]. The shell acts as a physical barrier between the developing embryo and the outside environment, as a source

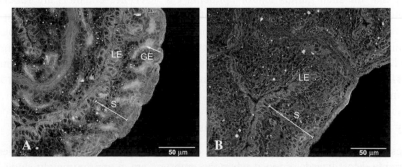

Fig. 1. Ca^{2+} ATPase immunofluorescent images of uterine tissue of the oviparous skink, *Lampropholis guichenoti*. (A) Uterus of a female that contained shell eggs. Note apical staining (arrow) of glandular epithelial cells (GE) in the stroma (S). Luminal epithelial cells (LE). (B) Negative control with no staining.

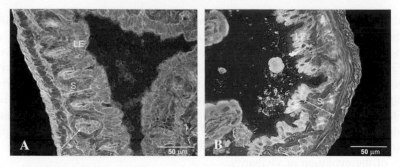

Fig. 2. Fluorescent immunohistochemical images of uterine tissue of the matrotrophic skink, *P. spenceri*. (A) Uterus of a nonreproductive female. Note shell glands (arrow) in the stroma (S). Luminal epithelial cells (LE). (B) Uterus of a pregnant female. Note the absence of glands in the stroma.

of calcium for the developing embryo and to mediate exchanges between the embryo and its environment. In viviparous species, the incubation environment of the egg is not hostile, so the need for a physical barrier is reduced, or absent, and the mediation functions of an eggshell are different. Indeed, arguably, there is no need to retain an eggshell at all, and indeed none is apparent in eutherian mammals. Nevertheless, components of an eggshell are retained in most viviparous squamates [11], regardless of the degree of reduction in yolk, although it is apparently lost as development proceeds in some species [12]. There is no indication, however, that the eggshell of any viviparous squamate contains a calcareous component.

Deposition of the calcareous component of the eggshell of oviparous lizards results from the transport of calcium via Ca^{2+} ATPase channels from the stromal compartment to the uterine lumen and/or the lumen of stromal shell glands [13, personal communication] (Fig. 1). Interestingly, structurally similar shell glands occur in the uterine stroma of viviparous species [14], although we have seen them only in non-pregnant female *Pseudemoia spenceri*, where they have little Ca^{2+} ATPase channel activity (Fig. 2).

The calcium content of egg yolks of viviparous and oviparous squamates is insufficient to meet the needs of the developing neonates, although the total calcium in neonates of both groups is similar (summarized by Stewart and Thompson [2]). Consequently, we postulate that the shell glands and/or epithelial Ca^{2+} ATPase channels are functional in viviparous species. However, the activity of the shell glands is much less than that of oviparous species because the quantity of calcium that is transported is less as there is no calcareous eggshell, and the rate of delivery less because the timing of transport is extended throughout pregnancy. Hence, as viviparity evolves, the timing and magnitude of Ca^{2+} ATPase function change to meet the reduced needs for calcium transport and the change in the timing of delivery of calcium.

3. Delay of expulsion of conceptus and vascularisation of the uterus

Interestingly, the timing of the expulsion of the conceptus in squamate reptiles is not very variable. Most lizards oviposit when the embryos are at approximately stage 30 [15] of the 40-stage embryonic staging scheme of Dufaure and Hubert [16], or they give birth to free-living neonates. Very few species oviposit when embryos are in advanced stages of development between stages 30 and 40, as one might expect in a transition from oviparity to viviparity. Similarly, very few species oviposit at very early embryonic stages (but see Blackburn [15] for list of exceptions, e.g., *Chamaeleo lateralis*).

If an eggshell has been reduced to the point of no longer providing an adequate barrier between the embryo and a nest environment, as is necessary to allow intrauterine development, then expulsion of the egg prior to completion of development to stage 40 would result in considerable risk to the embryo, and presumably be selected against in the population. Considerable research has gone into understanding the roles of the key hormones argenine vasotocin (AVT) and prostaglandins (PG), both of which result in contraction of oviductal tissues during oviposition and parturition (reviewed by Girling [17]). Both hormones are implicated in oviposition or birth, but their impacts are moderated by other hormones, particularly sex steroids, and uterine innervation, in ways that are not understood. Indeed, the picture that is emerging is one of a variety of responses among different taxa, but too few comparative studies on key lineages have been made to synthesise a coherent picture in the context of the evolution of viviparity.

Regardless of the apparent variations, it is likely that the mechanisms are not substantially different, but it is timing that differentiates oviparous and viviparous species. Although the details are not fully understood, the signals that determine the timing of oviposition in oviparous and birth in viviparous squamates are fundamentally the same [17]. With the reduction of an eggshell to allow exchange of substances between the mother and embryo in viviparous species, the opportunity for communication between the embryo and mother is greatly enhanced, providing the opportunity for the embryo to suppress triggering of the maternal mechanisms to expel the conceptus or, indeed, to trigger the mechanisms when is it ready to be born.

Vascular supply to the uterus of oviparous and viviparous squamates is fundamentally similar. Presumably the process of eggshelling, where there is a rapid up-regulation of Ca^{2+} ATPase channels in the stroma of the uterus, requires a substantial blood supply. In contrast, the timing of an increase in vascularity of the uterus is likely to be different in viviparous species compared to oviparous species, although details of increasing vascularity in viviparous species are poorly known [14]. The detail of development of capillaries is, however, likely to be different with the need to provide an adequate supply of oxygen to the embryo, particularly in the latter part of pregnancy when oxygen demand is likely to be highest [18].

4. Placental functions: *Pseudemoia entrecasteauxii* omphaloplacenta, placentome and paraplacentome

In its simplest form, viviparity requires gas exchange, and the uptake of water and some inorganic ions by the embryo from the mother. As the chorioallantoic placenta is well supported by a vascular supply, but the omphaloplacenta is not, it was long considered that the chorioallantoic placenta is the site for gas exchange and nutrient uptake, while the omphaloplacenta had little function other than uptake of water [8]. Recent detailed histology and electron microscopy on the placentae of viviparous squamates, however, seriously question this simplistic conclusion [2]. In addition, the chorioallantoic placenta of highly matrotrophic species, such as *P. entrecasteauxii*, the focus of the following descriptions, is further regionalised into a highly complex placentome and a simpler paraplacentomal region [19,2].

4.1. The chorioallantoic placenta

The placenta of all squamate reptiles is epitheliochorial [20,21], meaning that there is no breaching of the uterine epithelium by embryonic tissue. Nevertheless, for gas exchange, there must be close apposition of maternal and embryonic vasculature. Given the lack of blood supply in the omphaloplacenta [2,7], the most likely site for gas exchange is the chorioallantoic placenta. Close association of maternal and embryonic vascular beds occurs in the chorioallantoic placenta of all viviparous species (e.g., Stewart and Thompson [19,7], except where there is regional specialisation of the chorioallantoic placenta, especially in the form of a placentome [7]. In species with a placentome (e.g., *P. entrecasteauxii*, Fig. 3), close vascular apposition is maintained in the paraplacentomal region [7] (Fig. 3A).

The placentome of species in the genera *Pseudemoia* and *Mabuya* has enlarged cuboidal cells in the epithelium (e.g., Biazik [7]), so that the maternal blood supply is no longer closely apposed to the embryonic vessels. Instead, large cuboidal epithelial cells that lack secretory vesicles occur in the maternal epithelium, so that histotrophic nutrient transport may occur, but not via apocrine secretion [7]. The mechanism of transport and the substances that may be being transported are, however, not known.

4.2. Omphaloplacenta

In oviparous species, the extraembryonic yolk sac splanchnopleure and isolate yolk mass are the anatomical homologue of the embryonic contribution to the omphaloplacenta of viviparous species [2]. Given the close association of the yolk sac splanchnopleure and isolated yolk mass with the egg yolk, it is likely that these structures are intimately involved in nutrient supply to the embryo. The question then arises: how are they co-opted

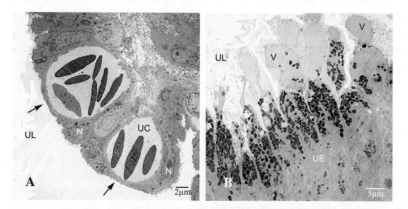

Fig. 3. TEM images of paraplacentome (A) and omphaloplacenta (B) in the matrotrophic skink, *P. entrecasteauxii*. (A) Uterine epithelial cells showing attenuated apical cytoplasm (arrows) caused by invaginating uterine capillaries (UC) and displacing nuclei (N). Uterine lumen (UL). (B) Uterine epithelial cells (UE) associated with large vesicles (V) protrude into the uterine lumen (UL).

in nutrient transport from the mother to the embryo? Most viviparous species have simple placentae and are essentially lecithotrophic [6]. Thus, there is little, if any, transport of organic nutrients from the mother to the embryo. However, several lineages have significant dry matter uptake by the embryo. In *P. entrecasteauxii*, the maternal epithelium consists of large columnar cells that contain secretory vesicles, which are apparently transferred to the embryo via histotrophic exchange. Hence, the function of the omphaloplacenta, at least in species with uptake of dry matter, is probably in histotrophic nutrient transport from the mother to the embryo via apocrine secretion, and not just as an avenue for water uptake. The adjacent embryonic cells of the omphaloplacenta are cuboidal [2].

4.3. Nutrient exchange

Anatomy of the structures present in the placentae of oviparous, lecithotrophic viviparous and matrotrophic viviparous squamates suggests that the omphaloplacenta is a major site for nutrient transfer from mother to embryo, and not just water uptake. That nutrient transfer is via histotrophic uptake of substances secreted into the uterine lumen by vesicles of the columnar epithelial cells of the uterus (Fig. 3B). By contrast, the unelaborated areas of the chorioallantoic placenta function as a major site for gas exchange between the mother and embryo. In some species, the blood to blood barrier is reduced to as little as 5 μm [7], the same as in mammalian lung [22]. Regional elaboration of the chorioallantoic placenta on both the maternal and embryonic side, especially where a placentome develops, results in an increase in the blood to blood barrier, reducing the efficiency of gas exchange. At the same time, the placentome takes on features of nutrient transport, such as large cuboidal epithelial cells, with secretory vesicles, but there is no evidence of histotrophic exchange. It is noteworthy that only the most matrotrophic species have a placentome, and that the placentome has evolved in at least three lineages independently. Consequently, the demand for nutrient transport in species with a placentome is higher than in species that lack a placentome, and it seems that both the omphaloplacenta and placentome function in nutrient transport in these species, but with different mechanisms.

5. Conclusions

Few changes are required to make the evolutionary transition from oviparity to viviparity in lizards, which is reflected in the extraordinary number of independent times the transition has occurred. Nevertheless, we have currently only characterised at a very crude level the features involved in the transition. There is a reduction in the thickness of the eggshell, and ultimately a loss of eggshell, at least in the later stages of pregnancy in species with complex placentae. In the simplest forms of viviparity, the calcareous eggshell is lost, and that probably is associated with changes in the mechanisms that transport calcium across the uterine surface. Nevertheless, eggshell glands similar to those that occur in the oviparous species also occur in at least some viviparous species, but we know nothing about the dynamics of their calcium transport.

We know even less about the differences in the uterine vascular beds of oviparous and viviparous species, and very little about the timing of expulsion of the conceptus.

However, the morphological data are now providing tantalizing clues to the functions of placental structures at the gross level for a small number of species.

What is required now are systematic and detailed functional and molecular studies of species of lizards that span the oviparity–viviparity transition, and that have different placental complexities. We are currently making detailed studies of some proteins of potential transport regulators, in particular tight junction proteins and the aquaporin family of water channels. We have also initiated studies of Hox genes that may be associated with the transition to viviparity. The superb model systems that have resulted in the multiple origins of viviparity in lizards, the relative ease with which the transformation seems to have occurred, and the new availability of excellent physiological and molecular techniques make the task of understanding this fundamental transition achievable.

Acknowledgements

All work was approved by the University of Sydney Animal Ethics Committee. Lizards were collected under license from the New South Wales National Parks and Wildlife Service, and funding was from ARC Discovery grants to MBT and CRM. Thank you to L. Lindsay for her helpful comments on the manuscript.

References

[1] D.G. Blackburn, Reptilian viviparity: past research, future directions, and appropriate models, Comp. Biochem. Physiol., A 127 (2000) 391–409.

[2] J.R. Stewart, M.B. Thompson, Evolution of placentation among squamate reptiles: recent research and future directions, Comp. Biochem. Physiol., A 127 (2000) 411–431.

[3] C.R. Murphy, M.J. Hosie, M.B. Thompson, The plasma membrane transformation facilitates pregnancy in both reptiles and lizards, Comp. Biochem. Physiol., A 127 (2000) 433–439.

[4] M.J. Hosie, et al., The viviparous lizard, *Eulamprus tympanum*, shows changes in the uterine surface epithelium during early pregnancy that are similar to the plasma membrane transformation of mammals, J. Morphol. 258 (2003) 346–357.

[5] D.G. Blackburn, Evolutionary origins of viviparity in the Reptilia: I. Sauria, Amphib.-Reptil. 3 (1982) 185–205.

[6] M.B. Thompson, J.R. Stewart, B.K. Speake, Comparison of nutrient transport across the placenta of lizards differing in placental complexity, Comp. Biochem. Physiol., A. 127 (2000) 469–479.

[7] J.M. Biazik, A structural study of the uterine epithelium in the viviparous lizard, *Pseudemoia entrecasteauxii*. B.Sc (Hons) Thesis. University of Sydney, NSW. (2003).

[8] H.C. Weekes, A review of placentation among reptiles with particular regard to the function and evolution of the placenta, Proc. Zool. Soc. Lond. 2 (1935) 625–645.

[9] M.J. Packard, K.F. Hirsch, Scanning electron microscopy of eggshells of contemporary reptiles, Scanning Electron Microsc. 4 (1986) 1581–1590.

[10] H.H. Schleich, W. Kästle, Reptile Eggshells: SEM Atlas, Gustav Fischer Verlag, Stuttgart, 1988.

[11] M.B. Thompson, B.K. Speake, Egg morphology and composition, in: D.C. Deeming (Ed.), Reptilian Incubation. Environment, Evolution and Behaviour, Nottingham University Press, Nottingham, 2004, pp. 45–74.

[12] A.F. Flemming, W.R. Branch, Extraordinary case of matrotrophy in the African skink *Eumecia anchietae*, J. Morphol. 247 (3) (2001) 264–287.

[13] B.D. Palmer, V.G. DeMarco, L.J. Guillette Jr., Oviductal morphology and eggshell formation in the lizard, *Sceloporus woodi*, J. Morphol. 217 (1993) 205–217.

[14] D.G. Blackburn, Structure, function, and evolution of the oviducts of squamate reptiles, with special reference to viviparity and placentation, J. Exp. Zool. 282 (1998) 560–617.

[15] D.G. Blackburn, Saltationist and punctuated equilibrium models for the evolution of viviparity and placentation, J. Theor. Biol. 174 (1995) 199–216.

[16] J.P. Dufaure, J. Hubert, Table de developpement du lezard vivipare *Lacerta* (*Zootoca*) *vivipara* Jacquin, Arch. Anat. Microsc. Morphol. Exp. 50 (1961) 309–328.

[17] J.E. Girling, The reptilian oviduct: a review of structure and function and directions for future research, J. Exp. Zool. 293 (2002) 141–170.

[18] K.A. Robert, M.B. Thompson, Energy consumption by embryos of a viviparous lizard, *Eulamprus tympanum*, during development, Comp. Biochem. Physiol., A 127 (2000) 481–486.

[19] J.R. Stewart, M.B. Thompson, Evolution of reptilian placentation: development of extraembryonic membranes of the Australian scincid lizards, *Bassiana duperreyi* (oviparous) and *Pseudemoia entrecasteauxii* (viviparous), J. Morphol. 227 (1996) 349–370.

[20] H.W. Mossman, Structural changes in vertebrate fetal membranes associated with the adoption of viviparity, Obstet. Gynecol. Annu. 3 (1974) 7–32.

[21] W.P. Luckett, Ontogeny of amniote fetal membranes and their application to phylogeny, in: M.K. Hecht, P.C. Goody, B.M. Hecht (Eds.), Major Patterns in Vertebrate Evolution, Plenum Press, New York, 1977, pp. 439–519.

[22] M.H. Ross, G.I. Kaye, W. Pawlina, Histology: A Text and Atlas, 4th ed., Lippincott Williams and Wilkins, USA, 2003.

International Congress Series 1275 (2004) 226–233

www.ics-elsevier.com

The influence of incubation temperature on post-hatching fitness characteristics of turtles

David T. Booth*, Elizabeth Burgess, Julia McCosker, Janet M. Lanyon

Department of Zoology and Entomology, School of Life Sciences, The University of Queensland, St. Lucia, Queensland 4072, Australia

Abstract. Turtle eggs collected immediately after oviposition were incubated in the laboratory at several different constant temperatures and fitness-related hatchling attributes measured at hatching, and in freshwater turtle species at 12 months after hatching. In green sea turtles, incubation temperature was found to influence sex, size, and amount of yolk material converted to hatchling tissue as well as swimming performance during the 24 h frenzy swimming period that occurs within 48 h of hatching. In freshwater turtles, incubation temperature influenced swimming performance, post-hatch survival, and post-hatch grow. These results clearly indicate that incubation temperature can have an important influence on hatchling fitness by influencing post-hatch mortality (sea turtles) and growth rates (freshwater turtles). © 2004 Elsevier B.V. All rights reserved.

Keywords: Incubation temperature; Phenotypic plasticity; Turtle; Fitness; Hatchling

1. Introduction

Many studies have reported that incubation temperature influences hatchling attributes of reptiles including turtles [1]. The range of these effects is diverse and can include determining a hatchling's sex, body shape, colouring, size, amount of yolk converted to tissue during embryonic development, locomotor performance, and behaviour. Variation in these traits is most likely to have consequences for the hatchling's fitness [2], and although studies documenting this type of phenotypic variation are numerous, only a relative few have attempted to relate such variation to

---

* Corresponding author. Tel.: +61 7 3365 2138; fax: +61 7 3365 1655.
E-mail address: DBooth@zen.uq.edu.au (D.T. Booth).

0531-5131/ © 2004 Elsevier B.V. All rights reserved.
doi:10.1016/j.ics.2004.08.057

hatchling fitness in a quantitative way [2]. Direct measurements of fitness in hatchling turtles is made difficult because of their relatively long life spans (>20 years for most species). In this article, we summarize the results from two recent studies on how incubation temperature induced phenotypic variation in hatchling traits influence attributes (size, swimming performance and growth rates) that are correlates of fitness in hatchling turtles.

2. Methods

We studied two species of chelonian, the Green turtle *Chelonia mydas* that has temperature dependent sex determination, and Brisbane river turtle *Emydura signata* that has genetic sex determination.

2.1. Green turtles

Sixty eggs were collected immediately after oviposition from each of four nesting Green turtles at the Heron Island rookery in November 2000. These eggs were immediately chilled to 10–15 °C for transport to the laboratory in Brisbane. On arrival in the laboratory, 20 eggs from each clutch were incubated at 26, 28, and 30 °C in moist perlite® (water potential ~−100 kPa). At hatching, hatchlings were marked with white paint on their carapace for individual identification, and left with other hatchlings in a darkened container at their incubation temperature for 48 h to simulate the time hatchlings usually spend digging out of natural nests. After this period, hatchlings were weighed and had their carapace length and front flipper length and width measured with calipers. A front flipper area index was calculated from the product of flipper length and width. A sub-sample from each incubation temperature (10 from 26 °C, 9 from 28 °C, and 16 from 30 °C) was killed by cooling and then freezing, and once thawed the residual yolk was dissected free. Both the residual yolk and yolk-free carcass was dried to constant mass at 60 °C. Most of the remaining turtles underwent swimming trials. Hatchlings were swum individually in a glass aquarium filled with seawater at 28 °C (the average seawater temperature at Heron Island during the hatching season). A monofilament nylon line was glued to the carapace and the line attached to bracket suspended above the middle of the tank. A low intensity light was placed at one end of the tank, and the other sides of the tank covered with black plastic to encourage unidirectional swimming. The length of the tether was adjusted so that hatchlings could swim freely below the water or on the surface but could not touch the bottom or sides of the tank. Hatchlings were videotaped for 10 min at time intervals of 0.5, 2, 6, 12, 18 and 23 h after being introduced to the tank. Power stroke rate was later calculated for each time interval from the videotapes by manual counting with a stopwatch and hand-held counter. After swimming trials had concluded, a sample of hatchlings from 26 and 30 °C and all hatchlings from 28 °C were killed by a 1 ml injection of barbiturate (Nembutal) into the brain, and the kidney with gonad attached dissected free and preserved in Bouin's fixative. The fixed gonad was imbedded in wax and serially sectioned. Sections were stained with hematoxylin and eosin and examined using light microscopy. Males and females were identified by the different cellular structure of testis and ovaries according to the criteria of Miller and

Limpus [3]. Single factor ANOVA and ANCOVA in which initial egg mass was the covariate was used to analyze Green turtle morphological characteristics. Repeat measures ANCOVA in which initial egg mass was the covariate was used to analyze stroke rate data.

2.2. Brisbane river turtles

Fifteen gravid females were collected during September 1999 and oviposition induced via the administration of oxytocin [4]. A sample of eggs from each clutch was incubated in moist vermiculite ($\sim$−150 kPa) at 24, 27, and 30 °C. On hatching, hatchlings were placed in individual plastic jars at their incubation temperature for a further 48 h to insure complete absorption of the yolk sac and allow the carapace to take on its natural shape. After 48 h, hatchlings were weighed and had their carapace length and width measured, and had their swim speed measured. Swim speed was measured by placing turtles in the middle of a tank containing 6 cm of 24 °C water with its bottom marked with concentric circles 2 cm apart. The turtle was videotaped while it swam away from the centre. This procedure was repeated 30 times for hatchling turtles and 10 times for yearling turtles. These trials were when analyzed for swimming over 12 cm and a mean swim speed calculated from the fastest 10 trial for hatchling turtles and all 10 trials for yearling turtles. Hatchling turtles were scute marked so individuals could be identified and released into a large outside tank and feed to satiation with nutra max™ turtle pellets every second day during the non-winter months. Turtles were not fed over winter because they were not active. Once per month turtles were weighed. After 12 months, swim speed was measured again by the previously described method. Two-factor mixed model (clutch random factor, incubation temperature fixed factor) ANOVA was used to analyze morphological and swim speed results.

3. Results

3.1. Green turtles

Of the 80 eggs set at each incubation temperature, 59, 60 and 56 eggs produced healthy hatchlings from 26, 28 and 30 °C, respectively. Samples of 20, 51, and 20 hatchlings from eggs incubated at 26, 28 and 30 °C had their gonads examined histologically. All hatchlings examined from 26 °C were males, all hatchlings examined from 30 °C were female, while 37% of hatchlings from 28 °C were female and 63% were male. Egg sizes did not differ between the incubation treatments (ANOVA, $P=0.200$) but sibling hatchings from 26 °C were larger in terms of mass, carapace length and front flipper size (Table 1). These differences are due to the effect of temperature and are independent of sex because males that hatched from eggs incubated at 28 °C had similar morphology to females hatched from eggs incubated at 28 and 30 °C (Table 1).

The proportion of yolk converted into hatchling tissue during incubation was greater in 26 °C males, resulting in larger yolk-free mass and smaller residual yolk compared to hatchlings from 28 and 30 °C (Table 1). All hatchlings fatigued during the swimming trials, with the largest drop-off in performance occurring within the first 2 h (repeat measures ANOVA with incubation treatment a fixed factor, time a repeated

Table 1
Incubation times and hatchling morphological parameters of Heron Island Green turtle (*C. mydas*) eggs incubated at different temperatures

Variable	26 °C, males $n=59$	28 °C, females $n=19$	28 °C, males $n=32$	30 °C, females $n=56$	Significant treatment effect?	Comparisons between temperature treatments
Incubation time (days)	80.6±0.2	62.5±0.1	62.8±0.1	52.6±0.1	yes $P<0.001$	26 ♂>28 ♂= 28 ♀>30 ♀
Hatchling mass (g)	26.3±0.2	25.6±0.2	25.6±0.2	25.4±0.2	yes $P<0.001$	26 ♂>28 ♂= 28 ♀=30 ♀
Carapace length (mm)	49.3±0.2	49.0±0.2	49.1±0.2	49.2±0.1	no $P=0.824$	26 ♂=28 ♂= 28 ♀=30 ♀
Carapace width (mm)	39.2±0.1	38.0±0.2	38.1±0.2	38.0±0.2	yes $P<0.001$	26 ♂>28 ♂= 28 ♀=30 ♀
Front flipper area index (mm²)	757±7	722±15	713±12	707±6	yes $P<0.001$	26 ♂>28 ♂= 28 ♀=30 ♀
Yolk-free carcass dry mass (g)	7.28±0.25 $n=10$	sex not known 5.43±0.52 $n=9$		5.10±0.54 $n=16$	yes $P<0.001$	26 ♂> 28 ♂/♀=30 ♀
Residual yolk dry mass (g)	0.57±0.12 $n=10$	sex not known 1.48±0.08 $n=9$		1.61±0.12 $n=16$	yes $P<0.001$	26 ♂< 28 ♂/♀=30 ♀

It was assumed that all hatchlings from 26 °C were male, and all hatchlings from 30 °C were female as all hatchlings examined histologically from these temperatures conformed with this assumption. Sex of hatchlings from 28 °C was determined by gonad histology. Statistical comparisons made between treatments with ANCOVA with initial egg mass as the covariate followed by a post hoc Tukey's honest significant difference test for unequal sample sizes. Data are presented as mean±standard error of the mean.

factor, and stroke rate as the dependent variable: $P<0.0001$; see Fig. 1). Males incubated at 26 °C were consistently poorer swimmers than males and females from the warmer incubation treatments in terms of power stroke rate. This finding was consistent across clutches. Once again this difference can be attributed to a temperature

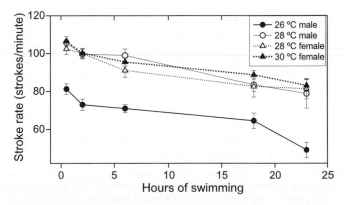

Fig. 1. Power stroke rate of Green turtle hatchlings incubated at different temperatures from Heron Island rookery during the frenzy swimming phase immediately after hatchlings were placed in water. Data are means±standard errors.

effect as males from 28 °C had a similar power stroke rate to females from 28 and 30 °C (*P*=0.506).

3.2. Brisbane river turtles

Incubation temperature influenced incubation length, while clutch of origin influenced all hatchling morphological characteristics, while incubation temperature influenced some hatchling morphological characteristics (Table 2). Incubation period was shortest at 30 °C, intermediate at 27 °C and longest at 24 °C. Hatchlings from eggs incubated at 30 °C were smaller in terms of mass, carapace width, and plastron width than those incubated at 27 and 24 °C. Swimming speed at hatching and also at 1 year was influenced by incubation temperature, but not by clutch (Table 2). Curiously, although turtles were larger at 1 year old, they did not swim any faster than when they were hatchlings. Relative swim performance was not repeatable between hatching and 1 year, i.e. within a temperature treatment, the fastest swimming turtles at hatching were not the fastest swimming at 1 year. Survival during the first year post-hatch was similar across all incubation temperature treatments and averaged 87% (Table 2). Growth patterns were similar across all incubation temperature treatments, with rapid growth during summer and autumn (November–May) little growth over the winter period (June–August) and rapid grow recommencing in Spring and Summer (September–January) (Fig. 2). Hatchlings from the 30 °C incubation treatment grew fast and were significantly larger after 12 months that hatchings from the

Table 2

Incubation times and hatchling morphological parameters of Brisbane river turtle (*E. signata*) eggs from 15 clutches incubated at different temperatures

Variable	24 °C, $n=70$	27 °C, $n=74$	30 °C, $n=77$	Significant temperature effect?	Significant clutch effect?	Comparisons between temperature treatments
Incubation time (days)	76±2	56±2	44±2	yes $P<0.001$	no $P=0.824$	24>27>30
Hatchling mass (g)	4.4±0.1	4.3±0.1	4.1±0.1	yes $P<0.001$	yes $P<0.001$	24=27>30
Carapace length (mm)	27.7±0.3	28.0±0.3	27.6±0.3	yes $P=0.021$	yes $P<0.001$	27>24=30
Carapace width (mm)	27.0±0.3	27.1±0.2	26.5±0.2	yes $P<0.001$	yes $P<0.001$	24=27>30
Plastron length (mm)	22.9±0.2	23.0±0.2	22.8±0.2	no $P=0.383$	yes $P<0.001$	24=27=30
Plastron width (mm)	13.0±0.1	13.1±0.1	12.8±0.1	yes $P=0.002$	yes $P<0.001$	24=27>30
Head width (mm)	9.2±0.1	9.2±0.1	9.2±0.1	no $P=0.441$	yes $P<0.001$	24=27=30
Hatchling swim speed (cm/s)	16.2±0.4	20.7±0.5	14.9±0.4	yes $P=0.032$	no $P=0.13$	27>24=30
Yearling swim speed (cm/s)	$n=61$ 15.3±0.5	$n=64$ 21.5± 0.6	$n=67$ 15.5±0.4	yes $P<0.001$	no $P=0.22$	27>24=30
Yearling mass (g)	$n=61$ 31.3±1.3	$n=64$ 34.1±1.8	$n=67$ 49.5±2.8	yes $P<0.001$	yes $P=0.048$	30>27=24
First year survival (%)	87	86	87			

Statistical comparisons made between treatments with a two-factor mixed model (temperature fixed factor, clutch random factor) ANOVA followed by a post hoc Tukey's honest significant difference test for unequal sample sizes. For all hatchling morphological attributes except plastron width there was a significant interaction between incubation temperature and clutch. For yearling attributes there was no significant interaction between incubation temperature and clutch. Data are presented as mean±standard error of the mean.

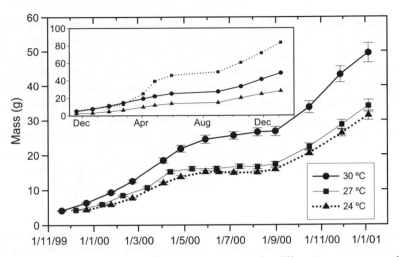

Fig. 2. Growth of Brisbane river turtles hatchlings from eggs incubated at different temperatures over the first 12 months post-hatching. Data are means±standard errors. Insert: growth of hatchlings from 3 of the 15 clutches from eggs incubated at 30 °C.

24 and 27 °C incubation treatment (Fig. 2; Table 2). Within a temperature treatment, hatchlings from different clutches grew at different rates (Fig. 2).

4. Discussion

Incubation temperature clearly has potential influence on hatchling fitness in both Green turtles and Brisbane river turtles, but the mechanism of by which fitness is influenced differ in the two species.

In Green turtles, incubation temperature influences sex determination, the amount of residual yolk converted to hatchling tissue, and swimming performance during the frenzy swimming period. The fitness consequence of temperature-sensitive sex determination has been extensively reviewed [5–8] and will not be discussed further. Conversion of more yolk to tissue during embryonic development at lower temperatures has been noted previously in the Green turtle [9], and in some other reptiles [10]. A larger hatchling with a smaller yolk reserve may be advantageous to hatchling entering an environment where food is easily obtained. The larger size may allow hatchlings to escape gape-limited predators, swim faster, and to successfully handle larger prey items hatchlings, i.e. the bigger is better hypothesis [11,12]. On the other hand, if the hatchling is entering an environment where food is scarce or difficult to locate, then a smaller body size and large residual yolk may be advantageous as the larger yolk could supply the hatchling with energy for a longer period of time than a smaller yolk. However, the difference in hatchling size/yolk reserve caused by differences in incubation temperature, although statistically significant are relatively small in Green turtles and is thus unlikely to play a major role in contributing differential fitness amongst hatchlings. By far the most important potential fitness outcome is the influence of incubation temperature on hatchling swimming performance during the frenzied swimming period when hatchlings are making their way from the natal beach to the open ocean.

In Green turtle hatchlings making their way from the nest to the open ocean, the highest rate of predation occurs in the water within the first 30–60 min of swimming as they pass through the gauntlet of predators found in the shallow water surrounding natal beaches [12–14]. Despite their larger body and front flipper size, 26 °C male hatchlings were consistently poorer swimmers than males and females from warmer incubation treatments, in terms of power stroke rate, and we anticipate that as a consequence predation of male hatchlings would be greater than females during this critical period. Curiously, nesting beach sand temperatures from Green turtle rookeries worldwide suggest a female-biased hatchling sex ratio [15–17]. Our results indicate that low temperature nest produce males of inferior swimming ability, and as a consequence the female-biased sex ratio of hatchling leaving nests may become even more skewed towards females in hatchlings that reach the open ocean.

The effect of incubation temperature on body size of hatchling Brisbane river turtles is small compared to interclutch differences in body size, so it probably has little or no ecological relevance. However, incubation temperature did influence swimming speed at both hatching and 1 year and also strongly influenced growth during the first year post-hatch, and both these traits could have significant effects of hatchling fitness. The faster burst swimming ability of hatchlings from 27 °C may enhance their fitness compared to hatchlings from 24 and 30 °C as these turtles may be more successful at avoiding predation [18]. Interestingly, clutch of origin did not influence swimming ability probably because the chief influence of clutch is on hatchling size, and there was no relationship between turtle size and swimming speed in our experiments. The absence of a correlation between swim speed at hatching and swim speed at 1 year also suggests that swim speed is not a good predictor of hatchling fitness in Brisbane river turtles.

The most significant influence of incubation temperature on Brisbane river turtles in terms of fitness outcomes is its effect on post-hatch growth rate. Hatchlings from 30 °C hatched earlier and grew faster than hatchlings from 24 and 27 °C. There are several potential advantages to having a faster growth rate. Firstly, predation rates on small turtles is thought to be greater than larger turtles [19,20], so the faster growing turtle will spend less time at a size that they are most vulnerable to predation. However, recent studies on wild populations of hatchling turtles indicate that size per se is not a good predictor of survival [10,21]. Secondly, sexual maturation in freshwater turtles is size-dependent and not age-dependent [19] and therefore the faster the growth, the sooner sexual maturity is achieved and this may increase the number of breeding seasons experienced and thus increase the life-time reproductive output.

In summary, incubation temperature has the potential to influence the fitness of hatchling turtles. In Green turtles this influence is manifested through sex determination and swimming ability, while in Brisbane river turtles it is manifested through post-hatch growth rate.

Acknowledgements

Part of this work was sponsored by the SeaWorld Research and Rescue Foundation. Work was carried out under Queensland EPA scientific research permits C6/000100/00/ SAA and E5/000100/98/SAA and University of Queensland animal ethics approvals ZOO/408/00/H and ZOO/ENT/468/00/PHD.

References

[1] D.C. Deeming, Post-hatching phenotypic effects of incubation in reptiles, in: D.C. Deeming (Ed.), Reptilian Incubation: Environment, Evolution and Behaviour, Nottingham University Press, Nottingham, 2004, pp. 229–252.

[2] R. Shine, Adaptive consequences of developmental plasticity, in: D.C. Deeming (Ed.), Reptilian Incubation: Environment, Evolution and Behaviour, Nottingham University Press, Nottingham, 2004, pp. 187–210.

[3] J.D. Miller, C.J. Limpus, Incubation period and sexual differentiation in the green turtle *Chelonia mydas*, in: C.B. Banks, A. Martin (Eds.), Proceedings of the Melbourne Herpetological Symposium, The Royal Botanical Gardens, Melbourne, 1981, pp. 66–73.

[4] M.A. Ewert, J.M. Legler, Hormonal induction of oviposition in turtles, Herpetologica 34 (1978) 314–318.

[5] F.J. Janzen, Experimental evidence for the evolutionary significance of temperature-dependent sex determination, Evolution 49 (1995) 864–873.

[6] M.J. Elphick, R. Shine, Sex differences in optimal incubation temperatures in a scincid lizard species, Oecologia 118 (1999) 431–437.

[7] R. Shine, Why is sex determined by nest temperature in many reptiles? Trends Ecol. Evol. 14 (1999) 186–189.

[8] N. Valenzuela, Temperature-dependent sex determination, in: D.C. Deeming (Ed.), Reptilian Incubation: Environment, Evolution and Behaviour, Nottingham University Press, Nottingham, 2004, pp. 211–228.

[9] D.T. Booth, K. Astill, Incubation temperature, energy expenditure and hatchling size in the green turtle (*Chelonia mydas*), a species with temperature-sensitive sex determination, Aust. J. Zool. 49 (2000) 389–396.

[10] D.T. Booth, Incubation of eggs of the Australian broad-shelled turtle, *Chelodina expansa* (Testudinata: Chelidae), at different temperatures: effects on pattern of oxygen consumption and hatchling morphology, Aust. J. Zool. 48 (2000) 369–378.

[11] J.D. Congdon, et al., The relationship of body size to survivorship of hatchling snapping turtles (*Chelydra serpentine*): an evaluation of the "bigger is better" hypothesis, Oecologia 12 (1999) 224–235.

[12] E. Gyuris, The relationship between body size and predation rates on hatchlings of the green turtle (*Chelonia mydas*): is bigger better? in: N.J. Pilcher, M.G. Ismail (Eds.), Sea Turtles of the Indo-Pacific: Research, Management and Conservation, Academic Press, New York, 2000, pp. 143–147.

[13] E. Gyuris, The rate of predation by fishes on hatchlings of the green turtle, Coral Reefs 13 (1994) 137–144.

[14] N.J. Pilcher, et al., Nearshore turtle hatchling distribution and predation, in: N.J. Pilcher, M.G. Ismail (Eds.), Sea Turtles of the Indo-Pacific: Research, Management and Conservation, Academic Press, New York, 2000, pp. 151–166.

[15] M.H. Godfrey, N. Sky, et al., Sex ratios of sea turtles in Suriname: past and present, in: J.A. Keinath, et al., (Eds.), Proceedings of the Fifteenth Annual Workshop on Sea Turtle Biology and Conservation, 100 NOAA Technical Memorandum NMFS-SEFSC-387, 1996, pp. 98–103.

[16] A.C. Broderick, et al., Metabolic heating and the prediction of sex ratios for green turtles (*Chelonia mydas*), Physiol. Biochem. Zool. 74 (2001) 161–170.

[17] D.T. Booth, K. Astill, Temperature variation within and between nests of the green sea turtle, *Chelonia mydas* (Chelonia: Cheloniidae) on Heron Island, Great Barrier Reef, Aust. J. Zool. 49 (2001) 71–84.

[18] F.J. Janzen, The influence of incubation temperature and family on eggs, embryos and hatchlings of the smooth softshell turtle (*Apalone mutica*), Physiol. Zool. 66 (1993) 349–379.

[19] J. Cann, Australian Freshwater Turtles, Beaumont Publishing, Singapore, 1998.

[20] F.J. Janzen, et al., Experimental analysis of an early life-history stage: avian predation selects for larger body size of hatchling turtles, J. Evol. Biol. 13 (2000) 947–954.

[21] J.J. Kolbe, F.J. Janzen, The influence of propagule size and maternal nest-site selection on survival and behaviour of neonate turtles, Funct. Ecol. 15 (2001) 772–781.

International Congress Series 1275 (2004) 234–241

www.ics-elsevier.com

Thermoregulation in African chameleons

Albert F. Bennett*

Department of Ecology and Evolutionary Biology, University of California, Irvine, CA 92697-2525, USA

Abstract. Field active and laboratory preferred body temperatures and critical thermal limits were measured in six species of Kenyan chameleons: *Chamaeleo bitaeniatus, Chamaeleo dilepis, Chamaeleo ellioti, Chamaeleo hohnelii, Chamaeleo jacksonii,* and *Chamaeleo schubotzi*. Given the opportunity, all six species are very competent heliothermic thermoregulators. Individuals typically spend the night low in shrubby vegetation with body temperatures equal to ambient air, and then climb to the top or edges of their bushes to bask when the sun shines. For most species, body temperatures quickly stabilize between 29 and 32 °C, which they maintain while the sun shines (except *C. schubotzi* at 19 °C). Preferred temperatures in the laboratory average 30–33 °C, with voluntary minima of 27–29 °C and voluntary maxima of 34–36 °C. From the elaborate suite of behaviors undertaken and the distribution of environmental temperatures, it is clear that when solar radiation is available, these chameleon species do not passively accept environmental temperatures. Rather they regulate their body temperatures in the field, utilizing many of the behaviors that have become classically associated with heliothermic behavioral thermoregulation. All other chameleon species previously studied also have thermal preferenda around 30 °C.
© 2004 Elsevier B.V. All rights reserved.

Keywords: Chamaeleo; Chameleon; Lizard; Temperature; Thermoregulation

1. Introduction

Diurnal lizards of many different families have been shown to regulate body temperature behaviorally at high and stable levels by adjusting exposure to the sun [1,2]. In contrast, chameleons, members of the Old World family Chamaeleonidae, have previously been classified as having low activity temperatures [2], being thermoconformers [3] and thermally passive [4], and in fact preferring low body temperatures [5].

---

* Corresponding author. Tel.: +1 949 824 6930; fax: +1 949 824 2181.
E-mail address: abennett@uci.edu.

0531-5131/ © 2004 Elsevier B.V. All rights reserved.
doi:10.1016/j.ics.2004.09.035

However, relatively few body temperature measurements have actually been reported for these lizards, and many of these are only anecdotal accounts (e.g., Refs. [3–8]). Here, measurements on field active and laboratory preferred temperatures and critical thermal limits are reported for six species of Kenyan chameleons. These previously unreported data were gathered as part of a series of studies on functional aspects of feeding, locomotion, and color change in these chameleons [9–13].

2. Material and methods

The following six species of chameleons (genus *Chamaeleo*) were collected in Kenya under Research Permit No. OP.13/001/18C94/19 from the Office of the President and Collection and Export Permits Nos. 1945, 5563, and 5564 from the Department of Wildlife Conservation and Management and University of California Irvine ARC permit 88-805: *Chamaeleo bitaeniatus*, Rift Valley, vicinity Olepolos, approx. 2000 m above sea level; *Chamaeleo dilepis*, coastal plains, vicinity Kibwezi, 800 m; *Chamaeleo ellioti*, Western Highlands, Kapsabet, 1800 m; *Chamaeleo hohnelii* and *Chamaeleo jacksonii*, Nairobi, 1700 m; *Chamaeleo schubotzi*, Mt. Kenya, 3300 m. Taxonomy and spelling conventions follow Welch [14]. Measurements of field body temperatures were made on collection or on the following day with thermocouple implants. Laboratory measurements were made at the University of Nairobi within 3 or 4 days of capture. Animals were watered frequently and subsequently either released or exported to the United States for further research.

A very fine (40 gauge), teflon-coated copper-constantan thermocouple wire was implanted about 1 cm intraperitoneally into the posterior abdomen of an animal on the day prior to measurements. The wire was secured with superglue, leaving an external lead approximately 1 m in length. Chameleons were then placed in bushes from which they were collected within their natural habitats. Body temperatures were measured every half hour by attaching a Tegam Model 821 thermocouple thermometer to the end of the thermocouple wire. Body temperatures were thus monitored on individual animals over the course on an entire day without touching or disturbing the lizards. The chameleons appeared unaffected by these implants or measurements: during these observations, they undertook a variety of different natural behaviors in addition to thermoregulation, including frequent feeding, defecation, copulation, and intraspecific aggression. Simultaneously with measurements of temperatures in these freely moving lizards, temperatures of highly reflective and absorbtive painted copper models in full sun were determined, as well as that of a copper model in the shade.

Preferred body temperatures were measured in a linear thermal gradient created by suspending a 150-W photoflood lamp above one end of wooden dowel (8–10 mm in diameter, 2 m in length) upon which an animal was placed. Equilibrium temperature directly under the light was in excess of 50 °C, above the critical thermal limit of all species. The cold end of the gradient was 17–23 °C, temperatures below the voluntary minimum of all species. Bright illumination was maintained over the entire gradient. Lizards moved freely along the gradient, either choosing an intermediate position and establishing a very constant temperature or more usually shuttling back and forth between the heated and cooler areas of the gradient. In the latter case, the average temperatures at which an animal voluntarily left the heat or moved toward the heat were taken as the maximum and minimum voluntary temperatures, respectively. Animals were observed continuously from behind a cloth blind. A lizard was placed directly under the heat lamp at the beginning of an experiment, and observations were begun at the first sign of a movement of obvious thermoregulatory significance, usually retreat from the hottest portion of the gradient. Body temperatures were measured with an implanted intra-peritoneal thermocouple connected to a Tegam thermocouple thermometer, and recorded every minute for 1 h. The mean body temperature during this time was taken as the preferred body temperature.

Critical thermal limits and panting thresholds were determined by heating or cooling a lizard just until the righting response was abolished. A lizard was placed under a photoflood lamp or in a metal pan on ice water and rate of body temperature change was adjusted to approximately 1 °C per min. Body temperature was monitored continuously with intraperitoneal thermocouples. When an animal approached critical temperatures, it was placed on its side and the first failure to right itself determined. It was then immediately removed and heated animals were placed in cool water. All animals recovered completely within a few minutes after termination of the experiment.

Mean values and standard errors are reported. Intergroup comparisons are done by *t*-tests or ANOVA with posthoc Tukey-Kramer Multiple Comparisons Tests.

3. Results

All six species of chameleons examined proved to be very competent heliothermic thermoregulators. Individuals typically spent the night low in shrubby vegetation, with body temperatures of the ambient air. As soon as the sun rose, they climbed to the top or edges of their bush. Body temperatures rose rapidly above those of the ambient air. For most species (except *C. schubotzi*), these quickly stabilized around 30 °C, a value maintained as long as the sun shone. When the sun set or solid cloud cover and rain commenced, lizards moved to the bottom of the vegetation and body temperatures fell to ambient shade levels. Field body temperatures of each species during sunny periods and for the entire observation period are reported in Table 1. Figs. 1 and 2 show a typical pattern of body and environmental temperatures for an individual *C. jacksonii* and *C.*

Table 1
Field body temperatures (FBT) for six species of Kenyan chameleons (*Chamaeleo* spp.)

Species	n	Time of day	Mean Daily FBT (°C)	Mean Sun FBT (°C)
bitaeniatus	5	0945–1200	28.6+0.32	28.9+0.22
dilepis	6	0900–1730	31.7+0.34	32.0+0.36
ellioti	6	0930–1400	30.3+0.24	32.5+0.36
hohnelii	4	0930–1700	30.1+0.15	31.3+0.30
jacksonii	8	0930–1700	29.2+0.36	30.4+0.39
schubotzi	6	0800–1400	19.1+0.66	22.2+0.98

FBT for both the entire measurement period (time of day) and for only those periods of intermittent or continuous sunshine are reported. All temperature measurements for an individual animal were averaged and the mean and standard error of these averages is reported along with number of animals observed (n). Measurements were begun 30 min after animals were placed in the vegetation and continued until sunset or rain commenced.

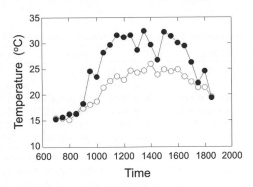

Fig. 1. Field body temperature of an individual *Chamaeleo jacksonii* (solid circles) and shade air temperature of a copper model (open circles). The day was cloudy and raining until 0845, when the first sun shone on the bush; sunshine was intermittent until sunset at 1820. The lizard illustrated had the median body temperature of all individuals measured.

ellioti, respectively. For all species except *C. schubotzi* (which are exceptionally difficult to locate during the day), body temperatures of other, previously undisturbed individuals were measured with a rapid registering cloacal thermometer, according to more traditional methods [2,15]. These temperatures were statistically undistinguishable ($p > 0.1$) from the daily averages reported in Table 1. Mean field body temperatures vary significantly among species [$p < 0.0001$ by ANOVA for both average daily ($F_{5,28} = 128$) and average sun temperatures ($F_{5,28} = 57$)]: *C. schubotzi* had lower field temperatures than all other species ($p < 0.001$); none of others were consistently different from all the rest. Mean field body temperatures are positively correlated with mean annual minimum ($p = 0.016$) and maximum ($p = 0.011$) air temperatures measured at weather stations closest to collection localities [16] and estimated for Mt. Kenya [17,18].

A suite of characteristic body temperatures for each species is reported in Table 2. Statistically significant ($p < 0.001$) interspecific differences occur in critical thermal

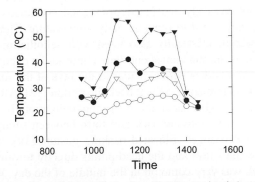

Fig. 2. Field body temperature of an individual *Chamaeleo ellioti* (open triangles) and associated environmental temperatures (copper model in shade: open circles; white painted copper model in sun: closed circles; black painted copper model in sun: closed triangles). Full sun shone on the site from 1035 to 1330, after which rain began at 1410 and the animal retreated to the base of the bush. Note that animal temperature is below the temperatures of both models in the sun. The lizard illustrated had the median body temperature of all individuals measured.

Table 2
Laboratory-determined body temperatures for six species of Kenyan chameleons (*Chamaeleo* spp.)

Species	CTMin	Vol Min	PBT	Vol Max	Pant Thresh	CTMax
bitaeniatus	4.4+0.67(5)	26.7+2.05(2)	31.1+0.29(5)	35.5+0.52(3)	34.7+0.87(5)	42.1+0.21(5)
dilepis	7.6+0.22(5)	–	32.8+0.14(6)	–	38.1+0.50(5)	43.6+0.05(5)
ellioti	3.5+0.50(6)	26.6+0.60(2)	33.4+0.70(6)	35.0+0.47(4)	37.8+1.27(6)	41.8+0.38(6)
hohnelii	5.1+0.73(6)	26.8+0.60(5)	30.2+0.36(6)	34.3+0.42(5)	37.2+0.62(5)	40.8+0.20(7)
jacksonii	5.3+0.50(8)	29.1+0.32(7)	32.1+0.24(7)	34.2+0.31(7)	36.2+0.67(5)	41.0+0.15(8)
schubotzi	1.4+0.27(6)	29.1+1.95(4)	32.6+0.63(8)	35.5+0.34(6)	36.7+0.74(6)	41.6+0.21(6)

CTMin=critical thermal minimum, Vol Min=voluntary minimum, PBT=preferred body temperature, Vol Max=voluntary maximum, Pant Thresh=panting threshold, CTMax=critical thermal maximum. Data in degrees Celsius are reported as mean ± SE (number of individuals); except for CTMin and CTMax, mean values for each individual were first obtained by averaging all observations for that animal and reported statistics are based on those means. *C. dilepis* did not have well defined Vol Min or Vol Max.

minima ($F_{5,30}$=14) and maxima ($F_{5,31}$=18) and in preferred body temperatures ($F_{5,32}$=5.6), but not in voluntary minima or maxima or panting thresholds (p>0.05).

The critical thermal minimum of *C. dilepis* is greater than those of all other species and that of *C. schubotzi* is lower than those of all other species except *C. ellioti*. Critical thermal maximum of *C. dilepis* is greater than that of all other species. No species was consistently different from all the others in preferred temperature. Mean critical thermal minima are significantly correlated with mean annual minimum (p=0.004) and mean annual maximum (p=0.018) air temperatures. Other thermoregulatory temperatures measured in the laboratory are not significantly correlated with air temperature.

4. Discussion

From the elaborate suite of behaviors undertaken and the distribution of environmental temperatures, it is clear that these chameleon species are not indifferent to body temperature and do not passively accept environmental conditions. Rather, when solar radiation is available, they use it to regulate body temperature. They utilize most of the behaviors that have become classically associated with heliothermic behavioral thermoregulation [1]. As soon as the sun comes out, they climb to the exposed side or top of the vegetation and orient their bodies perpendicular to the rays of the sun. At this time, body color is uniformly dark, maximizing radiant heat absorption [12]. After reaching preferred thermal levels (Table 2), lighter and more cryptic coloration is assumed, and body temperatures are stabilized by moving back and forth between sunny and shady areas of the bush and by postural changes. Elevated basking posture [19], in which the body is oriented parallel to the sun's rays and the head points directly toward the sun and radiant heat gain is minimized, was very common in the middle of the day. With the exception of *C. schubotzi*, natural thermoregulation in these species is apparently not simply a matter of thermal maximization, that is, of getting as hot as the environment permits. Several observations support this conclusion: the shade-seeking behavior already discussed, and the temperatures of both animals and thermal models placed in full sun. Body temperatures of tethered lizards given no access to shade rapidly rose above those of freely thermoregulating animals (when panting was initiated, they were immediately moved into the shade). Copper models placed in the sun, the same size and shape of the lizards and painted either white, gray, or black, attained equilibrium temperatures far in excess of those observed for freely thermoregulating animals (e.g., Fig. 2). All these observations suggest that, given access to solar radiation, these chameleon species are competent behavioral thermoregulators and not thermal maximizers.

Field body temperature regulation in *C. schubotzi* requires further comment. The moorland slopes of Mt. Kenya, the endemic habitat of this species, are frequently covered by cloud and fog [20,21], limiting thermoregulatory opportunities. Body temperatures of animals in the field were monitored on two days, one that was cloudy and rainy and the other that dawned cloudless and sunny (Fig. 3) (data from only the latter are reported in Table 1). On the cloudy day, cloud cover ranged from 60% to 100%, shade and exposed black body temperatures peaked at 10.9 and 22.1 °C, respectively. The four animals monitored reached a mean maximal body temperature of 20.4 °C. A heavy rain began at 1330 and the lizards retreated into their bushes. On the sunny day, unobstructed sunlight shone on the study site from 0740 to 1100. The six chameleons monitored, which had a mean body temperature at 0730 of 3.5 °C, climbed (slowly) to the topmost branches of their bushes and basked perpendicular to the sun's rays. Body temperatures rose to a mean maximum of 29.2 °C at 1000–1030, when black body temperatures exceeded 50 °C. Clouds began to move in at 1,100 and a steady rain started at 1400, whereupon the lizards retreated into their bushes. Although sunny periods of intense insolation do occur on Mt. Kenya [19], they appear to be very restricted temporally and the weather may be cloudy for many days at a time [18]. Even on an exceptionally clear day, the resident chameleons were able to attain preferred temperatures for only about an hour. On many days, they never approach these levels, but are nevertheless field active. Given the opportunity, *C. schubotzi* will regulate higher body temperatures under field conditions. Six animals were placed in natural vegetation in the vicinity of Nairobi (the same location used to monitor field body temperatures of *C. hohnelii* and *jacksonii*), an area receiving considerably more insolation (black body temperature during trial=55.9 °C). They

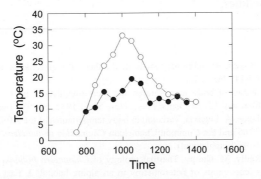

Fig. 3. Field body temperatures of two individual *Chamaeleo schubotzi* in the moorlands near the top of Mount Kenya, one on a cloudy day (22 Feb 1990, closed circles) and one on a sunny day (12 March 1990, open circles). Lizards illustrated had the median body temperature of individuals measured on each day.

maintained an average temperature of 31.3 °C (range of individual means=30.4–34.0 °C) throughout the sunny part of the day. These observations indicate that this species has low field body temperatures because of environmental temperature conditions, not an innately low behavioral preference for such temperatures.

The species investigated here and other previously examined chameleons have the ability to be active at low body temperatures. In the field, *C. schubotzi* climbed up into the sunlight with body temperatures of less than 5 °C. Feeding was observed at 18.4 °C in *C. jacksonii*, 24.2 °C in *C. ellioti*, and 26.4 °C in *C. schubotzi*. In the laboratory, *C. jacksonii* could feed, walk, and climb competently with a body temperature of 10 °C. Other workers have reported feeding in *C. pumilus* at 3.5 °C [8] and *C. hohnelii* at 7 °C [4]. Most other lizards are not active at such temperatures, and these scattered anecdotal observations of chameleon activity in the field have given the erroneous impression that they are indifferent to temperature or actually prefer low temperatures (e.g., Refs. [4,5]). While chameleons do have the ability to maintain limited activity in the cold, they nevertheless seem to prefer to be warmer. Given access to heat, chameleons are effective and fairly careful thermoregulators. The six species studied here have preferred temperatures of 30–33 °C, and other species of *Chamaeleo* studied similarly fall into this rather narrow range (*C. namaquensis*, 33 °C, *C. dilepis*, 31 °C [6]; *C. africanus*, 31 °C, *C. chamaeleon*, 32 °C [3]). Preferred temperatures of 25 and 29 °C have been reported for *C. pumilus* and *C. namquensis* [8], respectively, but these may be 24 h measurements and include inactive periods. Inclement weather, strong diurnal thermal fluctuations, and/or high altitude habitation may force them to spend part or even all of their day at low body temperatures, but given access to solar radiation, they seem little different than most other lizards in their preference for warm and constant body temperatures.

Acknowledgments

Supported by National Science Foundation research grants DCB88-12028, IBN-9118346, and IBN-0091308. I thank Jonathan Losos, Stephen Reilly, Peter Wainwright, and Michael Walton for assistance in collecting and observing these animals. I also thank Drs. Gabriel Mutungi and Titus Kanui of the University of Nairobi for their assistance and use of University facilities.

References

[1] R.B. Cowles, C.M. Bogert, A preliminary study of the thermal requirements of desert lizards, Bull. Am. Mus. Nat. Hist. 83 (1944) 265–276.

[2] R.A. Avery, Field studies of body temperatures and thermoregulation, in: C. Gans, F.H. Pough (Eds.), Biology of the Reptilia, vol. 12, Academic Press, New York, 1982, pp. 93–166.

[3] M. Dimaki, E.D. Valakos, A. Legakis, Variation in body temperatures of the African Chameleon *Chamaeleo africanus* Laurenti, 1786 and the Common Chameleon *Chamaeleo chamaeleon* (Linnaeus, 1758), Belg. J. Zool. 130 (2000) 89–93 (Supplement).

[4] J.J. Hebrard, S.M. Reilly, M. Guppy, Thermal ecology of *Chamaeleo hohnelii* and *Mabuya varia* in the Aberdare Mountains: constraints of heterothermy in an alpine habitat, J. East Afr. Nat. Hist. Soc. Mus. Kenya 176 (1982) 1–6.

[5] S.M. Reilly, Ecological notes on *Chamaeleo schubotzi* from Mount Kenya, J. Herpetol. Assoc. Afr. 28 (1982) 1–3.

[6] R.C. Stebbins, Body temperature studies in South African lizards, Koedoe 4 (1961) 54–67.

[7] H.R. Bustard, Observations on the life history and behaviour of *Chamaeleo hohnelii* (Steindachner), Copeia 1965 (1965) 401–410.

[8] B.R. Burrage, Comparative ecology and behaviour of *Chamaeleo pumilus pumilus* (Gmelin) and *C. namaquensis* A. Smith (Sauria: Chamaeleontidae), Ann. S. Afr. Mus. 61 (1973) 1–158.

[9] K.K.J. So, P.C. Wainwright, A.F. Bennett, Kinematics of prey processing in *Chamaeleo jacksonii*: conservation of function with morphological specialization, J. Zool. Lond. 226 (1992) 47–64.

[10] P.C. Wainwright, A.F. Bennett, The mechanism of tongue projection in chameleons: I. Electomyographic tests of functional hypotheses, J. Exp. Biol. 168 (1992) 1–21.

[11] P.C. Wainwright, A.F. Bennett, The mechanism of tongue projection in chameleons: II. Role of shape changes in a muscular hydrostat, J. Exp. Biol. 168 (1992) 23–40.

[12] B.M. Walton, A.F. Bennett, Temperature dependent color change in Kenyan chameleons, Physiol. Zool. 66 (1993) 270–287.

[13] J.B. Losos, B.M. Walton, A.F. Bennett, Trade-offs between sprinting and clinging ability in Kenyan chameleons, Funct. Ecol. 7 (1993) 281–286.

[14] K.R.G. Welch, Herpetology of Africa: A Checklist and Bibliography of the Orders Amphisbaenia, Sauria, and Serpentes, Krieger, Malabar, FL, 1982.

[15] B.H. Brattstrom, Body temperatures of reptiles, Am. Midl. Nat. 73 (1965) 376–422.

[16] Anonymous, Climatological Statistics for Kenya, Kenya Meteorological Department, Nairobi, 1984.

[17] Anonymous, Temperature Data for Stations in East Africa. Part 1, East African Meteorological Department, Nairobi, Kenya, 1970.

[18] S.E. Brinkman, P. Wurzel, R. Jaetzold, Meteorological observations on Mount Kenya, Mem. East Afr. Meteor. Dept. 4 (1968) 1–44.

[19] G.A. Bartholomew, A field study of temperature relations in the Galapagos Marine Iguana, Copeia 1966 (1966) 241–250.

[20] M.J. Coe, The Ecology of the Alpine Zone of Mount Kenya, W. Junk, The Hague, 1967.

[21] M.J. Coe, Microclimate and animal life in the equatorial mountains, Zool. Afr. 4 (1969) 101–128.

International Congress Series 1275 (2004) 242–249

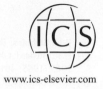

www.ics-elsevier.com

Cardiovascular mechanisms during thermoregulation in reptiles

Frank Seebacher[a],*, Craig E. Franklin[b]

[a]*Integrative Physiology, School of Biological Sciences A08, University of Sydney, N.S.W. 2006, Australia*
[b]*School of Life Sciences, University of Queensland, St. Lucia, Qld 4072, Australia*

Abstract. Vertebrates may control heat transfer with the environment by differentially changing heart rate and blood flow during heating and cooling. In reptiles, the ecological benefit of this physiological thermoregulation is a pronounced increase in the time spent at a "high" body temperature during the day. During heating and cooling in a lizard, the cardiovascular system is controlled by prostaglandins and to a lesser extent by the autonomic nervous system. There are, however, pronounced phylogenetic differences in cardiovascular control mechanisms of thermoregulating reptiles. Additionally, the characteristic heart rate "hysteresis" pattern also occurs in a crustacean, pointing towards parallel evolution of control mechanisms alongside increasing vascularisation. © 2004 Elsevier B.V. All rights reserved.

Keywords: Heart rate; Blood pressure; Nitric oxide; Prostaglandins; Heat transfer; Autonomic nervous system; Basking

1. Introduction

Temperature is the most pervasive physical parameter determining biological functions. The rate of enzyme catalyzed biochemical processes increases with temperature up to the denaturation temperature beyond which proteins lose their catalytic function. It may, therefore, be of selective advantage for body temperature to be within the range of biochemical performance [1,2]. The co-adaptation of body temperature and biochemical/physiological performance is most likely a combination of selecting body temperature within the range of optimal biochemical performance, and a change in the thermal sensitivity of physiological systems. The latter phenomenon is well demonstrated in reversible phenotypic plasticity of enzymatic functions where reaction optima change with

---

* Corresponding author. Tel.: +61 2 93512779; fax: +61 2 93514119.
E-mail address: fseebach@bio.usyd.edu.au (F. Seebacher).

0531-5131/ © 2004 Elsevier B.V. All rights reserved.
doi:10.1016/j.ics.2004.08.050

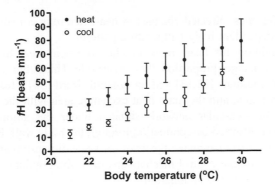

Fig. 1. A typical heart rate hysteresis pattern observed in the agamid lizard *Pogona vitticeps* (mean±S.E.; *n*=8; data redrawn from [10] where heart rates (f_H) during heating are significantly greater than during cooling at any given body temperature.

a change in average body temperatures [3,4]. Similar shifts of reaction optima exist also on an evolutionary scale whereby populations or species living at different latitudes have evolved different optima in biochemical and physiological rate processes that correspond to their different mean body temperatures [1,5].

Often, however, physiological performance is optimised within a tightly regulated body temperature range, and "thermoregulation" and optimisation of biochemical processes must at least have been correlated in evolutionary history. The most extreme examples of thermoregulators are endotherms which regulate body temperature within a range that is a fraction of environmental temperature fluctuations.

Terrestrial endotherms and ectotherms respond behaviourally to their thermal environment and seeking shade, panting, and basking are typical thermoregulatory behaviours. Rates of heat transfer between the animal and its environment may be controlled by regulation of blood flow between the core and periphery of the animal body. In reptiles, the term 'physiological thermoregulation' has been coined primarily to refer to cardiovascular changes in response to heating and cooling [6]. The notion of physiological mechanisms in reptilian thermoregulation is based on the striking pattern of differential heart rates during heating and cooling in lizards [7]. Heart rates during heating are significantly greater than during cooling at any given body temperature [7–9; Fig. 1]. This "heart rate hysteresis" presumably is of selective advantage by allowing the animal to heat faster when cool, and cool slower when hot so that body temperatures remain "high" and within preferred ranges for longer during the day. Similar patterns of cardiovascular control of heat exchange are widespread among ectothermic reptiles that regulate their body temperature behaviourally by moving between thermally different environments [6,8].

2. Function

Do changes in heart rate translate into an ecologically tangible benefit that may represent a selective advantage? The obvious ecological benefit is an increase in time per day spent at a body temperature within a range that allows physiological functions to proceed at biologically significant rates. Animals that are active in a thermally heterogeneous environment will rarely reach thermal equilibrium [11], and by altering transient heat transfer rates, directed changes in heart rate may convey ecological benefit by modifying time-dependent body temperature patterns.

A necessary condition for heart rates to alter transient heat transfer rates is that peripheral circulation changes proportionally to heart rate. This is the case for local rates of skin perfusion in crocodilians [12,13] and an iguanid lizard [14]. Heat transfer by blood flow occurs by convection, and the main heat exchange area with the environment is the three dimensional microvascular network situated under the animal surface [15,16]. Additionally, heat is transferred by conduction through the body wall. Rates of conduction will be similar in living and inanimate objects of the same dimension and material, and the significance of cardiovascular control mechanisms in thermoregulation lies in the relative contributions of blood flow and conduction.

The importance of convective heat transfer increases logistically with increasing heart rate in the lizard *Pogona barbata* (Fig. 2); the asymptote reached at high heart rates may reflect maximum perfusion rates of surface tissues. The range of heart rates within which convective heat exchange varies most rapidly corresponds to independently measured median heart rates in this species during heating and cooling (45 and 25 beats min^{-1}, respectively; [7]).

Changes in heart rate during heating and cooling may, therefore, significantly alter transient body temperature patterns. For example, agamid lizards usually emerge to bask in the morning, then move between heating and cooling environments during the day and cool in a shelter in the evening and overnight (Fig. 3). If differential heart rates were not displayed during the initial basking episode in the morning and the final cooling episode in the late afternoon/evening, the time during which body temperature was above 29.5 °C (the temperature the lizards heated to in the example) would be decreased as the ratio between heating and cooling heart rate decreases (Fig. 3). Even if only the initial heating and final cooling episodes are considered, lizards displaying the typical (observed) heart rate hysteresis pattern (heating/cooling f_H ratio=2) would have body temperature above 29.5 °C for an hour longer during the day compared with an animal whose heart rate was equal during heating and cooling (ratio=1; Fig. 3).

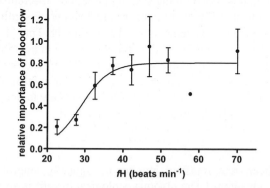

Fig. 2. The importance of blood flow relative to conduction in total animal heat transfer for different heart rates. The data were derived by calculating transient conduction during heating and cooling under field conditions in the agamid lizard *Pogona barbata* (mean±S.E.; *n*=6; [16,17]), and then comparing rates of conduction with measured rates of body temperature change at different heart rates.

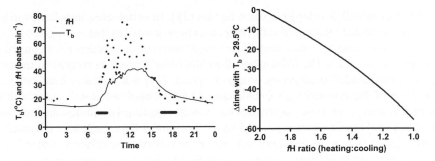

Fig. 3. A measured example of body temperature (T_b) and heart rate (f_H) records in the field (left panel). The decrease in time when body temperature >29.5 °C was calculated (using methods given in [16]) for different heating to cooling ratios of heart rate (right panel; observed heating/cooling f_H ratio=2) during the initial heating and final cooling episodes (indicated by the black bars, left panel).

Interestingly, the reverse pattern when heart rate during cooling is greater than during heating has been observed in animals that became heat stressed ([17], Franklin and Seebacher, unpublished data], and differential heart rates would provide a mechanism to avoid overheating as well as to accelerate heating.

3. Control

To be an effective mechanism of thermoregulation, differential heart rates during heating and cooling must be translated into changes in peripheral blood flow and be controlled by peripheral and central mechanisms. Incidence of heat at the animals' surface should lead to increased perfusion of peripheral tissue which, in turn, is likely to be maintained by increased cardiac output. Possibly, increased peripheral perfusion may be achieved by redistributing blood to the body surface while maintaining constant cardiac output. Such a pattern is not supported by experimental data, however, that clearly show an increase in heart rate (f_H) and cardiac output [18] in response to heat; it is, of course, possible that shunting and changes in cardiac output occur concomitantly. The central redistribution of flow blood via cardiac shunting could also influence flow patterns in the peripheral vasculature. Owing to their incompletely divided ventricle, non-crocodilian reptiles have the capacity to shunt blood between the pulmonary and systemic circuits, and both right to left, or left to right, shunting is possible [19]. In crocodilians, the complete separation of ventricles does not allow a left to right shunt, however, the exiting of the left aorta from the right ventricle permits a right to left shunt [20]. During heating, a right-to-left (i.e., pulmonary to systemic shunt) would facilitate an increase in blood flow to the body and possibly the periphery, whereas during cooling, a left to right shunt (systemic to pulmonary) would decrease blood flow to the periphery. Recent evidence of patterns of cardiac shunting in the freshwater turtle, *Trachemys scripta* during heating and cooling indicate however, that shunt patterns do not contribute to heat exchange [18].

In the marine iguana, *Amblyrhynchus cristatus*, peripheral blood flow changes immediately before heart rate [14] which would suggest that the 'hysteresis' pattern is initiated by local vasoactive compounds. Locally induced dilation or constriction of the peripheral vasculature may stimulate a compensatory response in heart rate via the baroreflex that is well developed in some reptiles [21]. In vertebrates, imbalances in blood pressure are regulated by a neural reflex response (the baroreflex) that is triggered by nerve endings in blood vessels sensing stretching (vasodilation) or contraction (vasoconstriction) of the vessel walls [22]. The information from the blood vessels is relayed to the central nervous system (medulla) triggering a reflex response [23] that modifies heart rate via the cardiac limb of the baroreflex [21]. Dilation of blood vessel walls will cause a drop in pressure that may elicit reflex adrenergic activation resulting in subsequent increases in heart rate. A cool reptile emerging to bask in the morning will gain selective advantages by increasing blood flow to its periphery, which may be achieved by dilation of blood vessels causing an increase in afferent baroreceptor discharge, and a subsequent increase in heart rate. This sequence of events would explain previous descriptions of heart rate hysteresis.

Adrenergic tone on the heart was three times as great during the initial phases of heating in *P. barbata* compared with during cooling at the same body temperature (Fig. 4). The increased sympathetic activity may partly explain the greater heart rates during heating, although cholinergic tone also increased initially during heating albeit to a lesser extent (Fig. 4). β-Adrenergic or muscarinic receptor induced modulation of heart rate does not, however, explain differential heart rates during heating and cooling, and the typical 'hysteresis' pattern persisted even when those receptors were blocked pharmacologically [9].

Potentially important non-neural vasoconstrictors or vasodilators include prostaglandins and nitric oxide. Prostaglandins are formed in vascular endothelium from arachidonic acid by cyclooxygenase (COX) enzymes of which there are two principle types: the constitutive COX 1, and the inducible COX 2 [24]. Interestingly, COX activity can be induced by nitric oxide and the interaction between these two systems may have far reaching physiological, including cardiovascular, implications [25]. A dramatic manifestation of prostaglandin vasoactivity is the disappearance of the typical heart rate 'hysteresis' pattern (see Fig. 1) in *Pogona vitticeps* when COX activity was inhibited (Fig. 5).

Hence, cardiovascular control during heating and cooling in this species is primarily driven by peripheral changes in resistance. Interestingly, however, there appears to be considerable variation in control mechanisms between species, and inhibiting COX

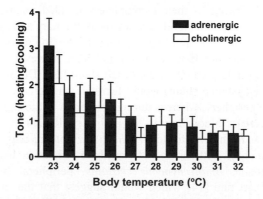

Fig. 4. The ratio between heating and cooling of adrenergic and cholinergic tones on the heart at different body temperatures in *Pogona barbata* (mean±S.E., $n=6$). Data were reanalysed and redrawn from [9].

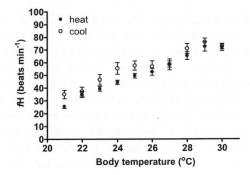

Fig. 5. Heart rate in *Pogona vitticeps* (mean±S.E., *n*=8) during heating and cooling after the prostaglandin synthesising cyclooxygenase (COX) enzyme was inhibited. There were no significant differences in heart rates between heating and cooling (data redrawn from [10]).

enzyme did not affect differential heart rates or blood pressure during heating and cooling in the crocodile *Crocodylus porosus* (Fig. 6). Additionally, inhibition of nitric oxide synthase did not affect the heart rate hysteresis pattern in *C. porosus* [26]. Crocodile cardiovascular responses are strongly controlled by cholinergic and adrenergic receptors [21] and it may be that cardiovascular control during heating and cooling in crocodiles is predominantly achieved by the autonomic nervous system.

4. Evolution

The pronounced differences in cardiovascular control during heating and cooling in reptiles beg the question of how the phenomenon of differential heart rates during heating and cooling ('heart rate hysteresis') has evolved. The question becomes particularly pertinent when considering that within the thermal neutral zone in endotherms thermoregulation is principally achieved by similar cardiovascular changes. An essential pre-requisite for control of blood flow is a vascular system, and it may be possible that 'hysteresis' evolved alongside vascularisation of circulatory systems. If this were the case, the phenomenon would not be a reptile or vertebrate specific trait, but it could potentially also be found in other groups with a high degree of vascularisation. This

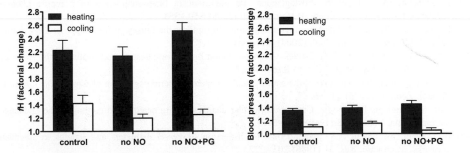

Fig. 6. Heart rate (left panel, mean±S.E., *n*=8) and blood pressure (right panel, mean±S.E., *n*=8) during heating and cooling in the crocodile *Crocodylus porosus* after administration of saline (control), or after inhibiting nitric oxide synthase (no NO), or NOS and COX enzymes (no NO+PG). Data are factorial changes from resting pre-heating heart rates (redrawn from [26]).

hypothesis was tested in a crustacean, the crayfish *Cherax destructor* [27]. Decapod crustaceans have a complex arterial system and return flow to the heart is via much reduced sinuses so that, while not a closed circulatory system, blood flow can be regulated [28]. Fascinatingly, *C. destructor* showed a strong pattern of heart rate hysteresis similar to that found in many reptiles (as exemplified in Fig. 1). Hence, heart rate hysteresis has evolved in lineages as evolutionarily distant as deuterostomes and protostomes. It seems unlikely that the trait is ancestral as the last common ancestor of crustaceans and reptiles, maybe a cnidarian-like organism, would not have had a circulatory system. It may be, however, that the principle components, such as neurons and a basic endocrine system present in modern cnidarians [29], in conjunction with physical constraints of fluid dynamics, led to similar outcomes in the parallel evolution of cardiovascular systems.

References

[1] D.L. Crawford, V. Pierce, J.A. Segal, Evolutionary physiology of closely related taxa: analyses of enzyme expression, Am. Zool. 39 (1999) 1–11.

[2] R.B. Huey, A.F. Bennett, Phylogenetic studies of coadaptation: preferred temperatures versus optimal performance temperatures of lizards, Evolution 41 (1987) 1098–1115 (120).

[3] J. St. Pierre, P.-M. Charest, H. Guderley, Relative contribution of quantitative changes in mitochondria to metabolic compensation during seasonal acclimatisation of rainbow trout *Oncorhynchus mykiss*, J. Exp. Biol. 201 (1998) 2961–2970.

[4] F. Seebacher, et al., Seasonal acclimatisation of muscle metabolic enzymes in a reptile (*Alligator mississippiensis*), J. Exp. Biol. 206 (2003) 1193–1200.

[5] H. Guderley, Metabolic responses to low temperature in fish muscle, Biol. Rev. 79 (2004) 409–427.

[6] G.A. Bartholomew, Physiological control of body temperature, in: C. Gans, F.H. Pough (Eds.), Biology of Reptilia, vol. 12, Academic Press, New York, 1982, pp. 167–212.

[7] G.A. Bartholomew, V.A. Tucker, Control of changes in body temperature, metabolism, and circulation by the agamid lizard, *Amphibolurus barbatus*, Physiol. Zool. 36 (1963) 199–218.

[8] G.C. Grigg, C.R. Drane, G.P. Courtice, Time constants of heating and cooling in the eastern water dragon, *Physignathus lesueurii*, and some generalizations about heating and cooling in reptiles, J. Therm. Biol. 4 (1979) 95–103.

[9] F. Seebacher, C.E. Franklin, Control of heart rate during thermoregulation in the heliothermic lizard, *Pogona barbata*: importance of cholinergic and adrenergic mechanisms, J. Exp. Biol. 204 (2001) 4361–4366.

[10] F. Seebacher, C.E. Franklin, Prostaglandins are important in thermoregulation of a reptile (*Pogona vitticeps*), Proc. Roy. Soc. Lond., B (Suppl.) 270 (2003) S50–S53.

[11] F. Seebacher, R. Shine, Evaluating thermoregulation in reptiles: the fallacy of the inappropriately applied method, Physiol. Biochem. Zool. (2004) (in press).

[12] E.N. Smith, S. Robertson, D.G. Davies, Cutaneous blood flow during heating and cooling in the American alligator, Am. J. Physiol. 235 (1978) R160–R167.

[13] G.C. Grigg, J. Alchin, The role of the cardiovascular system in thermoregulation of *Crocodylus johnstoni*, Physiol. Zool. 49 (1976) 24–36.

[14] K.R. Morgareidge, F.N. White, Cutaneous vascular changes during heating and cooling in the Galapagos marine iguana, Nature 223 (1969) 587–591.

[15] B. Dawant, M. Levin, A.S. Popel, Effect of dispersion of vessel diameters and lengths in stochastic networks, Microvasc. Res. 31 (1986) 203–222.

[16] F. Seebacher, Heat transfer in a microvascular network: the effect of heart rate on heating and cooling in reptiles (*Pogona barbata* and *Varanus varius*), J. Theor. Biol. 202 (2000) 97–109.

[17] G.C. Grigg, F. Seebacher, Field test of a paradigm: hysteresis of heart rate in thermoregulation by a free-ranging lizard (*Pogona barbata*), Proc. Roy. Soc. Lond., B 266 (1999) 1291–1297.

[18] G. Galli, E.W. Taylor, T. Wang, The cardiovascular responses of the freshwater turtle *Trachemys scripta* to warming and cooling, J. Exp. Biol. 207 (2004) 1471–1478.

[19] W.W. Burggren, Form and function in reptilian circulations, Am. Zool. 27 (1987) 2–19.

[20] M. Axelsson, C.E. Franklin, From anatomy to angioscopy: 164 years of crocodilian cardiovascular research, recent advances and speculations, Comp. Biochem. Physiol. 118A (1997) 51–62.

[21] J. Altimiras, C.E. Franklin, M. Axelsson, Relationship between blood pressure and heart rate in the saltwater crocodile *Crocodylus porosus*, J. Exp. Biol. 201 (1998) 2235–2242.

[22] P.A. Lafranchi, V.K. Somers, Arterial baroreflex function and cardiovascular variability: interactions and implications, Am. J. Physiol. 283 (2002) R815–R826.

[23] L.A. Henderson, K.A. Keay, R. Bandler, Caudal midline medulla mediates behaviourally-coupled but not baroreceptor-mediated vasodepression, Neuroscience 98 (2000) 779–792.

[24] H. Scholtz, Prostaglandins, Am. J. Physiol. 285 (2003) R512–R514.

[25] D. Salvemini, Regulation of cyclooxygenase enzymes by NO, Cell. Mol. Life Sci. 53 (1997) 576–582.

[26] F. Seebacher, C.E. Franklin, Integration of autonomic and local mechanisms in regulating cardiovascular responses to heating and cooling in a reptile (*Crocodylus porosus*), J. Comp. Physiol., B (2004) (in press).

[27] J.E. Goudkamp, et al., Physiological thermoregulation in a crustacean? Heart rate hysteresis in the freshwater crayfish *Cherax destructor*, Comp. Biochem. Physiol., A 138 (2004) 399-403.

[28] B. McMahon, Control of cardiovascular function and its evolution in Crustacea, J. Exp. Biol. 204 (2001) 923–932.

[29] R.T. Hinde, The cnidaria and ctenophora, in: D.T. Anderson (Ed.), Invertebrate Zoology, Oxford Univ. Press, Melbourne, 1999, pp. 28–57.

ELSEVIER

www.ics-elsevier.com

Do TSD, sex ratios, and nest characteristics influence the vulnerability of tuatara to global warming?

Nicola J. Nelson[a,*], Michael B. Thompson[b], Shirley Pledger[c], Susan N. Keall[a], Charles H. Daugherty[a]

[a]School of Biological Sciences, Victoria University of Wellington, P.O. Box 600,
Wellington, New Zealand
[b]Integrative Physiology Research Group, School of Biological Sciences (A08),
University of Sydney, Australia
[c]School of Mathematical and Computing Sciences, Victoria University of Wellington, New Zealand

Abstract. Tuatara (*Sphenodon punctatus*) are threatened New Zealand reptiles with temperature-dependent sex determination (TSD). Higher incubation temperatures produce males, and less than 1 °C separates production of males and females. We investigated variability in nesting ecology to assess whether global warming is likely to result in increasingly male-biased populations. We examined nesting seasons during 1998/1999 and 2002/2003 in New Zealand's largest tuatara population on Stephens Island, and collected hourly temperature recordings and physical descriptions from 70 nests. Nest depths were not significantly different between years, and ranged from 10 to 230 mm from the soil surface to the top egg. Incubation temperatures in successful nests throughout the year-long incubation period ranged from 1.6 to 38.4 °C. Sex ratios of nests were correlated with incubation temperature: 64% males were produced in 1998/1999, a relatively warm season, but we predict an equal sex ratio was produced in 2002/2003. Although temperatures varied over the 2002/2003 season with respect to monthly long-term averages, 2002 was the second warmest year on record. Stephens Island supports a wide range of nesting habitat, a relatively large population of tuatara, and nest characteristics are highly variable. As such, this population is likely to be resilient to global warming in the short term because an equal sex ratio was predicted from a relatively warm season. However, most other islands where tuatara occur are smaller, have smaller populations, and have fewer open areas for nesting and/or shallower soils. These conditions are more likely to produce a male bias in hatchlings because female

---

* Corresponding author. Tel.: +64 4 463 7443; fax: +64 4 463 5331.
E-mail address: nicola.nelson@vuw.ac.nz (N.J. Nelson).

0531-5131/ © 2004 Elsevier B.V. All rights reserved.
doi:10.1016/j.ics.2004.08.093

tuatara do not appear to vary construction of nests with respect to temperature or location. In the extreme, this could lead to the extinction of small populations. © 2004 Elsevier B.V. All rights reserved.

Keywords: Temperature-dependent sex determination; TSD; *Sphenodon*; Reptilia; Sex ratio; Nest variability; Global warming

1. Introduction

Reptiles with temperature-dependent sex determination (TSD), where embryonic sex is determined by incubation temperatures, have survived extreme climate change before [1]. However, the short time frame and the scale of global temperature increase predicted (+1.4–5.8 °C in the next 100 years)[2] may result in sex ratio imbalances that will threaten population persistence. Species with narrow transitional ranges (the range of incubation temperatures that produce 100% of one sex to 100% of the other sex) and long generation times (indicating limited potential to respond to rapid changes in climate) have four alternatives: to modify their geographic range, to convert to genetic sex determination, to go extinct, or to modify their nesting behaviour [3,4]. Biased sex ratios are already known for reptiles with TSD [5]. A general warming trend is already evident in sea turtle nests (*Chelonia mydas* at Ascension Island) over the past 100 years [6]. In addition, findings so far point to nest site selection by female reptiles for hatching success rather than sex ratio manipulation (e.g. Refs. [4,7,8]).

Tuatara (*Sphenodon*), long-lived sole surviving members of the reptilian Order Sphenodontia, are restricted to small off-shore islands of New Zealand [9]. The two species (*S. guntheri* and *S. punctatus*) both have the rare Type 1b pattern of TSD, where males are produced from nests with higher incubation temperatures [10,11]. There is no evidence so far to suggest they exhibit the type II pattern of TSD where females are produced at both extremes and males at intermediate incubation temperatures [11]. The pivotal temperature of the largest population of tuatara (21.7 °C, *S. punctatus* on Stephens Island) is relatively low for reptiles [12]. In addition, sex determination of embryos from this population occurs over a narrow transitional range of less than 1 °C [11]. The adult sex ratio on Stephens Island is estimated to be 50% males [13]. The only extant population of *S. guntheri* on North Brother Island comprises 60% adult males [14].

Nesting occurs in spring from early November, and female tuatara lay a clutch of eggs only about every 2–5 years [15,16]. Shallow subterranean nests are constructed in open areas, not in forest habitat where temperatures are too low for successful development of embryos. On Stephens Island, nesting occurs in paddocks grazed by sheep, open cliff faces and rocky outcrops, and paths [16].

We investigate whether the tuatara's rare pattern of TSD, biased sex ratios, and diversity of nest characteristics and habitat influence the likelihood of male-biased populations that potentially threaten population persistence as a result of global warming. As the first step towards an inventory we ask the following questions: (1) What is the hatchling sex ratio? (2) Are there between-year variations in hatchling sex ratio? (3) Are there between-year variations in nest construction or time of laying?

2. Methods

Nests of tuatara were investigated during the annual nesting seasons in 1998 (3 weeks, November 1–21)[11] and 2002 (6 weeks, October 28–December 7) on Stephens Island (150 ha), New Zealand. Temperature data loggers (waterproof Stowaway® TidbiT®, dimensions: $30 \times 41 \times 17$ mm, Onset Computer, MA, USA) set to record hourly measurements were inserted into nests spread throughout rookeries in sheep paddocks and on rocky outcrops (25 nests in 1998 and 45 nests in 2002). Back-fill of nests was excavated, and the data logger was placed beside the eggs. Nests were carefully re-filled and left intact until the following nesting season (October 1999 (11 months incubation) and December 2003 (13 months incubation), respectively). Physical descriptions were recorded for each nest, including depth to the top layer of eggs and location/rookery (for example, winch house paddock, house #3 paddock). The number of eggs and hatching success for each nest were recorded upon excavation of nests to retrieve data loggers. All hatchlings and/or eggs were collected from nests monitored during the 1998/1999 season and taken to Victoria University of Wellington to complete incubation at 22 °C (sex had already been determined in nests). Hatchlings were reared in captivity and sexed by laparoscopy at approximately one year of age [11]. Temperature recordings during the middle period of development were used to estimate the sex ratio of hatchlings from each nest in 2002/2003. The period of sex determination for tuatara is not known, but the middle third of development is when sex determination occurs in other reptiles [17].

Temperature records were summarised by calculating mean, minimum and maximum throughout incubation, and the constant temperature equivalent (CTE) during the middle period of development for each nest. The CTE is defined as the temperature above which half of embryonic development occurs [18,19]. In calculating the CTE, the models take account of the variance in temperatures, providing a more meaningful representation of the nest environment than the mean temperature. The inputs used for the Georges' model were developmental zero of 11.1 °C, reference temperature 18 °C with incubation period of 264 days, pivotal temperature 21°C, and hourly temperature records for each nest [11]. Outputs from the model include CTE and developmental progress (expressed as a proportion) for each 24-h period. Mean CTE during 0.45–0.55 of development was estimated to be within the period of sex determination for tuatara. Sex ratios predicted using CTE during 0.45–0.55 of development matched closely with known sex ratios of hatchlings from nests in 1998/1999. For tuatara, males are predicted to be produced if the CTE of a nest exceeds the threshold temperature for sex determination of males in artificial conditions, and females are predicted to be produced if the CTE is lower than the threshold. Previously, CTEs during February had been used due to the good correlation with known sex ratios in the 1998/1999 nesting season [11]. However, we did not want to make the assumption that 0.45–0.55 of development falls during February in all years. The narrow period of 0.45–0.55 of development was selected as this covered up to a month depending on the nest. A wider period, for example the middle third of development (0.33–0.66), would have resulted in inclusion of temperature data covering several months (and in some cases over winter), potentially introducing biases into sex ratio estimates for cooler nests.

Analyses of variance were performed using SAS on the following: nest depth as the dependent variable with nesting season (year), date of laying and rookery location as predictors; temperature of nest including minimum, maximum, mean or CTE as dependent variables with nest depth and year as predictors; and hatching success as the dependent variable and nest depth as the predictor.

Akaike's information criteria (AIC) [20,21] were used to compare logistic and asymmetric logistic models [22] for the proportion of male tuatara produced from nests in 1998/1999 with respect to nest CTE (mean during 0.45–0.55 of development) in R [23]. Proportions of males produced from nests in 2002/2003 were predicted using these models with input values of mean CTE during 0.45–0.55 of development for each nest in 2002/2003 and clutch size. Unless otherwise stated, all values presented are means±1 SE.

3. Results

Mean depth of nests was 103.5±9.2 mm (range 40–200 mm) in 1998/1999, and was not significantly different from 111.0±6.3 mm (range 10–230 mm) in 2002/2003 (Table 1; $F_{(1,60)}$=0.55; P=0.459). Nest depths were not significantly correlated with the date of laying or rookery location ($F_{(1,60)}$=0.36; P=0.551 and $F_{(8,53)}$=1.10; P=0.377). Depth significantly influenced variability of nest temperatures (minimum: $F_{(1,60)}$=28.45; P<0.001; maximum: $F_{(1,60)}$=17.25; P<0.001; CTE: $F_{(1,60)}$=5.50; P=0.022) but not mean temperatures ($F_{(1,60)}$=0.16; P=0.689). Nest depth influenced hatching success ($F_{(21,40)}$=2.35; P<0.01). For example, nests shallower than 50 mm were less than 50% successful.

Mean minimum and maximum temperatures in November 1998 during the laying season (measured at the meteorological station on Stephens Island; 10.3 and 14.9 °C, respectively) were higher than over the same period in 2002 (9.6 and 14.4 °C, respectively). Mean temperature throughout the lengthy incubation period in nests was higher in 1998/1999 (16.5±0.1 °C) than 2002/2003 (15.8±0.1 °C; $F_{(1,60)}$=24.93; P<0.001), but the range of temperatures experienced by successful nests was wider in the second season (2.9–34.4 °C in 1998/1999; 1.6–38.4 °C in 2002/2003). Minimum temperatures (but not maximum or CTE) were lower in 2002/2003 ($F_{(1,60)}$=9.38;

Table 1
Characteristics and temperatures of tuatara nests over two seasons: 1998/1999 (25 nests) and 2002/2003 (45 nests)

Incubation period	Depth (mm)	No. of eggs	Hatching success (%)	Temperature (°C)			CTE 0.45–0.55 Dev.
				Mean	Min.	Max.	
1998/1999							
Mean	103.5	9	66	16.5	7.1	27.6	22.1
Min.	40	3	0	15.3	2.9	23.3	18.5
Max.	200	13	100	17.6	8.7	34.4	25.7
SE	9.2	0.1	8	0.1	0.3	0.6	0.4
2002/2003							
Mean	110.9	8.8	55	15.8	5.6	28.7	21.4
Min.	10	0	0	14.1	1.6	20.1	17.1
Max.	230	22[a]	100	17.0	10.4	38.4	25.1
SE	6.3	0.6	6	0.1	0.2	0.6	0.2

[a] May include more than one clutch. CTE refers to constant temperature equivalent of nests.

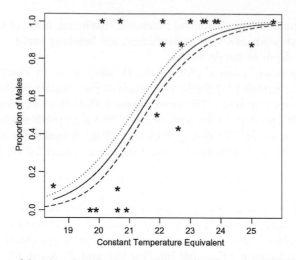

Fig. 1. A logistic curve of the proportion of males (±1 SE) produced from the 1998/1999 season tuatara nests with respect to constant temperature equivalents (CTE) during the middle (0.45–0.55) of development (°C). Individual nest CTEs are represented by stars. This curve was used to estimate the proportion of males in nests from the 2002/2003 season using CTE for those nests.

P=0.003). Mean temperatures of nests were significantly different across rookeries ($F_{(8,53)}$=3.07; P=0.006).

Mean clutch size did not differ between years: 9±0.6 eggs in 1998/1999 and 8.8±0.6 eggs in 2002/2003. Hatching success was significantly higher in the first season (66% compared to 55%; X_1^2=7.271, P=0.007).

Nests in 1998/1999 produced 64% males. The asymmetric logistic model (AIC 124.9; # parameters=3) was not a significantly better predictor of the pattern of sex determination than the logistic model (AIC 124.2; # parameters=2; X_1^2=1.275), so the logistic model (pivotal temperature=21.3°C; steepness parameter=0.97) was used to predict the sex ratio of hatchlings from the 2002/2003 season nests (Fig. 1). We predict an equal sex ratio of hatchlings was produced from nests incubated during the 2002/2003 season, comprising 111.3±7.1 males and 105.7±7.1 females. Sex ratios and numbers of nests varied across the rookeries, with only the winch house and house #3 paddocks having reasonable numbers of nests in both seasons. The winch house paddock produced a preponderance of male-biased nests from both seasons, while the house #3 paddock produced an equal sex ratio in 1998/1999 and a female-biased sex ratio from 2002/2003. No rookeries produced female-biased sex ratios in 1998/1999.

4. Discussion

We found a male-biased sex ratio in our first season of monitoring tuatara nests, but estimated an equal sex ratio from the second season. Several differences exist between the two seasons. Although we encompassed the preponderance of nesting in each instance, nests in the first season in 1998/1999 were marked over 3 weeks compared to 6 weeks in the second season (2002/2003). Temperatures during November, the primary period for laying, were higher in the first season. Warmer weather during nest construction may have resulted in the shortened nesting season. Deposition of eggs earlier in the season may result in higher average temperatures of nests due to nest exposure to a longer summer period. Mean incubation temperature of nests was higher in the first season. However, we do not know whether individual female tuatara that lay eggs only every 2–5 years [15] were the same (or different) between the two seasons, and whether individuals characteristically lay at a certain time during a season (for example early or late). Another difference between seasons was the number of nests. Almost twice as many nests were monitored in the second season. However, nests in the first season were a sample selected to represent the diversity of nest site characteristics observed during that season. Not all nests were monitored in 1998/1999 as during that study eggs were also collected for artificial incubation [11,24]. Lastly, the sex ratio in the first season was measured directly by laparoscopy of hatchlings, compared to estimation of sex ratios from the second season using TSD models developed using the first season's data. Direct measurements of sex ratio cannot be conducted on all individuals in all seasons due to logistics and restrictions involved in collecting hatchlings of a protected species and holding them for a year to enable laparoscopies to be conducted. We will continue to refine our estimates of the sex determining period for tuatara and techniques for modelling temperatures of natural nests to estimate sex ratios.

Nest depths were not significantly different between seasons, among rookeries, or with respect to date of egg deposition, suggesting female tuatara on average do not construct nests according to environmental cues during nesting (e.g. relative temperature or day length) or nest site location (e.g. aspect or soil structure). However, the location of nests (rookery) affected temperatures, probably as a result of thermal properties of soil and aspects of rookeries. Variability of temperatures and hatching success in a nest were correlated with nest depth, suggesting that individual females have the potential to manipulate success and sex ratio of hatchlings depending on which rookery they choose and how they construct nests. Other species of reptiles demonstrate both species-specific and female-specific differences in nest site selection, to maximise embryonic survival and potentially to manipulate sex ratio (e.g. Ref. [7]). We do not know whether female tuatara construct similar nests in similar locations every time they nest. However, we have observed nesting in the same rookeries and the same areas within rookeries since 1986. Many of the nesting females have individual marks (toe-clips [25] or passive integrated transponders) that will allow us to investigate whether variability of sex ratios among years is a consequence of year to year variation in temperatures during egg deposition and/or incubation season, and hence likely to be influenced by global warming, or of nest construction and site selection of individuals depositing eggs in any particular year.

Temperatures on Stephens Island throughout the 1998/1999 summer were warmer than average based on records covering the past 35 years, including the warmest February and March on record in 1999. The average temperature in 1998 was 0.47 °C warmer than usual in the Southern Hemisphere and the highest on record (NIWA National Climate Database). In contrast, temperatures on Stephens Island throughout the 2002/2003 summer were cooler than average in November, January and February, and warmer than average in December and March, although 2002 in the Southern Hemisphere was the second warmest year on record (0.36 °C warmer than usual; NIWA National Climate Database). Warmer periods during egg deposition are likely to result in greater nesting activity, but whether this translates into completion of nesting in a shorter period of time is uncertain. As female tuatara nest only every 2–5 years, we intend to investigate individual variation in nesting over time and patterns of nest variation over years where independence of females can be guaranteed.

Stephens Island supports a wide range of nesting habitat for tuatara, from artificially created areas like sheep paddocks to natural cliff edges. The variety and abundance of nesting habitat is proposed to be the reason this island supports the largest population of tuatara. Investigating how global warming may affect sex ratios of tuatara populations on Stephens Island is possible because nesting can be observed and relatively large amounts of data obtained. Results from two nesting seasons suggest sex ratios of tuatara populations will be resilient to global warming in the short term because an equal sex ratio was predicted from a relatively warm season. However, most other islands where tuatara occur are smaller, have fewer open areas for nesting and/or shallower soils. Additionally, nesting is comparatively difficult to monitor. As nest depth influences hatching success and sex ratio through temperature, and female tuatara do not appear to dig deeper nests in warmer years, a male bias in hatchlings may be more likely from tuatara nests on other islands. In the extreme, this could lead to extinction of small populations.

Acknowledgements

We thank the Marsden Fund and the Zoological Society of San Diego for funding, Arthur Georges, Brian Gartrell, and Alison Cree for help with techniques, and Victoria University of Wellington Animal Ethics Committee, Te Ngati Koata no Rangitoto ki te Tonga Trust and the New Zealand Department of Conservation for permitting the study.

References

[1] C.H. Daugherty, A. Cree, Tuatara: a survivor from the dinosaur age, N.Z. Geogr. 6 (1990) 66–86.
[2] IPCC, Climate Change 2001: The Scientific Basis. Inter-Governmental Panel on Climate Change, Cambridge University Press, 2001.
[3] F.J. Janzen, G.L. Paukstis, Environmental sex determination in reptiles: ecology, evolution, and experimental design, Q. Rev. Biol. 66 (1991) 149–179.
[4] C.L. Morjan, How rapidly can maternal behaviour affecting primary sex ratio evolve in a reptile with environmental sex determination, Am. Nat. 162 (2) (2003) 205–219.
[5] S. Freedberg, M.J. Wade, Cultural inheritance as a mechanism for population sex-ratio bias in reptiles, Evolution 55 (5) (2001) 1049–1055.
[6] G.C. Hays, et al., Climate change and sea turtles: a 150-year reconstruction of incubation temperatures at a major marine turtle rookery, Glob. Chang. Biol. 9 (4) (2003) 642–646.
[7] W.K. Bragg, J.D. Fawcett, T.B. Bragg, Nest-site selection in two eublepharid gecko species with temperature-dependent sex determination and one with genotypic sex determination, Biol. J. Linn. Soc. 69 (2000) 319–332.
[8] J.S. Doody, P. West, A. Georges, Beach selection in nesting pig-nosed turtles, Carettochelys insculpta, J. Herpetol. 37 (1) (2003) 178–182.
[9] A. Cree, D. Butler, in: Tuatara Recovery Plan (Sphenodon spp.). Threatened Species Recovery Plan Series, vol. 9, Department of Conservation, Wellington, New Zealand, 1993.
[10] A. Cree, M.B. Thompson, C.H. Daugherty, Tuatara sex determination, Nature 375 (1995) 543.

[11] N.J. Nelson, et al., Temperature-dependent sex determination in tuatara, in: N. Valenzuela, V. Lance (Eds.), Temperature-Dependent Sex Determination in Vertebrates, Smithsonian Institution Press, 2004, pp. 53–58.

[12] G.F. Birchard, Effects of incubation temperature, in: D.C. Deeming (Ed.), Reptilian Incubation: Environment, Evolution and Behaviour, Nottingham University Press, 2004.

[13] D.G. Newman, Tuatara, *Sphenodon punctatus*, and burrows, Stephens Island, in: D.G. Newman (Ed.), New Zealand Herpetology, Occasional Publication, vol. 2, New Zealand Wildlife Service, Department of Internal Affairs, Wellington, 1982.

[14] N.J. Nelson, et al., Male-biased sex ratio in a small tuatara population, J. Biogeogr. 29 (2002) 633–640.

[15] A. Cree, et al., Laparoscopy, radiography, and blood samples as techniques for identifying the reproductive condition of female tuatara, Herpetologica 47 (1991) 238–249.

[16] M.B. Thompson, et al., Analysis of the nest environment of tuatara, *Sphenodon punctatus*, J. Zool., Lond. 238 (1996) 239–251.

[17] C.L. Yntema, Temperature levels and periods of sex determination during incubation of eggs of *Chelydra serpentina*, J. Morph. 159 (1979) 17–28.

[18] A. Georges, Female turtles from hot nests: is it duration of incubation or proportion of development at high temperatures that matters? Oecologia 81 (1989) 323–328.

[19] A. Georges, C. Limpus, R. Stoutjesdijk, Hatchling sex in the marine turtle *Caretta caretta* is determined by proportion of development at a temperature, not daily duration of exposure, J. Exp. Zool. 270 (1994) 432–444.

[20] H. Akaike, Information theory as an extension of the maximum likelihood principle, in: B.N. Petrov, F. Caski (Eds.), Second International Symposium on Information Theory, Academiai Kiado, 1973.

[21] K.P. Burnham, D.R. Anderson, Model Selection and Inference. A Practical Information—Theoretic Approach, Springer-Verlag, NY, 1998.

[22] M.H. Godfrey, V. Delmas, M. Girondot, Assessment of patterns of temperature-dependent sex determination using maximum likelihood model selection, Ecoscience 10 (2003) 265–272.

[23] R. Gentleman, R. Ihaka, F. Leisch, R: A Language and Environment for Statistical Computing. Vienna, Austria, 2003.

[24] N.J. Nelson, Temperature-Dependent Sex Determination and Artificial Incubation of Tuatara, *Sphenodon punctatus*. [Unpublished PhD Thesis], Victoria University of Wellington, Wellington, 2002.

[25] E. Christmas, E. Coddington, A. Cree, A database for toe-clipped tuatara (*Sphenodon punctatus*) on Stephens Island (Takapourewa). University of Otago Wildlife Management Report Number 77, Otago, 1996.

International Congress Series 1275 (2004) 258–266

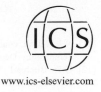

www.ics-elsevier.com

Thermal adaptation of maternal and embryonic phenotypes in a geographically widespread ectotherm

Michael J. Angilletta Jr.[a,*], Christopher E. Oufiero[a], Michael W. Sears[b]

[a]Department of Life Sciences, Indiana State University, Terre Haute, IN 47809, USA
[b]Department of Biology, University of Nevada, Reno, NV 89557, USA

Abstract. Current theories predict the thermal adaptation of both maternal and embryonic phenotypes such that the fitness of the entire life cycle is maximized. Our studies of the eastern fence lizard (*Sceloporus undulatus*) have generated evidence that maternal and embryonic phenotypes are designed to promote growth and development in cold environments. Females in colder environments allocate more energy per egg enabling offspring to grow faster and reach a larger size at hatching. Females in cold environments also nest exclusively in warm, open sites that maximize rates of embryonic growth and development, although this behavior involves risky migrations. Likewise, thermal adaptation of embryonic physiology also promotes growth and development in cold environments. When incubated in the laboratory under shared environmental conditions, embryos from colder environments developed faster and grew more efficiently than embryos from warmer environments, which is a pattern called counter-gradient variation. Because thermal adaptation can produce geographic variation in a suite of maternal and embryonic phenotypes, biologists should develop theories of coadaptation that consider costs and benefits of behavioral and physiological strategies at both stages of the life cycle. © 2004 Elsevier B.V. All rights reserved.

Keywords: Counter-gradient variation; Egg size; Embryo; Growth; Nesting; Temperature

1. Introduction

Spatial and temporal variation in environmental temperature is a challenge for all organisms. Growth and development are very sensitive to temperature such that extreme

---

* Corresponding author. Tel.: +1 812 237 4520; fax: +1 812 237 4480.
E-mail address: m-angilletta@indstate.edu (M.J. Angilletta).

0531-5131/ © 2004 Elsevier B.V. All rights reserved.
doi:10.1016/j.ics.2004.07.038

temperatures have significant consequences for the life histories of ectotherms [1,2]. The evolution of behavior, physiology, morphology and life history has enabled many species to span large portions of our planet despite the thermal gradients they encounter. Such adaptations might be required at all ontogenetic stages if a widespread species is to complete its life cycle in environments that differ not only in temperature but also in many other respects.

Thermal adaptation produces strategies that speed growth and development in cold environments, including modifications of maternal and embryonic phenotypes (Fig. 1). Mothers can speed the growth of their offspring by provisioning eggs with additional nutrients [3]. Viviparous females can thermoregulate during pregnancy [4,5] and oviparous females can construct nests that provide embryos with relatively warm conditions [6–8]. Finally, offspring can make more efficient use of resources by improving assimilation and reducing energy expenditure [9]. Here we consider the life-historical, behavioral, and physiological strategies available to ectotherms, and present evidence from our studies of lizards that these strategies facilitate growth and development in cold environments.

2. *Sceloporus undulatus*: a model for studies of thermal adaptation

The *Sceloporus undulatus* species group—a monophyletic group of phrynosomatids that includes *S. undulatus*, *S. belli*, *S. cautatus*, *S. exul* and *S. woodi* [10]—is ideal for studies of thermal adaptation. This group is widely distributed in the United States and northern Mexico, where it occupies a diversity of habitats including forests, prairies and canyons. Consequently, *S. undulatus* encounters a broad range of environmental

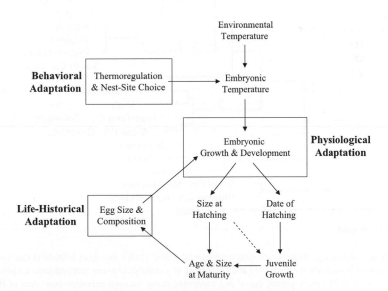

Fig. 1. A conceptual model relating life history, maternal behavior and embryonic physiology. Development and growth are enhanced by the thermal adaptation of these phenotypes.

temperatures and exhibits considerable variation in life history [11,12]. Phylogeographic evidence suggests *S. undulatus* expanded its range latitudinally at least four times [10], making it a good subject for comparative studies. Such studies have begun to shed light on the mechanisms by which this species has responded to thermal challenges.

3. Thermal adaptation of maternal and embryonic phenotypes

3.1. Life-historical adaptation: reproductive allocation across space and time

Reproductive allocation by females is an obvious mechanism by which the growth of offspring is promoted. A larger allocation of resources results in a larger hatchling [3] or a greater potential for growth after hatching [13]. Because low temperatures retard the growth of offspring, optimization theories predict females should allocate a greater quantity of energy per offspring in colder environments [14,15]. In seasonal environments, the same argument can be applied to temporal variation in temperature. Offspring produced later in the season will experience a shorter duration before environmental temperatures drop and brumation ensues; therefore, females should produce larger eggs later in the reproductive season [16].

We have investigated both spatial and temporal variation in the reproductive allocation of *S. undulatus*. Egg size varies considerably within each of the four major

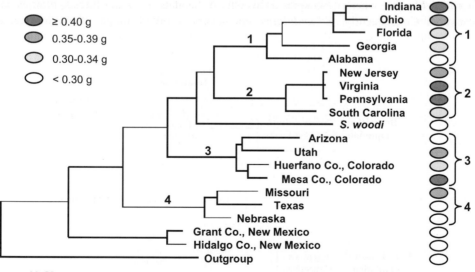

Fig. 2. In *S. undulatus*, egg mass varies considerably within four clades that span latitudinal thermal gradients. Egg masses from Niewiarowski et al. [11] and Oufiero et al. (unpublished) are mapped onto a cladogram from Angilletta et al. [12]. The phylogenetic signal (K), computed using the randomization procedure of Blomberg et al. [17], was only 0.1 (Niewiarowski et al., unpublished); a phylogenetic signal of 1.0 is expected for a trait that has evolved according to a model of Brownian motion.

clades of *S. undulatus* (Fig. 2), enabling powerful comparative studies of thermal adaptation. As predicted by theory, females in colder environments tend to produce larger eggs (Fig. 3). Lizards in Nebraska are a major exception to this trend because they produce relatively small eggs despite a very low environmental temperature. This exception is understandable considering females in Nebraska suffer unusually high rates of mortality as juveniles and thus mature early at an extremely small body size. The small body size of females in Nebraska probably constrains the size of eggs that can be produced [18].

Conversely, temporal variation in egg size provides mixed support for theories of reproductive allocation. Angilletta et al. [16] observed seasonal variation in egg mass that was inconsistent with the prediction of optimization theory. Females in New Jersey produce two clutches of eggs per year, and the offspring from the second clutch have about 40% less time to grow before brumation [16,19]. Theory predicts that a female should allocate more energy per egg in her second clutch than she allocated per egg in her first clutch. Yet, eggs of the second clutch were 10% smaller than those of the first clutch [16]. In contrast, *S. woodi* produced larger eggs later in the season some years, but not others [20]. One possible cause of these discrepancies is temporal variation in food availability. The clutch size of a lizard is fixed during mid-vitellogenesis, after which no additional recruitment occurs and atresia is rare [21,22]. If a female encounters a surplus of resources between mid-vitellogenesis and the point at which eggs are shelled, she could not add follicles but could increase her reproductive output by allocating additional energy to each of her developing follicles. Indeed, females of *S. undulatus* that consumed more food during vitellogenesis produced larger eggs (Pringle and Angilletta, unpublished). Thus, temporal variation in resources can be a confounding factor that produces counterintuitive patterns of reproductive allocation.

3.2. Behavioral adaptation: selection of nesting sites

The embryonic growth and development of *S. undulatus* can be greatly enhanced by nesting behavior. When incubated at constant temperatures, embryos hatch successfully in

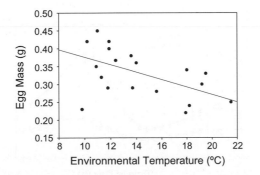

Fig. 3. Among 19 populations of *S. undulatus*, females in colder environments tend to produce larger eggs (robust regression: $F_{1,15.7}=6.90$, $P=0.02$, $r^2=0.30$). Egg sizes for 15 populations are from Ref. [11] and those for four populations are from Oufiero et al. (unpublished). Environmental temperatures are from Ref. [12].

the range of 23–34 °C [23–25]. Relatively high temperatures reduce the duration of incubation without affecting the body size at hatching [24,25], but survival is poor if the temperature is too high [23,25]. Angilletta et al. [25] combined data from the laboratory and the field to define sites that offered the most favorable thermal conditions for offspring. Specifically, they predicted that females in New Jersey—a locality at the northern limit of *S. undulatus*'s range—should nest in unshaded soil at a depth of ≥4 cm. Their reasoning was simple. Shaded soil, regardless of depth, offers relatively low temperatures that retard growth and development. By nesting at warmer sites, females could ensure that their offspring hatched earlier and had longer access to resources after hatching, potentially resulting in a higher survivorship, earlier reproduction, or a larger size at maturity [26]. Still, females that nest in unshaded soil must place their eggs sufficiently deep to prevent them from reaching lethally high temperatures.

In both natural and artificial environments, the nesting behavior of *S. undulatus* accorded extremely well with our expectation. Angilletta et al. (unpublished) used radiotelemetry to observe the nesting behavior of lizards in New Jersey. Nests were constructed at sites that were less shaded than randomly selected sights (canopy coverage of nests and random sites were 49±5.4% and 79±3%, respectively). Moreover, eggs were placed at mean minimal and maximal depths of 4.7 and 6.4 cm, respectively. Nests provided mean temperatures between 28 and 32 °C for approximately 8 h per day, whereas the mean temperature at random sites was below 25 °C at all times of the day (Fig. 4). Although eggs of *S. undulatus* can hatch successfully at temperatures below 25 °C [24], incubation would be greatly extended, possibly having major consequences for the fitness of offspring. These observations correspond remarkably with those of Warner and Andrews [27], who observed the nesting behavior of *S. undulatus* in an artificial thermal gradient; females in their gradient selected mean temperatures between 23.8 and 28.2 °C, and females in New Jersey selected mean temperatures between 23.2 and 29.1 °C. Collectively, these observations are strong evidence that the nesting behavior of *S. undulatus* provides offspring with thermal conditions that speed embryonic growth and development.

Although the benefits of nesting behavior are clear, the potential costs have not been documented. A major cost of nesting could be a greater exposure of gravid females to

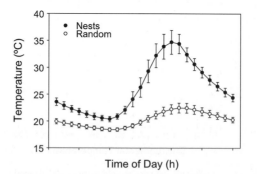

Fig. 4. At all times of the day, nests of *S. undulatus* were much warmer than randomly selected locations. Error bars are 95% confidence intervals. Data are from Angilletta et al. (unpublished).

predators. Nesting involved rapid migrations between habitats, which appeared risky for females. Just prior to nesting, females in New Jersey made sudden shifts from the forest to open terrain. These excursions appeared to be solely related to nesting because females returned to the forest immediately after nesting. On average, only 1% (range=0–8%, $n=19$ females) of the area used by a female during nesting was contained within her home range (i.e., the area used before and after nesting). Similar shifts in habitat have been observed for gravid fence lizards in Virginia (Andrews, pers. comm.). Gravid females probably experience a higher risk of mortality because of poor locomotor capacity [28], and migrations associated with nesting could further amplify this risk. Nesting behavior is possibly characterized by a considerable degree of philopatry because females from various regions of the forest migrated directly and rapidly to a rather restricted nesting area. If females were homing in on a known location [29], the risk of migration might have been less than if the nesting area was completely unfamiliar.

3.3. Physiological adaptation: embryonic growth and development

In many species, individuals from colder environments exhibit faster intrinsic rates of growth and development, which tend to counteract the effects of environmental temperature on these physiological processes [2,30]. Rapid growth can be achieved by higher rates of consumption, higher efficiencies of production, or both [31]. Embryos cannot use both of these strategies because their mother supplies them with nutrients and this supply cannot be supplemented through feeding. Still, the growth efficiency of embryos can be increased through modifications of metabolic functions that lead to greater assimilation and less expenditure of available energy [32].

Common garden experiments have revealed thermal adaptation of embryonic physiology in *S. undulatus*. The existence of multiple clades distributed along a latitudinal gradient enabled Oufiero and Angilletta (unpublished) to investigate parallel evolution of growth and development. They incubated eggs from populations belonging to two clades separated by the Appalachian Mountains (clades 1 and 2 in Fig. 2). Incubation temperatures were chosen to match thermal cycles of natural nests (see Section 3.2). In both clades, embryos from colder environments grew more efficiently and hatched earlier when incubated in the laboratory at realistic thermal cycles (Fig. 5). More efficient growth enabled embryos to reach a larger size before hatching, and a shorter incubation period provided more time for growth after hatching. Thus, embryos of *S. undulatus* exhibited counter-gradient variation in growth and development similar to that observed in juveniles of other ectothermic species [31]. The parallel evolution of counter-gradient variation in *S. undulatus* indicates strong selection of body size in cold environments.

Why don't lizards in all environments grow as efficiently and develop as rapidly as possible? We presume that rapid embryonic growth and development impose some cost to the embryo that arises from one or more tradeoffs [31,33]. Rapid growth might come at the expense of cellular maintenance, including protein turnover, ion transport and other ATP-consuming functions [34]. Since development is thought to occur at the expense of growth [35], the faster growth and development of embryos from colder environments must impose a complex set of tradeoffs, which presumably results in a lower survivorship of embryos or hatchlings. The consequences of these tradeoffs for fitness can be tested

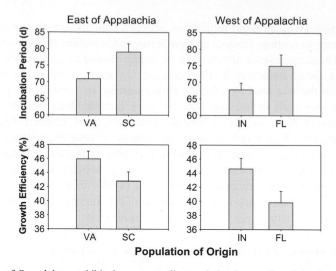

Fig. 5. Embryos of *S. undulatus* exhibited counter-gradient variation in growth and development. Top panels: embryos from colder environments (Virginia and Indiana) had shorter incubation periods than those from warmer environments (South Carolina and Florida). Bottom panels: embryos from colder environments grew more efficiently than those from warmer environments. Error bars are 95% confidence intervals. Data are from Oufiero and Angilletta (unpublished).

through reciprocal transplants of offspring. In cold environments, residents should have higher survivorship than lizards transplanted from warmer environments. However, lizards transplanted from cold environments to warmer environments should have lower survivorship than residents. Importantly, experimental reduction of yolk can be used to equalize the energy available to embryos from different populations, enabling one to tease apart the contributions of reproductive allocation and embryonic physiology to the success of offspring.

4. Conclusion

Using *S. undulatus* as a model, we have shown that ectotherms use a suite of strategies to enhance growth and development in cold environments. These strategies are manifested at both embryonic and adult stages of the life cycle. Because the survivorship and fecundity of a genotype is determined by its performance at all stages, fitness is a multivariate function of embryonic and maternal phenotypes [36,37]. Natural selection should produce a combination of strategies that maximizes fitness given genetic, developmental and functional constraints [38]. Because thermal adaptations impose tradeoffs, particular suites of strategies should arise in particular environments [31]. Although our work has highlighted potential responses to a thermal challenge, we should like to know why certain strategies evolve in a given environment and why others do not. Undoubtedly, we shall only achieve this goal through detailed studies of the costs and benefits of life-historical, behavioral and physiological strategies.

Acknowledgments

We thank the Indiana Academy of Sciences for supporting our research, and Indiana State University for an International Travel Grant, which enabled the senior author to participate in this symposium.

References

[1] R.B. Huey, R.D. Stevenson, Integrating thermal physiology and ecology of ectotherms: a discussion of approaches, Am. Zool. 19 (1979) 357–366.

[2] M.J. Angilletta, P.H. Niewiarowski, C.A. Navas, The evolution of thermal physiology in ectotherms, J. Therm. Biol. 27 (2002) 249–268.

[3] B. Sinervo, The evolution of maternal investment in lizards: an experimental and comparative analysis of egg size and its effects on offspring performance, Evolution 44 (1990) 279–294.

[4] J. Rock, A. Cree, R.M. Andrews, The effect of reproductive condition on thermoregulation in a viviparous gecko from a cool climate, J. Therm. Biol. 27 (1) (2000) 17–27.

[5] M.B. Charland, Thermal consequences of reptilian viviparity: thermoregulation in gravid and nongravid garter snakes (*Thamnophis*), J. Herpetol. 29 (3) (1995) 383–390.

[6] R. Shine, P.S. Harlow, Maternal manipulation of offspring phenotypes via nest-site selection in an oviparous lizard, Ecology 77 (6) (1996) 1808–1817.

[7] T. Madsen, R. Shine, Life history consequences of nest-site variation in tropical pythons (*Liasis fuscus*), Ecology 80 (3) (1999) 989–997.

[8] R. Shine, Some like it hot: effects of forest clearing on nest temperatures of montane reptiles, Ecology 83 (10) (2002) 2808–2815.

[9] S.J.W. Robinson, L. Partridge, Temperature and clinal variation in larval growth efficiency in *Drosophila melanogaster*, J. Evol. Biol. 14 (2001) 14–21.

[10] A.D. Leaché, T.W. Reeder, Molecular systematics of the eastern fence lizard. (*Sceloporus undulatus*): a comparison of parsimony, likelihood and Bayesian approaches, Syst. Biol. 51 (2002) 44–68 [2001].

[11] P.H. Niewiarowski, M.J. Angilletta, A. Leaché, Phylogenetic comparative analysis of life history variation among populations of the lizard *Sceloporus undulatus*: an example and prognosis, Evolution 58 (2004) 619–633.

[12] M.J. Angilletta, et al., Bergmann's clines in ectotherms: illustrating a life-historical perspective with sceloporine lizards, Am. Nat. 164 (2004) (in press).

[13] J.D. Congdon, Proximate and evolutionary constraints on energy relations of reptiles, Physiol. Zool. 62 (1989) 356–373.

[14] N. Perrin, Why are offspring born larger when it is colder? Phenotypic plasticity for offspring size in the cladoceran *Simocephalus vetulus* (Müller), Funct. Ecol. 2 (1988) 283–288.

[15] L.Y. Yampolsky, S.M. Scheiner, Why larger offspring at lower temperatures? A demographic approach, Am. Nat. 147 (1996) 86–100.

[16] M.J. Angilletta, M.W. Sears, R.S. Winters, Seasonal variation in reproductive effort and its consequences for offspring size in the lizard *Sceloporus undulatus*, Herpetologica 57 (2000) 365–375.

[17] S.P. Blomberg, T. Garland Jr., A.R. Ives, Testing for phylogenetic signal in comparative data: behavioral traits are more labile, Evolution 57 (2003) 717–745.

[18] J.D. Congdon, J.W. Gibbons, Morphological constraint on egg size: a challenge to optimal egg size theory? Proc. Natl. Acad. Sci. 84 (1987) 4145–4147.

[19] P.H. Niewiarowski, Understanding geographic life history variation in lizards, in: L.J. Vitt, E.R. Pianka (Eds.), Lizard Ecology: Historical and Experimental Perspectives, Princeton University Press, Princeton, 1994, pp. 31–49.

[20] V.G. DeMarco, Annual variation in the seasonal shift in egg size and clutch size in *Sceloporus woodi*, Oecologia 80 (1989) 525–532.

[21] B.A. Shanbhag, B.S.K. Prasad, Follicular dynamics and germinal bed activity during the annual ovarian cycle of the lizard *Calotes versicolor*, J. Morphol. 216 (1993) 1–7.

[22] B. Sinervo, P. Licht, Proximate constraints on the evolution of egg size, number, and total clutch mass in lizards, Science 252 (1991) 1300–1302.

[23] O.J. Sexton, K.R. Marion, Duration of incubation of *Sceloporus undulatus* eggs at constant temperature, Physiol. Zool. 47 (1974) 91–98.

[24] R.M. Andrews, T. Mathies, D.A. Warner, Effect of incubation temperature on morphology, growth, and survival of juvenile *Sceloporus undulatus*, Herpetol. Monogr. 14 (2000) 420–431.

[25] M.J. Angilletta, R.S. Winters, A.E. Dunham, Thermal effects on the energetics of lizard embryos: implications for hatchling phenotypes, Ecology 81 (2000) 2957–2968.

[26] F.J. Qualls, R. Shine, Post-hatching environment contributes greatly to phenotypic variation between two populations of the Australian garden skink, *Lampropholis guichenoti*, Biol. J. Linn. Soc. 71 (2000) 315–341.

[27] D.A. Warner, R.M. Andrews, Nest-site selection in relation to temperature and moisture by the lizard *Sceloporus undulatus*, Herpetologica 58 (2002) 399–407.

[28] D.B. Miles, B. Sinervo, W.A. Frankino, Reproductive burden, locomotor performance, and the cost of reproduction in free ranging lizards, Evolution 54 (2000) 1386–1395.

[29] E.W. Hein, S.J. Whitaker, Homing in eastern fence lizards (*Sceloporus undulatus*) following short-distance translocation, Great Basin Nat. 57 (1997) 348–351.

[30] D.O. Conover, E.T. Schultz, Phenotypic similarity and the evolutionary significance of countergradient variation, Trends Ecol. Evol. 10 (1995) 248–252.

[31] M.J. Angilletta, et al., Tradeoffs and the evolution of thermal reaction norms, Trends Ecol. Evol. 18 (2003) 234–240.

[32] B.L. Bayne, Phenotypic flexibility and physiological tradeoffs in the feeding and growth of marine bivalve molluscs, Integr. Comp. Biol. 44 (2004)2001 (in press).

[33] K. Gotthard, Growth strategies of ectothermic animals in temperate environments, in: D. Atkinson, M. Thorndyke (Eds.), Environment and Animal Development: Genes, Life Histories, and Plasticity, BIOS Scientific Publishers, Oxford, 2001, pp. 287–303.

[34] W. Wieser, Cost of growth in cells and organisms: general rules and comparative aspects, Biol. Rev. 68 (1994) 1–33.

[35] J.D. Arendt, Allocation of cells to proliferation vs. differentiation and its consequences for growth and development, J. Exp. Zool. 288 (2002) 219–234.

[36] C.A. Beuchat, S. Ellner, A quantitative test of life history theory: thermoregulation by a viviparous lizard, Ecol. Monogr. 57 (1987) 45–60.

[37] S.J. Arnold, C.R. Peterson, A model of optimal reaction norms: the case of the pregnant garter snake and her temperature-sensitive embryos, Am. Nat. 160 (2002) 306–316.

[38] S.J. Arnold, Constraints on phenotypic evolution, Am. Nat. 140 (1992) S85–S107.

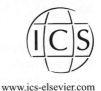

www.ics-elsevier.com

A comparative analysis of plasticity of thermal limits in porcelain crabs across latitudinal and intertidal zone clines

Jonathon H. Stillman*

Department of Zoology, 152 Edmondson Hall, 2538 McCarthy Mall, University of Hawaii, Manoa, Honolulu, HI 96822, USA

Abstract. The effect of thermal acclimation on cardiac thermal performance limits was examined in congeneric species of porcelain crabs (genus *Petrolisthes*) from temperate and subtropical habitats. In vivo heart rate was monitored using impedance electrodes during thermal ramps (0.1 °C/min) where temperature either increased or decreased from an intermediate temperature to thermal extremes. Arrhenius plots were used to define upper and lower critical temperatures of cardiac function (CT_{max} and CT_{min}, respectively). Across species and acclimation conditions, CT_{max} ranged from approximately 28.4 to 41.7 °C and CT_{min} from approximately -1.3 to 11.3 °C. Thermal acclimation had the greatest effect on CT_{max} in species from the coolest thermal microhabitat and the smallest effect on CT_{max} in species from the hottest thermal microhabitat. The opposite effect was observed on CT_{min}. The ecological consequences of these results are counterintuitive, as the most heat-tolerant species are predicted to be most susceptible to global warming. The results of this study will form the foundation of future studies designed to elucidate the mechanistic bases of thermal plasticity and eurythermy in porcelain crabs. © 2004 Elsevier B.V. All rights reserved.

Keywords: Thermal tolerance; Thermal acclimation; CT_{max}; CT_{min}; Porcelain crabs; Acclimation capacity; Cardiac thermal limits; Global climate change

1. Introduction

For ectothermic organisms, habitat temperature is a critically important environmental factor because of the effects of temperature on all biological processes [1]. Evolutionary responses of organisms to changes in temperature have been shown at a wide range of levels of biological organization, from molecular to physiological to behavioural [1,2]. Changes in

* Tel.: +1 808 956 9821; fax: +1 808 956 9812.
  E-mail address: stillman@hawaii.edu.

0531-5131/ © 2004 Elsevier B.V. All rights reserved.
doi:10.1016/j.ics.2004.09.034

habitat temperature can occur on a wide temporal range, from fluctuations that occur in hours as a result of day–night or tidal cycles [3–6] to those that might occur over many years as a result of global climate change [7–9]. To understand how the distribution and abundance limits of organisms might change as a result of changes in daily habitat temperature fluctuations associated with climate change [4], we must understand how much the thermal sensitivity of organisms can change, or acclimatize. The magnitude of effects of global warming on species distribution ranges will be a result of the proximity of organismal thermal limits to maximal habitat temperatures, and the capacity of those organisms to adjust their thermal limits through acclimation [10].

Thermal tolerance ranges, the range of temperatures between upper and lower thermal thresholds to normal biological performance (here referred to as upper and lower thermal tolerance limits, CT_{max} and CT_{min}, respectively), can be shifted through thermal acclimation. The degree to which organisms are able to adjust CT_{max} and CT_{min} has been referred to as acclimation flexibility [2], and capacity for acclimation [10].

In this study, the effects of thermal acclimation on cardiac CT_{max}, and CT_{min} have been investigated in six species of porcelain crabs in the genus *Petrolisthes*. Porcelain crabs are an excellent group of organisms for comparative studies of temperature adaptation because species exist across a large range in thermal microhabitat conditions as a result of differences in latitudinal and vertical (intertidal zone) distribution patterns [11], and because phylogenetic information for these crabs [12] facilitates selection of closely related species that live in different thermal microhabitats. Previous studies have shown that in over 20 *Petrolisthes* species, upper thermal tolerance limits are evolutionarily correlated with maximal habitat temperature [3,10,11,13], and cold tolerance varies across species from different vertical zones [3,10]. Differences in capacity for thermal acclimation of cardiac performance limits have been shown in four species of *Petrolisthes* from different thermal microhabitats [10]. *Petrolisthes* from the hottest habitats had the highest CT_{max}, but they also had the lowest acclimation capacity of CT_{max}, while the opposite pattern was true for CT_{min} [10].

2. Materials and methods

2.1. Species selection

Six species of *Petrolisthes* were selected for study. Four of the study species, *Petrolisthes cinctipes*, *Petrolisthes cabrilloi*, *Petrolisthes manimaculis* and *Petrolisthes eriomerus*, are within one phylogenetic clade of northern temperate species with a most recent common ancestor of about 16 million years ago (mya) [12], and two, *Petrolisthes gracilis* and *Petrolisthes hirtipes*, fall within one phylogenetic clade of species endemic to the northern Gulf of California with a most recent common ancestor of about 8 mya, and these two clades shared a common ancestor about 25 mya [12]. Both temperate and Gulf of California species have distinct vertical zonation patterns: *P. cinctipes* and *P. cabrilloi* inhabit the middle–upper intertidal zone, *P. eriomerus* and *P. manimaculis* inhabit the low intertidal and subtidal zones, and *P. gracilis* and *P. hirtipes* inhabit the high and middle intertidal zones, respectively [14].

The two species from the northern Gulf of California live in an extreme thermal habitat, as water temperatures can vary from 15 to 30 °C annually, and during low tide conditions, temperature fluctuations can be much greater. During low tide in the northern Gulf of California, under rock temperatures in *Petrolisthes* microhabitats have been measured at over 40 °C during summer months. In the cold north temperate, water temperatures fluctuate between 7 and 13 °C, and intertidal species of *Petrolisthes* experience fluctuating microhabitat temperatures (Fig. 1) that can be above 30 °C in summer months [3]. Thus, the species selected for study here are from a great range of thermal microhabitats, from *P. eriomerus*, which sees the coolest and least variable habitat temperatures, to *P. gracilis*, which sees the warmest and most variable thermal habitat.

2.2. Specimen collection

Specimens were collected by hand during low tide and transported to Hopkins Marine Station where they were maintained in flowing seawater at 12–15 °C (temperate species) or 25 °C (Gulf of California species) for approximately 5 weeks until the beginning of thermal acclimations. Crabs were fed SELCO-enriched *Artemia* and frozen copepods three times per week throughout the duration of the study.

2.3. Thermal acclimation experiments

Thermal acclimations were performed in recirculating aquaria with carbon and biological filtration (FLUVAL 304 canister filters) and weekly water changes. *P. cinctipes* and *P. eriomerus* were acclimated together for 8 weeks to 8, 13 and 18 °C, and *P. manimaculis* were also acclimated in the 8 and 13 °C tanks. *P. cabrilloi* were acclimated to 8 and 18 °C for 4 weeks. *P. cinctipes*, *P. hirtipes* and *P. gracilis* were acclimated together for 4 weeks to 15 and 25 °C (*P. eriomerus* cannot survive acclimation to 25 °C), and *P. gracilis* alone was acclimated to 35 °C (no other species in this study can survive acclimation to 35 °C). *P. cinctipes* were also acclimated to 22 and 4 °C, but none of the specimens survived for over 7 days at 4 °C, and no heart rate data were collected for those crabs.

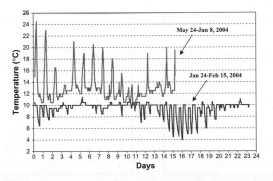

Fig. 1. Microhabitat temperatures of *P. cinctipes* at Cape Arago, OR during winter and summer months. Temperature data loggers ($n=5$; ibutton, Dallas Semiconductor) were placed underneath the same stones in winter and summer, 2004, and were set to collect temperature data every 15 min (summer) or 20 min (winter). Data shown is the average temperature of the recovered data loggers ($n=2$ (summer), $n=3$ (winter)), and variation between loggers was generally within 1–2 °C at any time-point.

2.4. Determination of cardiac thermal performance limits

Cardiac activity was monitored using impedance electrodes (as described elsewhere [10]) during thermal ramp experiments where temperature was increased (CT_{max}) or decreased (CT_{min}) at 0.1 °C min^{-1}. Briefly, crabs were suspended from a cork glued to their carapace in a water bath containing a heat exchanger connected to a recirculating temperature control device. Temperatures were held constant for 1 h prior to initiating the thermal ramp, and ramp experiments were generally completed within 5 h. Average heart rates (beats per minute) were calculated in bins of 30 s for the duration of the recording. Arrhenius break temperatures of heart rate (CT_{max} and CT_{min}) were determined from plots of the natural log of heart rate vs. inverse temperature by calculating the intersection point of regression lines fitted to the first 200 data points (before a transition in slope occurred) and the final 60 data points of each record (after the heart began to fail), as described elsewhere [10].

3. Results

3.1. Thermal acclimation of cardiac thermal performance limits

Thermal acclimation affected upper and lower thermal limits of cardiac function in all species; however, the magnitude of change of CT_{max} and CT_{min} differed among species. *P. eriomerus* and *P. manimaculis*, the temperate subtidal zone species, showed the greatest change in CT_{max} (~4 °C) and the smallest change in CT_{min} of all of the species tested (Fig. 2A). In *P. eriomerus* and *P. manimaculis*, CT_{max} changed by 2.1 and 3.5 °C, respectively, over the 10 °C acclimation temperature range of 8–18 °C (Fig. 2A). CT_{max} of *P. cinctipes* ranged from 32.6±0.2 °C (in 8 °C acclimated crabs) to 33.9±0.3 °C (in 18 and 22 °C acclimated crabs), and thus changed by 1.3 °C over the 10 °C acclimation temperature range of 8–18 °C (Fig. 2A). The CT_{max} of *P. cinctipes* changed the most between 8 and 18 °C (the largest jump was from 8 to 13 °C), and changed little from 18 to 25 °C (Fig. 2A). CT_{max} of *P. cabrilloi* was the same as *P. cinctipes* for 8 °C acclimated crabs, but increased by 2.3 °C in 18 °C acclimated crabs (Fig. 2A).

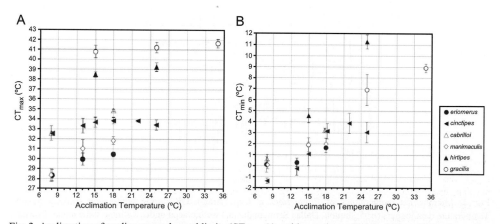

Fig. 2. Acclimation of cardiac upper thermal limits (CT_{max}, A) and lower thermal limits (CT_{min}, B) in six species of porcelain crabs (genus *Petrolisthes*) from different thermal habitats to a range of constant thermal regimes. Sample sizes are from $n=3$ to 11, and each point is the mean±one standard deviation.

In the warm-adapted crabs *P. gracilis* and *P. hirtipes* from the northern Gulf of California, small increases in CT_{max} were observed as the result of thermal acclimation over a 10 or 20 °C acclimation range (Fig. 2A). CT_{max} of *P. gracilis*, the high intertidal and most warm adapted species, increased by 0.4 °C from 15 °C acclimated crabs (40.8 ± 0.5 °C) to 25 °C acclimated crabs (41.2 ± 0.5 °C), and increased 0.4 °C further in 35 °C acclimated crabs (41.6 ± 0.4 °C). CT_{max} of *P. hirtipes* changed by 0.8 °C from 15 °C acclimated crabs (38.5 ± 0.2 °C) to 25 °C acclimated crabs (39.3 ± 0.4 °C) (Fig. 2A). *P. hirtipes* did not survive acclimation to 35 °C.

The interspecific differences in the effects of thermal acclimation on CT_{min} were opposite of those observed in CT_{max}. *P. gracilis* and *P. hirtipes*, the most warm adapted species, showed the largest change in CT_{min}, and *P. eriomerus* and *P. manimaculis*, the least warm adapted species, showed the smallest change in CT_{min} (Fig. 2B). CT_{min} of *P. gracilis* changed from 1.9 ± 0.5 °C in 15 °C acclimated crabs to 6.9 ± 1.3 °C in 25 °C acclimated crabs, a 5.0 °C change over this 10 °C temperature range, and increased by another 2 °C in crabs acclimated to 35 °C (Fig. 2B). In *P. hirtipes*, the change in CT_{min} was 6.7 °C over a 10 °C acclimation range, from 4.6 ± 0.5 °C in 15 °C acclimated crabs to 11.3 ± 0.4 °C in 25 °C acclimated crabs.

P. manimaculis and *P. eriomerus* had the same CT_{min} values across acclimation temperatures, and changed CT_{min} by 2 °C over the 10 °C acclimation temperature range from 8 to 18 °C (Fig. 2B). In *P. cinctipes*, CT_{min} changed by 4.3 °C from -1.4 ± 0.3 °C in 8 °C acclimated crabs to 3.9 ± 0.9 °C in 22 °C acclimated crabs, but did not increase further in crabs acclimated to 25 °C (Fig. 2B), and there was no significant difference between CT_{min} values of 18, 22 or 25 °C acclimated specimens of *P. cinctipes*. In *P. cabrilloi*, CT_{min} changed by 2.6 °C from 0.6 ± 0.4 °C in 8 °C acclimated crabs to 3.2 ± 0.2 °C in 18 °C acclimated crabs (Fig. 2B). CT_{min} values for *P. cinctipes* and *P. cabrilloi* were the same

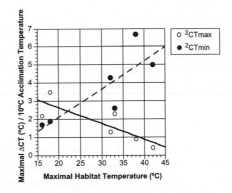

Fig. 3. Maximal plasticity of critical thermal limits of cardiac function during thermal acclimation in six species of porcelain crabs (genus *Petrolisthes*) from different thermal habitats. For each species, the maximal change in CT was calculated over a 10 °C acclimation temperature range using the above data for CT_{max} (Fig. 2A) and CT_{min} (Fig. 2B). From lowest to highest maximal habitat temperature, pairs of points for ΔCT are for *P. eriomerus*, *P. manimaculis*, *P. cinctipes*, *P. cabrilloi*, *P. hirtipes*, and *P. gracilis*. Linear regression indicated a significant relationship between ΔCT and maximal habitat temperature for both CT_{max} ($p=0.040$, $r^2=0.692$) and CT_{min} ($p=0.0396$, $r^2=0.694$). Maximal habitat temperature data from Ref. [13].

in 18 °C acclimated crabs, but in 8 °C acclimated crabs, P. cabrilloi had CT_{min} values that were about 2 °C higher than those of P. cinctipes. This is the opposite pattern observed for CT_{max} for these two species.

3.2. Maximal capacity for thermal acclimation of CT_{max} and CT_{min}

The maximal amount of change in CT_{max} and CT_{min} over a 10 °C acclimation range differs among species in a manner consistent with maximal microhabitat temperature ([10]; Fig. 3). The 10 °C range used was 8–18 °C for P. eriomerus, P. cinctipes, P. cabrilloi, and P. manimaculis, and 15–25 °C for P. gracilis and P. hirtipes. The change in CT_{max} of P. gracilis was the same across the 15–25 and the 25–35 °C acclimation temperature interval, but the change in CT_{min} was much greater across the 15–25 °C acclimation temperature interval for this species, and thus this interval was used in the analysis.

To remove the effects of phylogeny from these data, phylogenetic independent contrasts were generated following methods previously published for these crabs [13]. Independent contrasts of maximal habitat temperature were not significantly correlated with contrasts of ΔCT_{max} ($p=0.53$) or contrasts of ΔCT_{min} ($p=0.18$).

4. Discussion

4.1. Comparative analysis of thermal acclimation capacity

Functional analyses of the concomitant effects of thermal acclimation on both heat and cold tolerance have been made in many species (e.g., crabs [10], planarians [15], earthworms [16,17], flies [18], ticks [19], fish [20–23], crayfish [24], copepods [25]). However, few of these studies examined the relative effects of acclimation temperature on thermal tolerance in multiple species adapted to different thermal habitats. Thermal acclimation of three species of Drosophila from different thermal microhabitats had a greater affect on CT_{min} than on CT_{max}; however, this pattern did not vary among species and acclimation capacity was not clearly related to thermal habitat [18]. In porcelain crabs from different thermal habitats, this study shows that CT_{max} is inversely correlated with maximal habitat temperature, and the opposite is true for CT_{min} (Fig. 3). Although phylogenetics-based transformation of these data does not clarify the evolutionary significance of this relationship, the results suggest an evolutionary and/or functional trade-off between achieving extreme tolerance limits and maintaining plasticity of tolerance limits.

4.2. Ecological significance of thermal acclimation capacity

To assess the ecological consequences of the relationship between acclimation capacity of CT_{max} and maximal habitat temperature, it is necessary to also consider the proximity of thermal performance limits to maximal habitat temperatures. In the most warm adapted species, P. gracilis, CT_{max} of summer acclimatized crabs (25–30 °C) is within 1 °C of its maximal habitat temperature [13], whereas in the least warm adapted species, P. eriomerus, CT_{max} of summer acclimatized crabs (13 °C) is over 15 °C away from its maximal habitat temperature ([13]; Figs. 2A and 3). Since the acclimation capacity of CT_{max} of P. gracilis is only 1 °C across a 20 °C range of acclimation temperature (Fig. 2A), if maximal habitat temperatures that this species experiences change by more than 2

°C as a result of global climate change, it is likely that there will be a decline in abundance of this species. Thus, it is the most heat-tolerant species that will be most susceptible to global warming, a result that is counterintuitive.

References

[1] P.W. Hochachka, G.N. Somero, Biochemical Adaptation: Mechanism and Process in Physiological Evolution, Oxford University Press, New York, 2002.

[2] J.G. Kingsolver, R.B. Huey, Evolutionary analyses of morphological and physiological plasticity in thermally variable environments, American Zoologist 38 (3) (1998) 545–560.

[3] J. Stillman, G. Somero, Adaptation to temperature stress and aerial exposure in congeneric species of intertidal porcelain crabs (genus *Petrolisthes*): correlation of physiology, biochemistry and morphology with vertical distribution, Journal of Experimental Biology 199 (Pt 8) (1996) 1845–1855.

[4] B. Helmuth, et al., Climate change and latitudinal patterns of intertidal thermal stress, Science 298 (5595) (2002) 1015–1017.

[5] B. Helmuth, How do we measure the environment? Linking intertidal thermal physiology and ecology through biophysics, Integrative and Comparative Biology 42 (4) (2002) 837–845.

[6] J.E. Podrabsky, G.N. Somero, Changes in gene expression associated with acclimation to constant temperatures and fluctuating daily temperatures in an annual killifish *Austrofundulus limnaeus*, Journal of Experimental Biology 207 (2004) 2237–2254.

[7] L. Hughes, Climate change and Australia: trends, projections and impacts, Australian Ecology 28 (4) (2003) 423–443.

[8] L. Hughes, Biological consequences of global warming: in the signal already apparent? Trends in Ecology and Evolution 15 (2000) 56–61.

[9] J.P. Barry, et al., Climate-related, long-term faunal changes in a California rocky intertidal community, Science 267 (5198) (1995) 672–675.

[10] J.H. Stillman, Acclimation capacity underlies susceptibility to climate change, Science 301 (5629) (2003) 65.

[11] J.H. Stillman, Causes and consequences of thermal tolerance limits in rocky intertidal porcelain crabs, genus *Petrolisthes*, Integrative and Comparative Biology 42 (4) (2002) 790–796.

[12] J.H. Stillman, C.A. Reeb, Molecular phylogeny of eastern Pacific porcelain crabs, genera *Petrolisthes* and *Pachycheles*, based on the mtDNA 16S rDNA sequence: phylogeographic and systematic implications, Molecular Phylogenetics and Evolution 19 (2) (2001) 236–245.

[13] J.H. Stillman, G.N. Somero, A comparative analysis of the upper thermal tolerance limits of eastern Pacific porcelain crabs, genus *Petrolisthes*: influences of latitude, vertical zonation, acclimation, and phylogeny, Physiological and Biochemical Zoology 73 (2) (2000) 200–208.

[14] C.G. Romero, Sistematica, Biologia y Ecologia de Los Anomuros (Crustaceos: Decapodos) de Laguna Percebu, Alto Golfo de California [M.S.], Universidad Autonoma de Baja California, Ensenada, 1982.

[15] H. Tsukuda, K. Ogoshi, Heat and cold tolerance of the planarian, *Dugesia japonica*, in relation to acclimation temperature, Nippon Dobutsugaku Iho 51 (1978) 70–78.

[16] G.A. Nair, S.A. Bennour, Thermal reactions of the earthworm *Aporrectodea caliginosa* (Savigny 1826) (Oligochaeta: Lumbricidae), Proceedings of the Indian National Science Academy, Part B 63 (1977) 53–62.

[17] M.M. Hanumante, Thermal relations of the tropical poikilotherm, *Perionyx excavatus* (Oligochaeta: Megascolecidae), Geobios 4 (1977) 21–26.

[18] T. Ohtsu, C. Katagiri, M.T. Kimura, Biochemical aspects of climactic adaptations in *Drosophila curviceps*, *D. immigrans*, and *D. albicans* (Diptera: Drosophilidae), Physiological and Chemical Ecology 28 (1999) 968–972.

[19] M.M. Hanumante, P.M. Patil, R. Nagabhushanam, Thermobiology of the ixodid tick *Hyalomma anatolicus anatolicum*, Revista di Parasitologia 42 (1981) 67–78.

[20] R.M. Hernandez, R.L.F. Buckle, Temperature tolerance polygon of *Poecilia sphenops* Valenciennes (Pisces: Poeciliidae), Journal of Thermal Biology 27 (1) (2002) 1–5.

[21] F.E.J. Fry, J.R. Brett, G.H. Clawson, Lethal temperature limits of young goldfish, Revue Canadienne de Biologie 1 (1942) 50–56.

[22] J.R. Brett, Some principles in the thermal requirements of fishes, Quarterly Review of Biology 31 (1956) 75–87.

[23] O.A.M. Al-Habbib, M.P. Yacoob, Effects of acclimation and experience to changing heat and cold shock temperature on lethal temperature and thermal tolerance of *Gambusa affinis* (Baird and Girard) (Poeciliidae), Cybium 17 (1993) 265–272.

[24] J.R.J. Layne, M.L. Manis, D.L. Claussen, Seasonal variation in the time course of thermal acclimation in the crayfish *Orconectes rusticus*, Freshwater Invertebrate Biology 4 (1985) 98–104.

[25] B.P. Bradley, Increase in range of temperature tolerance by acclimation in the copepod *Eurytemora affinis*, Biological Bulletin 154 (1978) 177–187.

International Congress Series 1275 (2004) 275–282

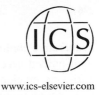

www.ics-elsevier.com

The eland and the oryx revisited: body and brain temperatures of free-living animals

A. Fuller[a,*], S.K. Maloney[a,b], G. Mitchell[a,c], D. Mitchell[a]

[a]School of Physiology, University of the Witwatersrand, Witwatersrand, South Africa
[b]Physiology, School of Biomedical and Chemical Science, University of Western Australia, Nedlands, WA, Australia
[c]Department of Zoology and Physiology, University of Wyoming, Laramie, WY, USA

Abstract. It is widely held that selective brain cooling, the lowering of brain temperature below arterial blood temperature, and adaptive heterothermy, the use of heat storage to reduce body water loss by evaporation, are crucial for the survival of large mammals in arid-zone habitats. These ideas arose 35 years ago as a consequence of work popularised on the eland and the oryx. However, brain temperature in these antelope was never measured. Also, the evidence that these large antelope use adaptive heterothermy was derived from experiments using captive animals. The development of miniature devices for remote sensing of body temperature now has allowed temperatures of free-living animals in their natural habitats to be recorded. With the exception of dehydrated Arabian oryx exposed to severe heat, free-living eland and oryx do not exhibit adaptive heterothermy, and have a mean body temperature at night higher than that during the day. Eland and oryx exhibit selective brain cooling of small magnitude (<0.5 °C) sporadically, at rest under moderate heat load. The view that eland and oryx routinely use adaptive heterothermy to save water and selective brain cooling to protect the brain is misleading, and arises from inadequate measurement or from depriving animals of access to thermoregulatory behaviour. © 2004 Elsevier B.V. All rights reserved.

Keywords: Body temperature; Heterothermy; Thermoregulation; Free-living; Selective brain cooling

1. Introduction

In arid-zone environments with high air temperature and solar radiation, evaporation is the most potent, and sometimes the only, means for an animal to dissipate heat. However,

* Corresponding author. Tel.: +27 11 7172162; fax: +27 11 6432765.
E-mail address: fullera@physiology.wits.ac.za (A. Fuller).

0531-5131/ © 2004 Elsevier B.V. All rights reserved.
doi:10.1016/j.ics.2004.08.092

evaporative cooling depletes body water stores with potentially lethal effects for an animal with limited access to drinking water. Thus, historical anecdotal accounts that two large arid-zone antelope, the eland and the oryx, could survive indefinitely without drinking were counterintuitive and prompted the late C. Richard Taylor to venture to Kenya to study these animals. His experiments, conducted more than 35 years ago, were carried out under challenging circumstances: Taylor had to capture and work with large, potentially dangerous African animals, and devise techniques for studying their thermal physiology. Following the practice prevalent at the time for smaller animals, he set up a laboratory environment simulating conditions that the animals would encounter naturally. That Taylor and his colleagues succeeded in making measurements of multiple physiological variables in eland (*Tragelaphus oryx*) and oryx (*Oryx gazella beisa*), and several other bovids, is testament to their tenacity, and a conviction that the animals must possess unique physiological adaptations for survival. The resulting data, popularised in a 1969 *Scientific American* account titled "The eland and the oryx" [1], led to the now widely accepted views that the eland and the oryx endure hot, arid environments by using two special mechanisms, namely adaptive heterothermy and selective brain cooling.

Adaptive heterothermy refers to an animal's ability to store heat during the day, in so doing reducing evaporative water loss, then to allow its body temperature to fall passively during the cool night without invoking the usual heat conservation or generation, reaching a low that allows scope for substantial heat storage the following day [2]. Largely as a result of Taylor's paper [1] and another on camels by Schmidt-Nielsen [3], the idea that large mammals use adaptive heterothermy as a crucial adaptation in warm, arid habitats has become widely entrenched in textbooks and popular biological literature. Selective brain cooling, that is, the ability to maintain brain temperature below the temperature of arterial blood perfusing the brain [4], is also thought to be critical for survival. Selective brain cooling is evident in artiodactyls (the order including the eland and oryx) and felids, both of which possess a carotid rete, a network of intertwining arteries in a venous lake at the base of the brain. Taylor [1] documented rectal temperatures as high as 45 °C in an oryx, a temperature he thought would be lethal for a mammal. He surmised that the apparent lack of ill effect on the animal could be attributed to an ability to cool the brain below core body temperature, in so doing protecting a supposedly thermally vulnerable brain during the rise in body temperature inherent to adaptive heterothermy.

Although he published data indicating that tame gazelles lower brain temperature below arterial blood temperature during exercise [5], Taylor never measured brain temperature in the eland or oryx. Indeed, until we measured brain temperature 30 years later in eland [6] and oryx [7], all claims that these animals could cool their brains, reportedly by as much as 3 °C, were based on conjecture. Also, body temperatures of the eland and oryx were obtained from experiments using tame, juvenile, or restrained animals housed in artificial laboratory environments or small paddocks. Only with the recent advent of miniature ambulatory thermometers, and advances in animal capture and surgery techniques, have we and others been able to measure body temperatures in free-living animals. These later studies have shown that the thermoregulatory responses of animals in their natural habitats differ from those of captive animals. It is timely, therefore, to address whether the reported patterns of adaptive heterothermy and selective brain cooling, derived from the seminal experiments of Taylor, hold true for free-living eland and oryx in their natural habitats.

2. Adaptive heterothermy

"One way the body can reduce evaporation under heat stress is to abandon the maintenance of a constant body temperature. Schmidt–Nielsen and his collaborators found that when the camel is confronted with a shortage of water, its body temperature rises during the course of the day by as much as seven degrees C. To see if the eland or the oryx had the same ability, I recorded their rectal temperature during the laboratory's hot 12-hour day. The animals had all the water they could drink, so that nothing prevented the maintenance of a constant body temperature by evaporation. Nonetheless, during 12 hours at 40 degrees C, the eland's temperature on occasion rose by more than seven degrees (from 33.9 to 41.2 degrees C) and the oryx's by more than six degrees (from 35.7 to 42.1 degrees) before increased evaporation prevented any further rise (although usually the temperature rise was less extreme). Thus instead of spending water to maintain a constant body temperature, the animals "stored" heat in their bodies" [1].

In contrast, when the eland and oryx were exposed to a constant 22 °C laboratory environment, body temperature fluctuated by only about 1 °C [1,8]. Taylor ascribed adaptive significance to his findings. Heat storage not only reduces the demand for evaporative cooling but, if body temperature exceeds air temperature, also creates a greater temperature gradient for dry heat loss to the environment. As an extreme example, he calculated that a 500-kg eland (his study eland actually weighed 100–150 kg) could save more than 5 l of water by allowing body temperature to rise 7.3 °C [1]. Typically, the eland, when allowed access to drinking water, had rectal temperatures of about 36.5 °C after 12 h overnight at 22 °C, and reached a maximum of almost 40 °C after 10-h exposure to 40 °C [8,9]. This body temperature fluctuation was much greater than that previously reported [10] for unrestrained eland exposed to cooler air temperatures in outdoor paddocks (Table 1). Rectal temperature of oryx in Taylor's study varied by about 2.5 °C, in this case less than that previously observed under outdoor conditions (Table 1). However, Taylor noted that the variation in rectal temperatures of both eland and oryx was greater than that for several other bovid species subjected to the same protocol [8].

If the heterothermy exhibited by eland and oryx indeed is adaptive, one would expect the fluctuations in body temperature to increase in dehydrated animals. Taylor, however, obtained conflicting results when he restricted water until animals reached 85% of original body mass. The average variation in rectal temperature of dehydrated oryx indeed was greater than that of hydrated oryx, but only by about 0.5 °C (in comparison, rectal temperature of smaller gazelles increased by up to 3 °C after dehydration [8]). In dehydrated eland, rectal temperature fluctuation was slightly less than that in hydrated eland (Table 1). These results appear anomalous, but Harthoorn et al. [11] made the same observation for free-living eland; body temperature varied no more in dehydrated than in hydrated animals (Table 1). The finding that the maximum body temperature of eland, at least, does not increase with dehydration (Table 1) is surprising because dehydration elevates the threshold skin temperature for sweating and panting, and reduces evaporative water loss [12,13].

In free-living animals, we believe the result may be attributed, at least in part, to animals employing behavioural thermoregulation to decrease heat gain from solar radiation and defend body temperature, particularly when dehydrated. Indeed, Taylor recognised the

Table 1
Eland and oryx: characteristics of study area and animal status, mean daily average, minimum, maximum and amplitude of body temperature, and mean range of air temperature

Study area	Animal status	Body temperature (°C)					Air temperature (°C)	Reference
		Mean	Minimum	Maximum	Amplitude	Site	Range	
Eland								
Laboratory	Hydrated	–	36.4	39.8	3.4	Rectal	22–40	[1,8]
Laboratory	Dehydrated	–	36.4	39.5	3.1	Rectal	22–40	[1,8]
Paddock	Free-living[a]	39.1	38.4	39.8	1.4	Tissue[b]	16–25	[10]
Paddock[c]	Hydrated	–	36.3	39.4	3.1	–	12–32	[11]
	Dehydrated	–	36.0	39.0	3.0	–	12–27	[11]
Game camp	Free-living[a]	38.2	37.1	39.4	2.3	Carotid	6–27	[6]
Oryx								
Laboratory	Hydrated	–	37.0	39.7	2.7	Rectal	22–40	[1,8]
Laboratory	Dehydrated	–	37.2	40.6	3.4	Rectal	22–40	[1,8]
Paddock	Free-living[a]	39.0	36.6	40.0	3.4	Tissue	12–26	[10]
Game camp	Free-living[a]	38.8	37.5	40.3	1.8	Carotid	11–33	[7]
Game camp	Free-living[a]	38.4	36.5	40.5	4.1	Abdominal	29–44[d]	[15]
Game camp	Free-living[a]	38.4	37.5	39.2	1.5	Abdominal	13–27[e]	[15]

[a] Animals had access to drinking water, but drinking patterns were not recorded.
[b] Various deep tissue sites used.
[c] Some animals were housed in larger game camp.
[d] Summer.
[e] Winter.

importance of allowing animals access to normal behaviours, but was constrained to using a laboratory setting. Using miniature thermometric data loggers, we have been able to measure body temperatures continuously in free-living large animals. We also have been able to measure temperatures at sites other than the rectum or abdomen, including central arterial blood temperature, which accurately reflects the general thermal status of an animal [14]. Although our free-living eland and oryx (gemsbok; *O. gazella*) were exposed to heat loads similar to those imposed artificially by Taylor [1,8,9], the patterns of body core temperature (Fig. 1A) were different [6,7]. The amplitude of the daily rhythm of body temperature was

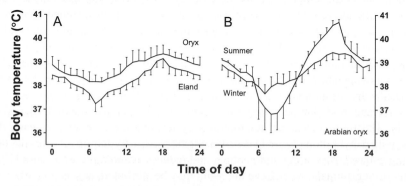

Fig. 1. Mean±S.D. of (A) 5-min arterial blood temperature in one eland and one oryx, and (B) 30-min abdominal temperature of six oryx in summer and winter. Redrawn from Refs. [6,7,15].

small (Table 1) and not related to the variation in environmental heat load. Also, body temperature at night was higher, on average, than body temperature during the day. Despite being subjected to cool nights (<15 °C), body temperature declined slowly, reaching a minimum of about 37 °C (Table 1); temperatures never fell as low (34–35 °C) as those reported by Taylor [1]. The low temperatures Taylor recorded may be artefacts arising from preventing intraspecific interactions or refuge seeking [6]. In our investigations of several large antelope, we have observed core body temperatures below 36 °C only on occasion, when animals, particularly juveniles, were housed in small paddocks without adequate nutrition or protection from cold (unpublished observations).

Unusually high body temperatures were also absent in our animals. At most, arterial blood temperature reached 40.5 °C, and we believe these temperatures were associated with exercise. However, Ostrowski et al. [15] have argued recently that our studies were conducted under moderate climatic conditions (air temperature <35 °C). They measured abdominal temperatures in free-living Arabian oryx (*Oryx leucoryx*) in Saudi Arabia where average maximum summer air temperature was 44 °C, and showed that body temperature fluctuated, on average, by more than 4 °C in summer but by less than 2 °C in winter (Fig. 1B). In summer, minimum body temperature was lower, while maximum body temperature was higher, than those in winter (Table 1), permitting the oryx to store additional heat on summer days and increase water savings [15]. Like our eland (Fig. 1A), body temperature of Arabian oryx continued to drop after dawn, despite a rising air temperature. The fall, however, was much more pronounced in the summer oryx, and was associated with a peculiar 1 °C drop between 05:00 and 06:00 when air temperature was ~30 °C (Fig. 1B). Data sampling in this study was sporadic and so this precipitous decrease in body temperature may partly reflect inadequate sampling over that period. Nevertheless, a morning fall in body temperature, a key event for adaptive heterothermy, also has been reported for other eland [11], and for camels [3] and kangaroos [16,17], and may be caused by peripheral vasodilation in response to solar radiation, or circulation of cold blood from peripheral tissues during sudden activity [6]. There is some evidence from kangaroos that the magnitude of the fall is linked to environmental cues and that body temperature is lowered preemptively in anticipation of hot ambient daytime conditions [17].

Ostrowski et al. [15] also reported a significant correlation between total heat stored by oryx (derived from body temperatures) and variation in daily air temperature, a relationship we investigated but found lacking in eland, oryx, and other large free-living African antelope [18]. However, the relationship reported for the Arabian oryx was weak; in summer, only about 17% of the variation in heat storage could be attributed to variation in air temperature. The Arabian oryx also attained higher body temperatures (up to 42 °C) than our larger oryx (~twice the body mass), which the authors ascribed to higher thermal loads. However, the high temperatures also may be attributed to a hyperthermia resulting from dehydration. Ostrowksi noted that the Arabian oryx had higher haematocrits and plasma osmolalities in summer than in winter. The high body temperatures therefore may reflect suppression of evaporative heat loss [13]. Also, because body temperature was measured intermittently from radio signals, the investigators had to be within 800 m of animals to obtain data; indeed, night measurements were terminated after obtaining modest data (only ~14 h per animal) because the animals were sensitive to the experimenter's presence. Nevertheless, Arabian oryx, like our eland, rested in shade during the day when body temperature was increasing, but this behaviour did not allow the animals to maintain homeothermy.

3. Selective brain cooling

"How do the oryx and gazelle survive these high internal temperatures? The brain, with its complex integrative functions, is probably the part of the body most sensitive to high temperatures. It is possible that in both animals the brain remains cooler than the rest of the body. As the external carotid artery, which supplies most of the blood to the brain in these animals, passes through the region called the cavernous sinus, it divides into hundreds of small parallel arteries. Cool venous blood from nasal passages drains into the sinus, presumably reducing the temperature of arterial blood on its way to the brain" [1].

Taylor referred to gazelle here, citing data from an earlier study where he had observed that the brain of an exercising gazelle was cooled as much as 3 °C below arterial blood temperature [5]. A similar magnitude of selective brain cooling never has been recorded subsequently in any other animal; typically, it is less than 1 °C even at brain temperatures exceeding 40 °C. Nevertheless, laboratory studies have shown that animal's possessing a carotid rete enveloped by cool blood of the cavernous (or pterygoid) sinus exhibit selective brain cooling when body temperature rises [4,18]. It was only logical, therefore, to infer that selective brain cooling functioned to protect the brain from thermal damage. However, data from free-living animals, including the eland and the oryx, are incompatible with that concept.

Contrary to what Taylor and others hypothesised, eland and oryx in their natural habitats seldom employed selective brain cooling [6,7]. On average, brain temperature, measured at 5-min intervals, always exceeded carotid blood temperature. Selective brain cooling occurred sporadically, sometimes when body temperature was decreasing, but usually when animals were at rest and body temperature was rising slowly in the late afternoon. Even then, brain temperature at most was 0.4 °C lower than arterial blood temperature, a difference unlikely to offer protection for the brain. Also, although selective brain cooling was more likely to occur when the animals had high body temperatures, high body temperatures were not always accompanied by selective brain cooling (Fig. 2). In particular, during high-

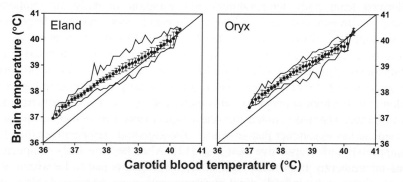

Fig. 2. Brain temperature as a function of blood temperature for one eland and one oryx. The curve shows mean, S.D., maxima and minima of brain temperature for each 0.1 °C class of blood temperature measured at 5-min intervals. The diagonal line is the line of identity. Redrawn from Refs. [6,7].

intensity exercise, when free-living animals are likely to experience their highest temperatures, selective brain cooling always was absent. This pattern in eland and oryx is similar to that observed in free-living springbok (*Antidorcas marsupialis*) [19] and black wildebeest (*Connochaetes gnou*) [20], suggesting there is no enhanced use of selective brain cooling in the arid-adapted oryx and eland. It might be argued that brain temperatures of our animals, which rarely exceeded 40 °C, were not high enough for significant selective brain cooling to be evoked. Arabian oryx exposed to severe heat had an average maximum abdominal temperature of 40.5 °C (Table 1). However, the threshold for selective brain cooling in all species studied lies within the range within which body temperature is regulated, usually near to the mode of blood temperature, and well less than 40 °C [6].

Despite Taylor's reservations, antelope appear to be able to tolerate high brain temperatures, at least up to 42 °C [20], without ill effect. Indeed, there is no evidence that the brain is the organ most sensitive to heat; during general body heating, the gut is the first organ to fail [18]. If eland and oryx do not use selective brain cooling to protect the brain from overheating, what is its function? Our current view is that selective brain cooling plays a role in whole body thermoregulation, but it is a role more subtle than first conceived [4,18]. By cooling the hypothalamus, and hence temperature sensors that drive heat loss, selective brain cooling inhibits evaporative heat loss. Selective brain cooling of only 0.5 °C, which typically is achieved, is sufficient to reduce evaporative heat loss substantially, and therefore conserve body water [21]. Selective brain cooling therefore may play a role in reducing body water loss in antelope under water stress and moderate heat stress. Jessen et al. [13] have shown that selective brain cooling occurred rarely in euhydrated Bedouin goats, but frequently and to a larger extent in dehydrated goats. The dehydrated goats had a maximum arterial blood temperature 0.5–0.9 °C higher than that of euhydrated goats, but did not exhibit adaptive heterothermy; minimum blood temperature was not lower than that in euhydration. Selective brain cooling also may provide another function during stressful situations, such as intense exercise to escape predation, when an animal's survival depends on rapid whole body heat loss. By abolishing selective brain cooling, which is what we have observed consistently in antelope during exertional hyperthermia [18], animals allow brain temperature to rise rapidly, which invokes evaporative heat loss mechanisms. So, contrary to what Taylor proposed, exercising antelope may survive by allowing brain temperature to rise, rather than by keeping it cooler than the rest of the body.

4. The eland and the oryx today

There is no evidence that adaptive heterothermy is employed by free-living eland or oryx when the animals have access to drinking water. Variations in body temperature of these antelope appear to reflect endogenous rhythms rather than reactions to environmental thermal load. Body temperature may be elevated during the day in dehydrated animals, but this elevation does not signal adaptive heterothermy. Adaptive heterothermy, by definition, is characterised by both a higher peak and a lower trough in the 24-h rhythm of body temperature. Only data obtained from apparently dehydrated Arabian oryx have yielded that pattern. However, the results need to be interpreted with caution because the investigators obtained limited, sporadic measurements of abdominal temperature. Measurements of brain and blood temperature obtained from captive animals also need to be interpreted carefully. Selective brain cooling is implemented by animals in their natural habitats in ways very different to that under laboratory conditions. At the time, Taylor and others did not conceive that selective brain cooling could be a means to save body water, rather than an adaptation to protect the brain. That realisation came about only after blood and brain temperatures had been obtained from large, adult free-living African mammals. Taylor recognised that behaviour, in addition to adaptive heterothermy and selective brain cooling, was an important adaptation for survival in hot, arid environments. Indeed, the keys to the success of the eland and the oryx may lie in their behaviour, particularly in the avoidance of the midday sun, social interactions, and the selection of succulent food. Thermoregulatory mechanisms that free-living animals use cannot be predicted accurately from animals in an artificial setting.

References

[1] C.R. Taylor, The eland and the oryx, Sci. Am. 220 (1969) 88–97.
[2] G. Louw, M. Seely, Ecology of Desert Organisms, Longman, London, 1982.
[3] K.B. Schmidt-Nielsen, et al., Body temperature of the camel and its relation to water economy, Am. J. Physiol. 188 (1957) 103–112.
[4] C. Jessen, Selective brain cooling in mammals and birds, Jpn. J. Physiol. 51 (2001) 291–301.
[5] C.R. Taylor, C.P. Lyman, Heat storage in running antelopes: independence of brain and body temperatures, Am. J. Physiol. 222 (1972) 114–117.
[6] A. Fuller, et al., Brain, abdominal and arterial blood temperatures of free-ranging eland in their natural habitat, Pflügers Arch. Eur. J. Physiol. 438 (1999) 671–680.
[7] S.K. Maloney, et al., Brain and arterial blood temperatures of free-ranging oryx (*Oryx gazella*), Pflügers Arch. Eur. J. Physiol. 443 (2002) 437–445.
[8] C.R. Taylor, Strategies of temperature regulation: effect on evaporation in East African ungulates, Am. J. Physiol. 219 (1970) 1131–1135.
[9] C.R. Taylor, C.P. Lyman, A comparative study of the environmental physiology of an East African antelope, the eland, and the Hereford steer, Physiol. Zool. 40 (1967) 280–295.
[10] J. Bligh, A.M. Harthoorn, Continuous radiotelemetric records of deep body temperature of some unrestrained African mammals under near-natural conditions, J. Physiol. 176 (1965) 145–162.
[11] A.M. Harthoorn, et al., Adaptation to solar radiation by African large herbivores, J. S. Afr. Vet. Med. Assoc. 41 (1970) 17–24.
[12] V.A. Finch, D. Robertshaw, Effect of dehydration on thermoregulation in eland and hartebeest, Am. J. Physiol. 237 (1979) R192–R196.
[13] C. Jessen, et al., Effects of dehydration and rehydration on body temperatures in the black Bedouin goat, Pflügers Arch. Eur. J. Physiol. 436 (1998) 659–666.
[14] G.L. Brengelmann, Dilemma of body temperature measurement, in: K. Shiraki, M.K. Yousef (Eds.), Man in Stressful Environments—Thermal and Work Physiology, Thomas, Springfield, 1987.
[15] S. Ostrowski, J.B. Williams, K. Ismael, Heterothermy and the water economy of free-living Arabian oryx (*Oryx leucoryx*), J. Exp. Biol. 206 (2003) 1471–1478.
[16] G.D. Brown, T.J. Dawson, Seasonal variations in the body temperatures of unrestrained kangaroos (Macropodidae: Marsupialia), Comp. Biochem. Physiol., A 56 (1977) 59–67.
[17] S.K. Maloney, et al., Variation in body temperature in free-ranging western grey kangaroos (*Macropus fuliginosus*), Aust. Mammal. 26 (2004) 135–144.
[18] D. Mitchell, et al., Adaptive heterothermy and selective brain cooling in arid-zone mammals, Comp. Biochem. Physiol., B 131 (2002) 571–585.
[19] D. Mitchell, et al., Activity, blood temperature and brain temperature of free-ranging springbok, J. Comp. Physiol., B 167 (1997) 335–343.
[20] C. Jessen, et al., Blood and brain temperatures of free-ranging black wildebeest in their natural environment, Am. J. Physiol. 267 (1994) R1528–R1536.
[21] G. Kuhnen, Selective brain cooling reduces respiratory water loss during heat stress, Comp. Biochem. Physiol., A 118 (1997) 891–895.

International Congress Series 1275 (2004) 283–290

www.ics-elsevier.com

Plasticity of the water barrier in vertebrate integument

Harvey B. Lillywhite*

Department of Zoology, University of Florida, Gainesville 32611, USA

Abstract. Water barrier function in vertebrates is typically relatively fixed and characteristic of species. However, both plasticity and genetic adaptation can account for covariation between environment and resistance to transepidermal water passage (R_s). The capacity to adjust R_s may involve phenotypic plasticity, acclimation, or developmental plasticity, and fundamental mechanisms include changes in barrier thickness, composition and physicochemical properties of cutaneous lipids, and/or geometry of the barrier within the epidermis. In amniotes, lipid barriers are structured within keratin complexes that, while important to efficacy of function, appear to constrain the possibilities and time course of plastic responses. Studies of the relative importance of plastic responses and genetic variation are few and inconclusive. © 2004 Elsevier B.V. All rights reserved.

Keywords: Vertebrate; Skin; Epidermis; Lipid; Water permeability

1. Introduction

Terrestrial environments pose numerous challenges to the physiology of animals, especially larger, more active species that interact conspicuously with the physical landscape and microclimate [1]. Survival dictates that animals acquire sufficient water and energy from the environment to maintain cellular function and to support a level of metabolism sufficient for maintenance, growth and reproduction. Water is key in providing an adequate milieu for biochemical transformations and is potentially lost across body surfaces and in secretions and excreta. Evaporation of water from permeable surfaces generally constitutes the greatest source of loss, key routes of transfer being the skin and respiratory surfaces.

* Tel.: +1 352 392 1101; fax: +1 352 392 3704.
E-mail address: hbl@zoo.ufl.edu.

0531-5131/ © 2004 Elsevier B.V. All rights reserved.
doi:10.1016/j.ics.2004.08.088

Clearly, features of integument that limit cutaneous water loss (CWL) are of key significance in the evolutionary radiation of vertebrates in terrestrial and especially xeric environments. Although numerous aspects of cutaneous morphology potentially influence CWL, it is well accepted that the principal barrier to transepidermal water flux consists of lipids having adaptive geometry and composition. Indeed, lipids provide a range of waterproofing mechanisms in terrestrial plants, arthropods, and vertebrates [2]. While a fair number of studies representing all three principal taxa demonstrate "adaptive" variation in CWL in the sense that lower rates are often associated with drier environments, less is known about the stimuli and mechanisms that are causally related to this variation, either in terms of genetic adjustments or of phenotypic responses to the environment. Even less is known relating these mechanistic issues to fitness consequences of plasticity in nature and potentially related genetic constraints.

This paper briefly reviews what is known concerning plasticity of water barrier function from a perspective that considers evolutionary trends and habitat demands of vertebrates. Understanding the water relations of vertebrate integument has benefited from technological advances and physicochemical studies of lipids from other systems such as arthropods and artificial membranes [3,4]. It is hoped that such advances and techniques from dermatological disciplines will find marriage with investigations that embrace comparative and evolutionary perspectives as well as application to understanding of pending environmental change [5].

2. Water barriers and morphology of integument

Although numerous attributes of skin have been proposed to influence skin resistance to evaporative water loss (R_s), it is widely accepted that lipids provide the principal barrier to transepidermal water loss (TEWL). In both plants and arthropods, lipids are associated with or deposited on a multilayered cuticle. These surface lipids constitute the principal resistance to water passage across the cuticle or integument of these organisms [2]. Importantly, the cuticle of these organisms is a rigid structure and provides a stable platform for stability of the lipid barrier.

Terrestrial vertebrates evolved from aquatic ancestors, and a permeability barrier was an important feature of integument that evolved in concert with increased mechanical resilience related to increasing size and terrestrial demands. Mechanical toughness of the integument was provided by the evolution of a stratum corneum comprised of multiple layers of fibrous keratins with crude correlations between degree of terrestriality and degree of keratinization. Living aquatic, semi-aquatic and terrestrial but dehydration-sensitive amphibians exhibit a stratum corneum comprised of but one or two cell layers of keratin. In contrast, reptiles, birds and mammals possess a much thicker stratum corneum having multiple layers of keratinized cells and, in sauropsids (reptiles and birds), added strength and rigidity due to presence of β-type keratins. The amphibian skin is an important site of gaseous and ionic exchange, and is highly permeable to bi-directional water flux in many species, whereas the amniotes have better developed lungs and generally do not exchange gases and ions extensively across the skin. The multilayered stratum corneum of amniotes also provides a structural template for sealing lipids that perform a water barrier function. Unlike plants and arthropods, the water barrier lipids of

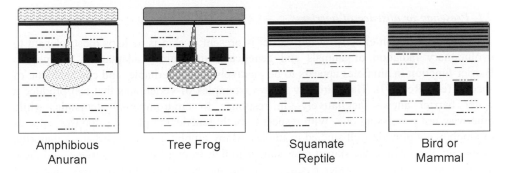

| Amphibious Anuran | Tree Frog | Squamate Reptile | Bird or Mammal |

Fig. 1. Schematic models of vertebrate integument illustrating fundamental dichotomy in means of preventing dehydration of epidermis and whole animal. In the amphibious anuran (left), either externally present moisture or aqueous mucus secreted from dermal glands maintains a wet exterior of epidermis, and therefore water evaporates from the external water film rather than from the underlying epidermis. Water is replenished from the environment, either directly or (in the case of mucus discharge) by means of cutaneous absorption across the ventral seat patch, then via blood circulation to the mucous secretions within mucous glands. In the arboreal frog (left center), lipids are secreted onto the skin surfaces from dermal glands and form a barrier to water evaporation once they dry on the exterior. A lipid barrier functions similarly in the squamate reptile (center right), bird and mammal (right) except the barrier lipids are structured internally within the stratum corneum. Lipids are shown in gray shading. The large bold broken lines represent stratum germinativum.

amniotes are contained within, not upon, the integument. In either case, however, the barrier is located superficially and distal to the vascularized tissues of the inner skin.

Among vertebrates, there is a fundamental dichotomy reflecting structure of integument and associated strategies for water balance. Either the epidermis is protected from excessive water loss by a lipid or keratin–lipid water barrier (amniotes and some amphibians), or the epidermis is maintained in a hydrated state by an overlying aqueous film or external moisture from an external source (many amphibians and some reptiles). In either strategy, the location of the lipid or aqueous film reflects the requirement for maintaining water balance of the skin itself as well as that of the entire organism (Fig. 1). Thus, when bullfrogs are basking in dehydrating environments, discharge of mucus onto the skin surfaces increases with increasing body temperature—a response interpreted to maintain a hydrated integument as well as evaporative cooling in the interest of thermoregulation [6]. These frogs do not bask or risk dehydration if water is unavailable to replenish body stores that contribute to the mucus secretions and TEWL. On the other hand, various arboreal frogs inhabiting yet drier environments secrete lipids onto the skin and wipe them over the body surfaces to form a protective water barrier that restricts losses of body water and protects the hydration status of underlying epidermis. In terrestrial amniotes, the skin is protected by a water barrier of variable effectiveness in the lipid–keratin complex of the stratum corneum (Fig. 1).

3. Mechanisms for renewal and regulation of the water barrier

There are numerous potential means by which water barriers associated with vertebrate integument can be adjusted to meet environmental demands. Fundamentally, these can be reduced to the categories of response that follow in the subsequent subsections.

3.1. Presence or absence of barriers

Whether or not an effective water barrier is present in skin is perhaps most relevant to evolutionary radiation of animals and genetically determined adaptations of species. Barrier function in amniotes appears to be relatively fixed, heritable, and characteristic of species (e.g. Ref. [7]). There are few known examples of vertebrates that can produce a water barrier anew—facultatively—in response to environmental demands, while otherwise not possessing one. With respect to both genetic and plastic responses, species of amphibians provide well-studied examples. Many amphibians, and perhaps a majority, evaporate water across the skin at rates similar to that from a free water surface, and there are no known barriers to water passage in these species. In contrast, various species of anurans inhabiting arid or semi-arid environments exhibit features of integument that pose well-known barriers to TEWL [8]. The more efficacious examples include cocoons that form in burrowing anurans during aestivation and epicutaneous lipids that are secreted from dermal glands and wiped over the body surfaces in elaborate behaviors thought to stimulate secretion and spreading of lipids over the entire body surface [9]. Such behaviors are observed prior to animals retiring from activity and assuming a water-conserving posture, or when frogs are subjected to gradual dehydration and disturbance by handling [9,10]. The stimulus that elicits the behavior is not clear, however, and it is not known how "clean" the skin becomes between bouts of wiping when R_s might potentially decrease as lipids wear away.

3.2. Barrier thickness

The amphibian examples also are relevant to mechanisms for increasing thickness of the water barrier. Characteristic cocoons consist of multiple single cell-thick layers of shed stratum corneum resulting from multiple shedding of the skin layers during periods of dormancy in drying soils. Such cocoons may consist of 40–60 layers of cornified cells with secreted lipids and proteinaceous materials sandwiched between them [11]. These structures impose considerable resistance to water movement, and the barrier efficacy presumably increases with the numbers of layers or thickness of the structure.

In frogs that wipe lipids over the body surface, tactile stimulation of the wiping elicits reflexive release of lipids from dermal glands, so the thickness of the final lipid layer could presumably be controlled to some extent by the duration and nature of the wiping [9]. The externally wiped layer of lipid was estimated to be about 0.2 μm in phyllomedusine frogs [12], but nothing is known about its variability either among or within species of anurans.

In amniotes, the barrier region of the stratum corneum provides a tough and resilient framework for intercellular lamellar lipids, and the laminated feature of the entire lipid–keratin structure is a means by which thickness of the barrier might be altered. Hypothetical proliferation of additive layers would enhance R_s to water permeation if the requirement was increased in response to increased drying power of the ambient atmosphere. Is there evidence this mechanism is utilized?

Recently, it was demonstrated that R_s essentially doubles following the first postnatal ecdysis in California king snakes (*Lampropeltis getula*), and the increased resistance correlates nicely with a doubling in thickness and number of strata of the specialized mesos layer of epidermis that constitutes the water barrier in this and other species of squamates [13]. This response is interpreted as an adaptive adjustment of R_s during the natal transition from aqueous environment of the embryo to atmospheric air that surrounds the newborn. Some lizards also exhibit upregulation of the cutaneous water barrier as a response to changes in environmental conditions, and changes in cutaneous lipids are known to be involved [14]. However, it remains unclear as to whether such changes in R_s might be correlated with changes in thickness of the water barrier. Chicks of the Japanese Quail (*Coturnix c. japonica*) exhibit a 43% decrease in skin water permeability and approach adult values within 13 days post-hatching. Histological data suggest that increased barrier efficacy is attributable to epidermal thickening, as in snakes [15].

In other studies, reptilian skin responds to trauma such as tape stripping with a "thickening" response involving hyperplasia of the α-keratin keratinocytes [16]. Human disorders of cornification in various disease states can result in different densities or thickness of stratum corneum and intercellular bilayer structures [3]. However, comparative studies of possible adaptive modifications of such structures in relation to natural environments have not been undertaken.

3.3. Composition of barrier lipids

While a few generalizations are appropriate regarding composition of lipid classes in various water barriers of vertebrates, the subject is one that has amazing complexity. In every case examined, permeability barriers contain a complex mixture of lipid molecules. Longer chain-length hydrocarbons tend to comprise a dominant category of lipids in most barriers examined. These will tend to melt at higher temperatures and will result in reduced water permeation, whereas short chain length molecules reduce the intensity of van der Waals interactions between hydrocarbon molecules and create a more fluid structure that is more readily penetrated by water. Relative saturation of hydrocarbons also contributes to a tighter water barrier, whereas unsaturation and methyl branching tends to introduce kinks in molecules and disrupts packing. In some systems, however, chain elongation and unsaturation may offset one another, such that chain length alone is not necessarily a reliable indicator of water permeation [17]. Hydrocarbons and wax esters are both very nonpolar, which also assists in repelling water. Polar phospholipids and other classes of lipids having intermediate polarity, in addition to branching, might be important in structuring the geometry of a water barrier and providing a degree or specific orientation of fluidity important with respect to potential mechanical distortion or disruption of the barrier structure.

Detailed information on cutaneous lipids of amphibians can be found in relatively few published studies. Analyses of the epicutaneous lipids secreted during wiping behaviors of phyllomedusine frogs demonstrate a mixture of hydrocarbons, triacylglycerols, cholesterol, cholesterol esters, free fatty acids and wax esters [12]. Wax esters are dominant and average about 46 carbons in length. Other studies demonstrate a cocktail of lipids that can be extracted from skin of frogs that do not exhibit wiping behaviors, and there is generally no correlation between these lipid properties and rates of evaporative water loss [18]. However, lipid mixtures extracted from whole skin undoubtedly include elements of membrane lipids not associated with a water barrier as well as precursor molecules that might be converted to other components when a barrier is present. There is no information that sheds light on how composition of barrier lipids are altered in relation to facultative waterproofing of skin by wiping or formation of a cocoon.

Studies of squamates demonstrate a complex mixture of lipids including hydrocarbons, wax and sterol esters, di- and triacylglycerols, free fatty acids, alcohols, cholesterol, ceramides, and a variety of phospholipids present in skin, with concentration shown histochemically in the mesos layer of epidermis [19–21]. Analyses of lipids extracted from the skin of snakes are complicated potentially by presence of lipid classes important as sex attractant pheromones, in addition to barrier lipids that might be present. Again, there is no information regarding possible regulation of compositional features of lipids in relation to plasticity of barrier function.

The cutaneous lipids of mammals have been studied extensively, but largely in humans and laboratory rodents and in contexts of disease and cosmetic interests in skin. Lamellar bodies provide precursor lipids consisting mainly of glycosphingolipids, free sterols and phospholipids that are delivered to the extracellular spaces in developing stratum corneum. Subsequently, these are enzymatically converted to nonpolar products and assembled into lamellar structures surrounding the corneocytes. The changes in lipid composition result in a barrier structure consisting largely of ceramides, free fatty acids, and cholesterol [22]. It is known in mammals that barrier structure and function is genetically determined and is rapidly restored following trauma. Furthermore, transformation of the precursor lipids to nonpolar-enriched barrier lipids of the stratum corneum is susceptible to disturbance by a number of factors, including essential fatty acid deficiency, genetic defects and enzyme deficiencies, environmental factors and hydration status [3]. These and various disease states are known to cause dysfunction of the water barrier and abnormally elevated TEWL. Barrier defects are indeed reflected in the lipid composition of the stratum corneum. Experimental studies of mammalian epidermis demonstrate that mechanical or chemical disruption of normal barrier morphology influences cellular kinetics, protein and lipid synthesis within 15–20 h that restore the barrier efficacy (reviewed in Ref. [23]). However, covariation of lipids and TEWL in relation to variation of natural stressors in the environment of mammalian species has not been investigated.

Recent investigations have demonstrated facultative waterproofing in the skin of birds. When subjected to conditions of dehydration, adult zebra finches are capable of rapid upregulation of the cutaneous water barrier. Within 16 h of water deprivation, TEWL decreases by 50%, and the skin barrier efficacy continues to improve until mammal-like values are achieved [24]. Similarly, hoopoe larks in extremely arid regions of the Arabian Peninsula are characterized by TEWL rates about 30% lower than that of larks from mesic environments, and these rates decrease significantly when birds are acclimated to high temperatures [25]. In these desert birds, adjustments of lipid ratios have been shown to favor ceramides over free fatty acids and sterols, and these changes correlate with reductions of TEWL [26]. The higher ratios of ceramides evidently allow the lipids of the permeability barrier to exist in a more highly ordered crystalline phase, which creates a tighter barrier to water vapor diffusion. Acclimation of water loss rates does not appear to occur in skylarks and woodlarks from mesic environments in Europe, nor in Dunn's larks from the Arabian desert [25]. Thus, capacity for plasticity of the permeability barrier appears to vary among species and, in the case of larks, is characteristic only of species inhabiting more extreme desert regions.

3.4. Physical properties and geometry

There is a great deal of information relating to physicochemical properties of lipids and lipid membranes, and it is well accepted that permeability can differ quantitatively because of the physical nature of the water movement pathway. It is important to note that in models of vertebrate barriers, lipids form a continuous barrier in the horizontal dimension parallel with the skin surface (Fig. 1). Either immobility of the animal (surface lipids of amphibians) or a tough, resilient lattice of keratin (stratum corneum–lipid complex of amniotes) appears to be important for optimal integrity of barrier function. It is not known to what degree physical disruption of the barrier structure necessitates repair or renewal during normal activity of animals that might bend or jar the skin.

Recent studies that employ molecular models suggest that resistance to water permeation of mammalian stratum corneum is related, in part, to tight, gel-like packing of hydrocarbon chains and changes in lipid phase behavior related to component ratios and molecular arrangement of cholesterol [27,28]. Additionally, fluid and crystalline phases of the lipid lattice alternate vertically in repetition with stacked lamellae [29]. The crystalline phase enhances barrier efficacy, while the presence and localization of fluid domains facilitate elasticity in relation to geometry of the barrier and lipid interactions with keratin components. Models further suggest that diffusion of water is limited in directions both parallel and perpendicular to the plane of the lipid bilayers due to their organization [28]. In avian skin, the efficacy of facultative waterproofing resides in a capacity to modulate the organization of secreted lipids, viz. non-bilayer, electron-lucent lipids under basal conditions, but lamellar lipid structures in response to xeric stress, leading to significantly decreased TEWL [24]. Both compositional features of cutaneous lipids and the hydration status of the skin will influence the phase properties of the barrier, which becomes disrupted as the skin becomes progressively hydrated. Unlike terrestrial mammals, the stratum corneum of marine mammals retains appreciable amounts of glycolipids [30].

4. Conclusion

In spite of extensive literature on membrane physiology and the structure and function of mammalian skin in relation to disease and cosmetics, there is comparatively little understanding of adaptive adjustments of permeability barriers in contexts of evolution, phylogeny and environment. Comparative and experimental approaches with goals of understanding mechanisms of plasticity in relation to adaptation will hopefully remedy this deficit of understanding in the future. Such investigations should include, or interface with, genetics, morphology, ecology and evolutionary disciplines, as well as physiology.

References

[1] W.P. Porter, et al., Calculating climate effects on birds and mammals: impacts on biodiversity, conservation, population parameters, and global community structure, Am. Zool. 40 (2000) 597–630.

[2] N.F. Hadley, Integumental lipids of plants and animals: comparative function and biochemistry, Adv. Lipid Res. 24 (1991) 303–320.

[3] G. Menon, R. Ghadially, Morphology of lipid alterations in the epidermis: a review, Microsc. Res. Tech. 37 (1997) 180–192.

[4] A.G. Gibbs, Water-proofing properties of cuticular lipids, Am. Zool. 38 (1998) 471–482.

[5] P.M. Kareiva, J.G. Kingsolver, R.B. Huey (Eds.), Biotic Interactions and Global Change, Sunderland, Sinauer Associates, Massachusetts, 1993.

[6] H. Lillywhite, Thermal modulation of cutaneous mucus discharge as a determinant of evaporative water loss in the frog, *Rana catesbeiana*, Z. Vgl. Physiol. 73 (1971) 84–104.

[7] F. Furuyama, K. Ohara, Genetic development of an inbred rat strain with increased resistance adaptation to a hot environment, Am. J. Physiol. 265 (Part 2) (1993) R957–R962.

[8] R.C. Toledo, C. Jared, Cutaneous adaptations to water balance in amphibians, Comp. Biochem. Physiol. 105A (1993) 593–608.

[9] H.B. Lillywhite, et al., Wiping behavior and its ecophysiological significance in the Indian tree frog *Polypedates maculatus*, Copeia 1997 (1997) 88–100.

[10] L.A. Blaylock, R. Ruibal, K. Plat-Aloia, Skin structure and wiping behaviour of phyllomedusine frogs, Copeia 1976 (1976) 283–295.

[11] R. Ruibal, S.S. Hillman, Cocoon structure and function in the burrowing hylid frog, *Pternohyla fodiens*, J. Herpetol. 15 (1981) 403–408.

[12] L.L. McClanahan, J.N. Stinner, V.H. Shoemaker, Skin lipids, water loss, and energy metabolism in a South American tree frog (*Phyllomedusa sauvagei*), Physiol. Zool. 51 (1978) 179–187.

[13] M.C. Tu, et al., Postnatal ecdysis establishes the permeability barrier in snake skin: new insights into lipid barrier structures, J. Exp. Biol. 205 (2002) 3019–3030.

[14] G.H. Kattan, H.B. Lillywhite, Humidity acclimation and skin permeability in the lizard *Anolis carolinensis*, Physiol. Zool. 62 (1989) 593–606.

[15] F.M.A. McNabb, R.A. McNabb, Skin and plumage changes during the development of thermoregulatory ability in Japanese quail chicks, Comp. Biochem. Physiol. 58A (1977) 163–166.

[16] P.F.A. Maderson, A.H. Zucker, S.I. Roth, Epidermal regeneration and percutaneous water loss following cellophane stripping of reptile epidermis, J. Exp. Zool. 204 (1978) 11–32.

[17] A.G. Gibbs, A.K. Louie, J.A. Ayala, Effects of temperature on cuticular lipids and water balance in desert *Drosophila*: is thermal acclimation beneficial? J. Exp. Biol. 201 (1998) 71–80.

[18] P.C. Withers, S.S. Hillman, R.C. Drewes, Evaporative water loss and skin lipids of anuran amphibians, J. Exp. Zool. 232 (1984) 11–17.

[19] J.B. Roberts, H.B. Lillywhite, Lipid barrier to water exchange in reptile epidermis, Science 207 (1980) 1077–1079.

[20] J.B. Roberts, H.B. Lillywhite, Lipids and the permeability of epidermis from snakes, J. Exp. Zool. 228 (1983) 1–9.

[21] R.R. Burken, P.W. Wertz, D.T. Downing, A survey of polar and nonpolar lipids extracted from snake skin, Comp. Biochem. Physiol. 81 (1985) 315–318.

[22] J.A. Bouwstra, et al., Structure of the skin barrier and its modulation by vesicular formulations, Prog. Lipid Res. 42 (2003) 1–36.

[23] E. Proksch, et al., Barrier function regulates epidermal lipid and DNA synthesis, Br. J. Dermatol. 193 (1993) 473–482.

[24] G.K. Menon, et al., Ultrastructural organization of avian stratum corneum lipids as the basis for facultative cutaneous waterproofing, J. Morphol. 227 (1996) 1–13.

[25] B.I. Tieleman, J.B. Williams, Cutaneous and respiratory water loss in larks from arid and mesic environments, Physiol. Biochem. Zool. 75 (2002) 590–599.

[26] M.J. Haugen, et al., Lipids of the stratum corneum vary with cutaneous water loss along a temperature–moisture gradient, Physiol. Biochem. Zool. (2003) 907–917.

[27] R.O. Potts, M.L. Francoeur, Lipid biophysics of water loss through the skin, Proc. Natl. Acad. Sci. 87 (1990) 3871–3873.

[28] T.J. McIntosh, Organization of skin stratum corneum extracellular lamellae: diffraction evidence for asymmetric distribution of cholesterol, Biophys. J. 85 (2003) 1675–1681.

[29] J.A. Bouwstra, et al., The lipid organization in the skin barrier, Acta Derm.-Venereol. Supp 208 (2000) 23–30.

[30] P.M. Elias, et al., Avian sebokeratocytes and marine mammal lipokeratinocytes: structural, lipid biochemical and functional considerations, Am. J. Anat. 180 (1987) 161–177.

International Congress Series 1275 (2004) 291–297

www.ics-elsevier.com

Water economy of free-living desert animals

Kenneth A. Nagy*

Department of Ecology and Evolutionary Biology, University of California Los Angeles, 621 Young Drive South, Los Angeles, CA 90095-1606, USA

Abstract. Deserts are relatively dry and dehydrating places, by definition, but desert animals are composed of 65–75% water, just like non-desert animals. Do desert animals maintain water balance and body hydration level by conserving water better (decreasing output, as compared with non-desert species) or by getting more water each day (increasing input), or both? These questions can be evaluated with measurements of daily water flux rates (in ml/day) as determined with isotopically labeled water through free-ranging animals that are maintaining constant body masses. Inspection of the many field measurements now available reveals great variation (10 million-fold among terrestrial vertebrates alone), due largely to differences in body mass, but also due to taxonomic affinity (endothermy vs. ectothermy), season, diet and age, as well as to variation in habitat aridity. Fortunately, water flux rates can be normalized for much of this variation by dividing them by field metabolic rates, to yield units of ml water used per kJ energy metabolized (termed Water Economy Index, WEI). The WEI values of desert-dwelling eutherian mammals are significantly lower than in non-desert eutherians, and (surprisingly) desert endotherms have lower WEIs than desert ectotherms. Year-round WEI measurements on desert kangaroo rats, which have the lowest index yet measured, revealed that they often obtained more water than was available just from dry seeds, not by drinking, but by eating young green vegetation when available in spring, and especially by hydrating dry seeds before consumption by storing them in humid burrows for a while. © 2004 Elsevier B.V. All rights reserved.

Keywords: Desert adaptation; Minimum water requirement; Water Economy Index; Water flux rate; Field metabolic rate; Doubly labeled water

* Tel.: +1 310 825 8771; fax: +1 310 206 3987.
E-mail address: kennagy@biology.ucla.edu.

0531-5131/ © 2004 Elsevier B.V. All rights reserved.
doi:10.1016/j.ics.2004.08.054

1. Introduction

Deserts are considered to be extreme environments, mainly due to their lack of water. Many deserts also have high temperatures, which contributes to the problem of water scarcity for animals. The aridity also reduces food availability, compared to other habitats, so food energy is often in short supply, as well as water. Despite these challenges to life, deserts are occupied by many species of animals. Most desert species studied have behavioral, physiological and morphological adaptations which facilitate survival and reproduction. In this review, the focus is on daily water requirements of free-living animals. Two questions are evaluated: do desert species of mammals, birds, and how reptiles get by with less water than do non-desert species; and which taxonomic group and which species conserves water "the best"? To evaluate these questions, daily water intake rates are considered in relation to the field metabolic rates of each species, in order to account for the influences of taxonomic group (endothermy, ectothermy), habitat effects of metabolic rates and differences in body mass.

2. Methods

2.1. Data sources

Measurements of water flux rates and field metabolic rates (via doubly labeled water [1–3]) of desert and non-desert animals living in their natural habitats were gathered from the literature. Only results representing animals that were in or near a steady-state regarding water balance were used. In most cases, this condition was not directly measured, but was assumed to exist when body mass remained constant during the measurement period. When animals are not eating or drinking enough to maintain weight, their rates of water intake are relatively low and not representative of their minimum maintenance needs (Fig. 1). Even when maintaining constant body mass, an animal may be taking in excess water and just excreting the excess, thus yielding a steady-state intake rate that is above minimum maintenance requirements. Accordingly, where several steady-state values were available for a species, I selected the one yielding the lowest WEI value (see definition below). Most data were obtained from two previous review articles [4,5], but some of the more recently

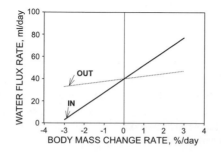

Fig. 1. Relationships among daily water influx and efflux rates and daily rate of body mass change. Vertical line indicates maintenance of constant body mass, an index of being in an energetic steady-state.

published results that are available were included. Unfortunately, many published reports did not state whether the animals were maintaining constant masses or not, so those results were not included in this analysis.

2.1.1. Water Economy Index (WEI)

Whole-animal rates of water influx, in units of milliliters per day under steady-state conditions, range over eight orders of magnitude [4], mainly in accord with differences in body size. Other important sources of variation are season, taxon, endothermy or ectothermy, age cohort, and habitat. This huge variation must be addressed before meaningful comparisons between species can be made. Many of these sources of variation are underlain by variation in metabolic rate. That is, larger animals use more energy per day (hence eat and drink more and have higher water intake per day) than do small ones, endotherms use more energy daily than do equivalent-sized ectotherms, animals often use energy faster when breeding than when not breeding or when very young or very old, and desert-dwelling eutherian mammals and birds have lower basal and field metabolic rates than do non-desert relatives. Thus, much of the variation in the raw water influx data may be accounted for by adjusting it for the "speed of living" or metabolic rate of the animal at the time its water influx rate was measured. The ratio of ml water "turned over" (equal to both intake rate and loss rate in a steady-state situation) per day to kJ energy metabolized per day in the field, or ml/kJ, represents an adjusted water flux value, or Water Economy Index (WEI), which is normalized to an animal's rate of living. This is similar, in a way, to the "water use efficiency" ratio of mol CO_2 fixed per mol water transpired by leaves of plants, and its reciprocal "transpiration ratio", expressing the water cost of obtaining atmospheric CO_2 for photosynthesis, with lowest being "best" for desert-dwelling plants. Doubly labeled water yields estimates of both water influx and field metabolic rate (FMR [2]). Results for many desert and non-desert species are available, and a table of data used herein is available from the author via e-mail.

2.1.2. Data analysis

Results were grouped into desert-dwelling and non-desert-dwelling species for subsequent analysis. Within taxa, habitat differences in WEI were tested for differences at the $P=0.05$ level using t-tests, or with Mann–Whitney rank sum tests when normality requirements were not met. Possible differences among desert taxa were evaluated using a Kruskal–Wallis one-way analysis of variance.

3. Results

There is much overlap in WEI values of desert and non-desert species among eutherian and marsupial mammals, birds and reptiles (Fig. 2). Nevertheless, some statistically significant differences (Table 1) emerged. Desert-dwelling eutherians had WEIs averaged only 55% of those of non-desert eutherian mammals. Marsupial mammals, on the other hand, showed no difference in WEI according to habitat, and two of the four desert species had quite high relative water intake rates. Birds, in general, do not use much water relative to their metabolic rate, but desert birds had WEIs averaging only 77% of those of non-desert birds. Surprisingly, desert reptiles had

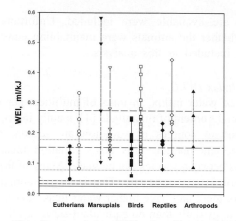

Fig. 2. Summary of minimum Water Economy Index (WEI) values for mammals, birds, reptiles and arthropods superimposed on a template indicating expected WEI values for animals maintaining constant body mass on three common diets without drinking water [herbivory, between horizontal long-dashed lines; carnivory, between dotted lines; granivory, between short-dashed lines; and for fat metabolism (no eating or drinking), solid line at bottom of graph].

rather high WEI values, which were not statistically distinguishable from those of non-desert reptiles. Desert arthropods showed a wide range of WEI values, which overlapped with those of the other taxa. In comparing all five groups of desert animals, there was no significant variation among them. However, small sample sizes available at present may preclude statistical detection of possibly lower WEI values among desert marsupial mammals and reptiles.

Table 1

Mean WEI values of desert and non-desert animals, along with probability values for differences within taxa due to habitat

Group	N	Mean WEI, ml/kJ	S.D.	P
Eutherian mammals				
Desert	6	0.111	0.036	0.033
Non-desert	6	0.203	0.084	
Marsupial mammals				
Desert	4	0.364	0.217	0.249
Non-desert	12	0.197	0.081	
Birds				
Desert	14	0.150	0.056	0.047
Non-desert	41	0.195	0.076	
Reptiles				
Desert	7	0.171	0.047	0.098
Non-desert	6	0.251	0.105	
Arthropods				
Desert	4	0.210	0.111	

There was no significant variation in WEI among the five desert groups ($P=0.100$).

4. Discussion

4.1. Desert adaptation

Eutherian mammals and birds that occupy deserts apparently require less water each day to achieve water balance than do their non-desert relatives. This reduction in daily water needs is in addition to the reduction that would be associated with the lower field metabolic rates [6] and feeding rates [7] that are found in desert species of eutherians and birds. The WEI ratio adjusts for these differences in metabolism, and the WEI values of desert eutherians and birds are still significantly lower than in non-desert species. Reduced metabolism itself is considered to be a desert adaptation, and it may even have evolved in response to selection by water restriction [5]. The further reduction in water needs indicates that at least some desert species of eutherians and birds have even lower water losses in the field, perhaps due to physiological adjustments (lower evaporation, more concentrated urine, drier feces) or behavioral adjustments (less time spent active above ground, being relatively more nocturnal) or both.

Interestingly, marsupial mammals that live in deserts do have lower field metabolic rates (by about 35% [8]), but not lower WEI values than do their non-desert relatives. However, desert marsupials do have reduced water flux rates (also by about 35%), and these reductions are apparently due entirely to their reduced metabolic rates. Thus, free-living desert marsupials may rely less on physiological and behavioral adaptations that specifically reduce water requirements than do eutherian mammals and birds. The lower water needs of desert marsupials can be accounted for entirely by their reduced metabolic rate. The wide range in WEI values of desert marsupials indicates that some species utilized water for drinking from the oasis near the study site.

Desert reptiles do not have unusually low field metabolic rates [6]. They tended to have low WEI values but the difference is not significant (Table 1). However, their water flux rates are substantially (50%) lower than in non-desert species [4]. These two observations indicate that desert reptiles exploited the strategy of reducing water needs mainly through direct physiological and behavioral adjustments influencing water loss, rather than indirectly through reducing energy metabolism. Compared to desert vertebrates, desert arthropods have moderately, but not spectacularly, low WEI values, despite having some remarkable physiological mechanisms (cryptonephridial excretory systems, water vapor absorption, very water-proof cuticles [9]) for conserving water. This group warrants more study.

4.2. WEI theoretical framework

It is possible to predict the WEI value for a specific diet, on the basis of that diet's chemical composition and digestibility. The water yield of a diet will be the sum of its "preformed" water content (its succulence) and its "metabolic" water, which is the product of its dry matter content, dry matter digestibility, and the water produced upon oxidation of that assimilated dry matter. The WEI numerator will be dietary water yield alone, if the animal does not drink water (which is usually unavailable to many desert animals). The WEI denominator will be the energy content of the assimilated dry matter, assuming the animal is in energetic steady-state, and is burning all dry matter absorbed from its food.

For a non-drinking herbivore maintaining constant body mass while eating green plant foods, typical WEI values range from about 0.16 to 0.27, WEIs for typical carnivore diets range from 0.08 to 0.17, and a seed diet (granivory) yields a WEI of 0.03–0.04 [4]. Oxidation of stored body fat alone, as occurs in a starving animal, has a WEI of about 0.025, and this should be the lower limit of feasible WEI values.

Superimposing the available WEI results on this theoretical framework is instructive (Fig. 2). Those species having WEI values above the range expected for their diet category are either selecting unusually wet foods, or more likely are drinking free-standing water. Drinking by free-ranging non-desert vertebrates seems to be more common than in desert vertebrates, but some desert marsupials and desert arthropods rely on drinking (or vapor absorption) to maintain themselves in the field. These observations illustrate the two main ways of achieving water balance in desert habitats: reduce water losses to minimize water requirements, or leave water losses unmodified but enhance water-obtaining skills to increase water intake to meet the higher water needs.

4.3. WEI champion

Water Economy Index, which relates an animal's water use under natural conditions to its "rate of living", is only one of several ways to look at water balance. Another is the absolute amount of water an animal needs each day. This is a very important factor in a practical sense. Also important is the form in which water is obtained (food or drink or fat metabolism or vapor). WEI offers a way to adjust for variables (size, taxon, etc.) that have very large effects on absolute water flux rates, so that species can be compared with each other more readily.

In this vein, we can ask the question "Who is the best?" The current world's champion water conserver is Merriam's kangaroo rat, which has the lowest WEI yet measured in animals maintaining weight in their natural habitats. The WEI of kangaroo rats reached low values in autumn and winter, before rains came, and when the soil was at its driest (Fig. 3). At that time, water intake by kangaroo rats could be completely accounted for by metabolic water, water vapor condensation in lungs from humidity in burrow air

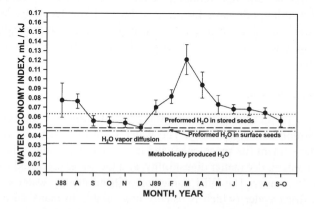

Fig. 3. Seasonal changes in WEI values of free-living desert kangaroo rats (*Dipodomys merriami*) in relation to their itemized water intake budget (from Ref. [10]).

(primarily), and the small amount of preformed water in dry, dehisced seeds in the soil "seed bank". In other seasons, WEIs were higher, indicating consumption of some succulent vegetation that became available in spring, and "hydration" of dry seeds by storage in humid places before consumption in spring and summer [10].

However, kangaroo rats may be outdone by granivorous desert birds that also do not drink, such as the Black-throated Sparrow in the Mojave Desert (as yet unstudied in the field). Unlike kangaroo rats, these birds do not use burrows, and they are diurnally active, so they experience the desert's daytime heat and low humidities that kangaroo rats avoid. Also, these birds apparently do not hydrate seeds before consumption, so they are eating drier food than kangaroo rats, and should have a lower WEI. The next lowest WEI known besides kangaroo rats (Fig. 3) is for Dune Larks in southern African deserts [11]. The Dune Lark is ecologically similar to Black-throated Sparrows, except that they are omnivorous, thereby having a wetter diet. Thus, a doubly labeled water study on Black-throated Sparrows should yield instructive insights.

References

[1] N. Lifson, R. McClintock, Theory of use of the turnover rates of body water for measuring energy and material balance, J. Theor. Biol. 12 (1966) 46–74.

[2] K.A. Nagy, The Doubly Labeled Water (^{3}HH^{18}O)Method: A Guide to Its Use. Los Angeles: University of California Publ. No. 12-1417, 1983.

[3] J.R. Speakman, Doubly Labelled Water: Theory and Practice, Chapman and Hall, London, 1997.

[4] K.A. Nagy, C.C. Peterson, Scaling of Water Flux Rate in Animals, University of California Press, Berkeley, 1988.

[5] B.I. Tielman, J.B. Williams, The adjustment of avian metabolic rates and water fluxes to desert environments, Physiol. Biochem. Zool. 73 (2000) 461–479.

[6] K.A. Nagy, I.A. Girard, T.K. Brown, Energetics of free-ranging mammals, reptiles, and birds, Annu. Rev. Nutr. 19 (1999) 247–277.

[7] K.A. Nagy, Food requirements of wild animals: predictive equations for free-living mammals, reptiles, and birds, Nutr. Abstr. Rev. Ser. B. Livest. Feeds Feed. 71 (2001) 21R–32R.

[8] K.A. Nagy, S.D. Bradshaw, Scaling of energy and water fluxes in free-living arid-zone Australian marsupials, J. Mammal. 81 (2000) 962–970.

[9] E.B. Edney, Water Balance in Land Arthropods, Springer-Verlag, Berlin, 1977.

[10] K.A. Nagy, M.J. Gruchacz, Seasonal water and energy metabolism of the desert-dwelling kangaroo rat (*Dipodomys merriami*), Physiol. Zool. 67 (1994) 1461–1478.

[11] J.B. Williams, Energy expenditure and water flux of free-living Dune Larks in the Namib: a test of the reallocation hypothesis on a desert bird, Funct. Ecol. 15 (2001) 175–185.

International Congress Series 1275 (2004) 298–305

www.ics-elsevier.com

A preliminary assessment of anuran physiological and morphological adaptation to the Caatinga, a Brazilian semi-arid environment

Carlos A. Navas[a],*, Marta M. Antoniazzi[b], Carlos Jared[b]

[a]Departamento de Fisiologia, Instituto de Biociências, Universidade de São Paulo, Rua do Matão, Travessa 14 no. 321, 05508-900 São Paulo, Brazil
[b]Laboratório de Biologia Celular, Instituto Butantan, Brazil

Abstract. Anuran amphibians exploit a variety of water-deprived environments, including the Caatinga, a semi-arid biome that is exclusive to Brazil. The Caatinga is characterized by seasonal but unpredictable rains and by droughts that might last from several months to more than a year, or various years with negligible rain. Despite expected ecophysiological challenges, the Caatinga is home to a significant anuran fauna represented by five families. Many species retain behaviors and ecological associations that are typical for their genera, and avoid the full challenge of the Caatinga climate by seasonal and opportunistic activity. Therefore, the ability to aestivate seems a requirement for the colonization of the Caatinga, but a deep dormant state might not be typical of all species, as the microecological conditions of the shelters might vary significantly. From the standpoint of the skin as barrier to evaporative water loss, Caatinga anurans range from species with reduced levels of water evaporation due to waxy secretions to species that favor water uptake and exhibit a fully permeable skin. Most species are seasonal and nocturnal, but the few diurnal species tolerate temperatures that would impair or kill typical tropical anurans. The Caatinga anuran community depends on diverse behaviors, ecological associations and physiological adaptations that vary from taxa to taxa. © 2004 Elsevier B.V. All rights reserved.

Keywords: Anuran; Aestivation; Caatinga; Semi-arid; Skin; Thermal physiology; Temperature

* Correspondence author. Tel.: +55 11 30917560; fax: +55 11 30917521.
E-mail address: navas@usp.br (C.A. Navas).

0531-5131/ © 2004 Elsevier B.V. All rights reserved.
doi:10.1016/j.ics.2004.08.061

1. Introduction

Anuran amphibians have radiated along extreme environments such as high elevations, high latitudes or deserts. Among these, semi-arid regions are considered particularly severe for anurans given well known aspects of their natural history such as skin permeability and consequent risk of dehydration in a dry milieu. One semi-arid setting occupied by anurans is the Caatinga, an exclusively North-Eastern Brazilian biome (Fig. 1). In addition to ecological characteristics that are well known to many arid regions, including low relative humidity, sparse vegetation, and high day temperatures, the Caatinga is characterized by rather unpredictable seasonality of rains [1]. A rainy season usually comes in January, but rain patterns are variable, leading to uncertainty in the length of aestivation periods and in the duration of temporary ponds. Despite these ecophysiological challenges, the Caatinga exhibits an anuran fauna that can be considered exuberant for a semi-arid environment: it is inhabited by more than 40 species in the families Hylidae (including Phyllomedusinae), Leptodactylidae, Bufonidae, Microhylidae, and Pipidae, being the first two mentioned the best represented [2]. Here we discuss the ecological associations and physiological adjustments of some Caatinga anurans to this semi-arid environment, stressing important differences in natural history that exist among taxa.

2. Aestivation in Caatinga anurans

Fully arid environments are not inhabited by amphibians, but aestivation allows anurans to occupy semi-arid environments that offer suitable conditions for activity and reproduction on a seasonal basis [3]. Specialized anurans tolerate droughts by means of water savings derived from adjustments of nitrogen metabolism [3,4], the formation of hygroscopic cocoons from the stratum corneum [5], depression of metabolic rate [6] and physiological mechanisms to avoid damage to bone or skeletal muscle due to inactivity [7,8]. The Caatinga dry season might last several months and most species of anurans are

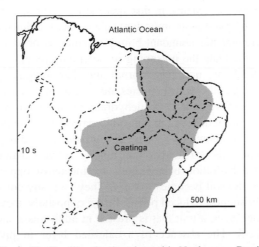

Fig. 1. The Brazilian Caatinga located in Northeastern Brazil.

rarely seen during the drought, thus some capacity for aestivation is likely to be a convergent trait for the taxa in this biome. Drastic dormant states appear to occur in at least some species. For example, it is possible to find *Proceratophrys cristiceps* buried deep in the soil along the dry season (up to 1 m) and exhibiting a modified skin (species in this genus do not build a cocoon comparable to those reported for *Ceratophrys* [9]).

Deep aestivation, however, might not be a norm for Caatinga anurans, given species-specific differences in natural history and microhabitat associations. During the dry season *Bufo paracnemis* and *B. granulosus* might be seen active, and *Pleurodema diplolistris* and the casque-head tree frog *Corythomantis greeningi* is found hiding but attentive. Regarding microhabitat selection, large water holes on rock outcrops, common in the Caatinga and inhabited by *C. greeningi* and *Phyllomedusa hypochondrialis*, might be humid most of the year. Monitoring the physical conditions of microhabitats used by caatinga anurans during the dry season is a first step necessary to propose hypotheses and generalizations regarding aestivation by Caatinga anurans.

3. Behavior and water conservation in non-aestivating Caatinga anurans

The ability to find and prefer appropriate microhabitats for aestivation is essential for the survival of many anurans species in arid environments [10], but hydric constraints are relaxed during the rainy season, particularly in species associated with large bodies of water. Given the characteristics of Caatinga rain patterns, however, some anuran species in this biome might be exposed to hot and dehydrating conditions during activity. In these species appropriate choice of retreat sites and good timing for retreat is fundamental for survival.

Selection of the most humid retreat available has been experimentally demonstrated in *C. greeningi*. This tree frog is notorious for exhibiting phragmotic behavior (hiding in holes baring access to the shelter with their co-ossified head), and individuals consistently choose for prhagmosis the only test tube (out of 10 choices) containing a humid cotton fluff [11]. The combination of phragmotic behavior and the ability to find humid crevices act together to improve water balance in this species. Phragmotic behaviors not only save water but also energy, by playing an important role in passive defense. The labial portion of the head of *C. greeningi* has abundant bonny spicules associated with venom glands, which are believed to facilitate the poisoning of potential predators [12].

Many species of toads are normally diurnal and thermoregulate during the juvenile dispersion phase [13–15], and caatinga species are no exception to this rule. They venture far from reliable sources of water and may dehydrate rapidly if exposed for long periods of time to the typical air conditions (even in non-rainy days within the rainy season, as shown by our field observations). Therefore, juvenile *B. paracnemis* and *B. granulosus* are likely to experience the highest risk of dehydration among active Caatinga anurans. Juvenile Caatinga toads avoid dehydration behaviorally, by means of opportunistic activity and retreat to shelter when the soil becomes too dry. They lack any conspicuous trait of skin morphology that might suggest reduced permeability; oppositely, they have a thin skin that lacks a calcified dermal layer, a trait that is present in adult toads and has been related to water conservation [16]. The absence of a calcified layer in juveniles might reflect physiological constraints in calcium allocation.

4. Skin morphology and water balance

A key aspect of anuran water balance, water uptake via ventral skin, has been well established since the 1790s [17]. Thereafter, a number of contributions have revealed diverse traits of ventral skin morphology that differ among species and affect water uptake, such as thickness, sculpturing, presence of verruca hidrophilica (protrusions that increase surface area and characterize the ventral integument of many anuran amphibians), or increased capillary bedding [5]. Furthermore, the ventral skin of some anurans have chemosensory properties and can detect salts, helping individuals to avoid hyper-osmotic sources of water [18].

The ecological significance of intraspecific differences in skin morphology, and their relationship with water ecology, are being studied in *Bufo granulosus*, a common species that is distributed along an ecological gradient from mesic habitats in the Atlantic Forest to the Caatinga. The preliminary data obtained so far suggests noticeable interpopulational morphological differentiation along this gradient, but the patterns observed are not of trivial interpretation. For example, the verruca hidrophilica, believed to increased water uptake [5], are much more pronounced in individuals from populations in the Atlantic Forest that in individual from the semi-arid Caatinga (Fig. 2). The skin of Caatinga individuals is about half as thick than that of toads from the Atlantic Forest, and is similarly thin both ventrally and dorsally, whereas the skin of individuals from the Atlantic Forest is thicker dorsally (Fig. 3). Caatinga toads also exhibit about twice as many capillary vessels. It is possible that a smoother, thinner and more vascular skin promotes opportunistic water uptake in Caatinga toads which, given other aspects of behavior and ecology, eventually increased fossoriality, might have evolved a morphology that prioritizes water uptake over water loss.

Body coating with diverse types of skin secretions has evolved various times in unrelated anuran taxa, not necessarily in the context of extreme environments [19]. However, it is largely acknowledged that the secretion of skin lipids contributes to a significant reduction of evaporative water loss and enhances anuran survival in arid habitats [5]. Tree frogs in the genus *Phyllomedusa*, which typically spend the day on leaves and exposed to sunshine, are know to produce waxy secretions that greatly reduce water loss during exposure to solar radiation [20,21]. Caatinga species in this genus (*P.*

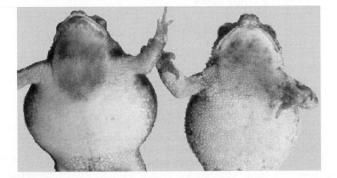

Fig. 2. Ventral view of adult male *Bufo granulosus* from the Caatinga (left) and the Atlantic Forest (right).

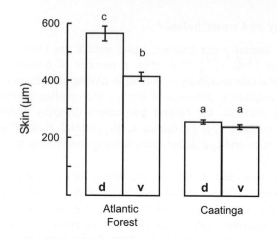

Fig. 3. Skin thickness in two populations of *Bufo granulosus*. The letters d and v indicate dorsal and ventral skin.

hypochondrialis) are often seen fully exposed on leaves, reaching body temperatures above 40 °C, and most likely exhibit similar traits of skin morphology to those reported by congener species.

Waxy secretions are not the only mechanisms that reduce water evaporation in anurans. Various degrees of skin permeability, from free water surfaces to the so-called "water-proof frogs" have been reported in this taxon [22]. One Caatinga species with morphologically reduced skin permeability is the above mentioned *C. greeningi*, that evaporates about half the water that agar models of similar size do (Fig. 4).

5. Tolerance to high temperatures

Whether or not challenging physiological conditions are experienced by Caatinga anurans during aestivation remains to be investigated, as we know little about the micro-climatic conditions experienced by dormant frogs. Most Caatinga anurans are nocturnal and active only during the rainy season, thus they have plenty of water available for evaporative cooling and are very unlikely to experience near-lethal temperatures. The

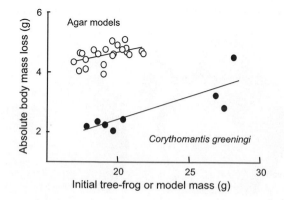

Fig. 4. Water loss in *Corythomantis greeningi* and agar models exposed to dehydrating conditions.

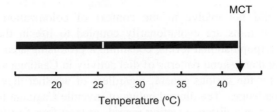

Fig. 5. Temperature selection and maximum critical temperature (MCT) in juvenile *Bufo granulosus* from a Caatinga population. The white line on indicates the median.

highest day temperatures among Caatinga anurans are probably endured by diurnal species, such as juvenile *B. paracnemis*, *B. granulosus* and *P. hypochondrialis*. Juvenile toads are of special interest because they are prone to rapid desiccation and have an unfavorable volume/area ratio. From a thermal biology point of view juvenile *B. granulosus* are quite atypical: they exhibit critical maximum temperatures bordering 45 °C, are often active near this temperature, and do not show thermal preferences, at least in humid laboratory gradients (Fig. 5). These patterns contrast dramatically with those reported in juveniles of other species such as *B. woodhousei*, which avoid high temperatures in an experimental gradient [23].

Further studies on the thermal ecology of Caatinga *P. hypochondrialis* are necessary to understand whether these species are exceptional within the genus in terms of color, reflectance and thermal tolerances, traits that are fundamental to other desert species of anurans that tolerate very intense solar radiation, such as *Hyperolius viridiflavus* [24].

6. Concluding remarks

Anuran adaptation to the Caatinga involves a complex array of physiological and behavioral traits that vary from taxa to taxa (Table 1). Many traits of the natural history of Caatinga anurans, for example nocturnality, decrease the impact of environmental physical variables in a semi-arid climate, but do not constitute formal adaptations to this

Table 1
Contrasts in natural history traits of five Caatinga anuran species representing the families Bufonidae, Hylidae and Leptodactylidae

TRAIT	Species			
	Bufo granulosus and B. paracnemis	*Corythomantis greeningi*	*Phyllomedusa hypochondrialis*	*Proceratophrys cristiceps*
Cutaneous morphological adaptations	Calcified dermal layer	Calcified dermal layer	Lipid secretion glands	Apparently none
Deep aestivation	No	No	No	Very likely
Strict microhabitat associations	Opportunistic search for hiding places during activity	To rock outcrops	To rock outcrops	Fossorial for aestivation
Tolerance to high temperatures	Yes	Yes	Yes	No
Phragmotic behaviors	No	Yes	No	No
Poison as a defense during inactivity	Yes	Yes	Yes	No

environment (i.e., did not evolve in the context of colonization of the Caatinga). Understanding which traits are evolutionarily coupled to life in the Caatinga at both interspecific and interpopulational levels, constitute a promising area for future research.

It is worth noting that general patterns of diel activity in Caatinga anurans appear to be those most typical for the various genera, regardless of whether they increase or reduce ecophysiological challenges. The diurnal habits of juvenile Caatinga toads exemplify this issue. A similar report in a different setting regards at least four families of tropical high-elevation anurans that are active at low and very variable temperatures [25]. Tropical high-elevation *Eleutherodactylus*, for example, retain a nocturnal and typically bimodal pattern of vocal activity that results in extremely low temperatures during calling, and therefore require significant evolutionary shifts in thermal physiology [26]. Together, these studies support the idea that keen microhabitat selection and remarkable evolutionary plasticity of physiology are key factors in anuran ecological radiations along extreme environments.

The skin, interface between the organism and the environment, plays a very significant role in anuran adaptation to semi-arid environments. However, contrasting strategies can be detected, from waterproofing to increased skin permeability, as seems the case of *B. granulosus*. This scenario illustrates that caution is needed before anticipating general adaptive trends of anurans from arid environments.

Given the unpredictability of the rainy season and the prolonged droughts that occur in the Caatinga, the ability to aestivate appears to be a requirement for anuran species to occupy this biome. Most likely, however, anuran aestivation in the semi-arid Caatinga involves diverse physiologically states that vary among taxa. Similar physiological diversity is expected also in the context of thermal tolerances, because life in a semi-arid environment is not necessarily associated with activity at high temperatures. Many species are nocturnal and seasonal, thus do not experience thermal stress during activity. Finally, it must be pointed out that, although this discussion has focused post-metamorphic states, tadpoles in the Caatinga are often exposed to very high temperatures and oxygen limitations in dehydrating ponds. Little is known about larval adaptation to such extreme microhabitats.

Acknowledgments

Work supported by grants from FAPESP (State of São Paulo Science Foundation 2003/01577-8), CNPq (Brazilian Research Council, 474208/2003-6) and Fundação Butantan. Specimens were collected under IBAMA permits 172/1999 and 193/2001.

References

[1] A.C.D. Souzareis, Climate of Caatinga, Anais da Academia Brasileira de Ciências 48 (1976) 325–335.

[2] M.T. Rodrigues, Herpetofauna da Caatinga, Ecologia e Conservação da Caatinga, Recife, Universidade Federal de Pernambuco, 2003, pp. 181–236.

[3] A.S. Abe, Estivation in south american amphibians and reptiles, Braz. J. Med. Biol. Res. 28 (11–12) (1995) 1241–1247.

[4] K.B. Storey, Life in the slow lane: molecular mechanisms of estivation, J. Comp. Physiol. 133 (3) (2002) 733–754.

[5] R.C. Toledo, C. Jared, Cutaneous adaptations to water balance in amphibians, Comp. Biochem. Physiol. 105A (1993) 593–608.

[6] P. Withers, Metabolic depression during estivation in the australian frogs, *neobatrachus* and *cyclorana*, Aust. J. Zool. 41 (5) (1993) 467–473.

[7] N.J. Hudson, M.B. Bennet, C.E. Franklin, Effect of aestivation on long bone mechanical properties in the green-striped burrowing frog, *Cyclorana alboguttata*, J. Exp. Biol. 207 (3) (2004) 475–482.

[8] N.J. Hudson, C.E. Franklin, Effect of aestivation on muscle characteristics and locomotor performance in the green-striped burrowing frog, *Cyclorana alboguttata*, J. Comp. Physiol. 172B (2) (2002) 177–182.

[9] L.L. McClanahan, R. Ruibal, V.H. Shoemaker, Rate of cocoon formation and its physiological correlates in a ceratophryd frog, Physiol. Zool. 56 (3) (1983) 430–435.

[10] F. Kobelt, K.E. Linsenmair, Adaptations of the reed frog *Hyperolius viridiflavus* (amphibia, anura, hyperoliidae) to its arid environment: VII. The heat budget of *Hyperolius viridiflavus nitidulus* and the evolution of optimized body shape, J. Comp. Physiol. 165 (2) (1995) 110–124.

[11] C.A. Navas, C. Jared, M.M. Antoniazzi, Water economy in the casque-headed tree-frog *Corythomantis greeningi* (hylidae): role of behavior, skin, and skull skin coossification, J. Zool. 257 (2002) 525–532.

[12] C. Jared, et al., Head, co-ossification, phragmosis and defence in the casque-headed tree frog *Corythomantis greeningi*, J. Zool. (2004) (In press).

[13] C. Carey, Factors affecting body temperature in toads, Oecologia 35 (1978) 179–219.

[14] J.G. Lambrinos, C.C. Kleier, Thermoregulation of juvenile andean toads (*Bufo spinulosus*) at 4300 m, J. Therm. Biol. 28 (1) (2003) 15–19.

[15] H.B. Lillywhite, P. Licht, P. Chelgren, The role of behavioral thermoregulation in the growth energetics of the toad *Bufo boreas*, Ecology 54 (1973) 375–383.

[16] R.C. Toledo, C. Jared, The calcified dermal layer in anurans, Comp. Biochem. Physiol. 104A (1993) 593–608.

[17] C.B. Jorgensen, 200 years of amphibian water economy: from robert townson to the present, Biol. Rev. Camb. Philos. Soc. 72 (2) (1997) 153–237.

[18] H. Koyama, et al., The spinal nerves innervate putative chemosensory cells in the ventral skin of desert toads, *Bufo alvarius*, Cell Tissue Res. 304 (2) (2001) 185–192.

[19] H.B. Lillywhite, et al., Integumentary structure and its relationship to wiping behaviour in the common indian tree frog, *Polypedates maculatus*, J. Zool. 243 (1997) 675–687.

[20] G. Delfino, et al., Serous cutaneous glands of argentine *Phyllomedusa wagler* 1830 (anura hylidae): secretory polymorphism and adaptive plasticity, Trop. Zool. 11 (2) (1998) 333–351.

[21] L.L. McClanahan, J.N. Stinner, V.H. Shoemaker, Skin lipids, water loss, and energy metabolism in a south american tree frog (*Phyllomedusa sauvagel*), Physiol. Zool. 51 (2) (1978) 179–187.

[22] F.H. Pough, et al., Herpetology, Prentice-Hall, New Jersey, 1998.

[23] M.P. Oconnor, C.R. Tracy, Thermoregulation by juvenile toads of *Bufo woodhousei* in the field and in the laboratory, Copeia 3 (1992) 865–876.

[24] F.L.K. Kobelt, Adaptations of the reed frog *Hyperolius viridiflavus* (amphibia, anura, hyperoliidae) to its arid environment: VI. The iridophores in the skin as radiation reflectors, J. Comp. Physiol. 162B (1992) 314–326.

[25] C.A. Navas, Implications of microhabitat selection and patterns of activity on the thermal ecology of high elevation neotropical anurans, Oecologia 108 (1996) 617–626.

[26] C.A. Navas, Metabolic physiology, locomotor performance, and thermal niche breadth in neotropical anurans, Physiol. Zool. 69 (1996) 1481–1501.

International Congress Series 1275 (2004) 306–312

www.ics-elsevier.com

Individual variation in the basal metabolism of Zebra finches *Taeniopygia guttata*: no effect of food quality during early development

Claus Bech*, Bernt Rønning, Børge Moe

Department of Biology, Norwegian University of Science and Technology, Trondheim, Norway

Abstract. We investigated the physiological background to individual variation in basal metabolic rate (BMR) in a laboratory population of a small passerine bird, the Zebra finch, *Taeniopygia guttata*. We especially explored whether food-quality during early development influenced the BMR later in life. Zebra finches were raised on two different food regimes; one ('low quality') involving only mixed seed diet, while the other ('high quality') in addition including a protein supplement and daily fresh hard-boiled eggs. The different diets were administrated to the birds only during the first 6 weeks of life. At an age of 1.5 to 2 years, and after a breeding period of their own, BMR was measured in all individuals. Food quality had a significant effect on body mass. Adult finches raised on high-quality protein-rich food were significantly heavier (2.2 g for males and 1.9 g for females) than their counterparts raised on low-quality food. Despite this, the BMR of the adult birds did not differ beyond that expected based on variation in body mass alone. Hence, the early feeding regimes, which induced a non-genetic phenotypic variability in body mass, did apparently not induce any long-term changes in body composition or in organ metabolic intensity. © 2004 Elsevier B.V. All rights reserved.

Keywords: Allometry; Basal metabolic rate; Diet quality; *Taeniopygia guttata*; Zebra finch

1. Introduction

The basal metabolic rate (BMR) represents the lowest sustainable aerobic metabolism of a resting, postabsorptive, endothermic organism at thermoneutral conditions [1]. The

---

* Corresponding author. Tel.: +47 7359 6297; fax: +47 7359 1309.
  E-mail address: claus.bech@bio.ntnu.no (C. Bech).

BMR differs greatly between endothermic organisms, both within and between species. The interspecific variation have been attributed to adaptations to either specific environmental conditions, or to certain behavioural traits of the species. In birds, for instance, a high BMR is characteristic of species living in colder climates and at higher latitudes [2–4], in species living in an aquatic environment [5] and in species with a high level of aerobic activity [6]. In contrast, low BMR is characteristic of birds living in the tropics [7,8], of birds living on islands [9], and of night-active birds [5].

Intraspecific variations in BMR may be of two types. Firstly, variation in BMR may occur between populations. Such variations usually correlate with different environments. In House finches (*Carpodacus mexicanus*), for example, those individuals living in Colorado and Michigan have a significantly higher winter-BMR compared to those individuals living in southern California, which experience much milder winters [10]. Secondly, BMR may also vary within populations. For instance, a significant repeatability of BMR, measured over two consecutive years, have been described within an arctic population of Black-legged kittiwakes (*Rissa tridactyla* [11]). Other studies have also shown BMR to be a repeatable parameter [12,13]. Hence, within populations, some individuals may be 'high-metabolic' while others may be 'low-metabolic'. The reasons to such differences in metabolic rate have hardly been studied. Some of the within-species BMR-variation may have a genetic component [14,15]. However, intraspecific variation in BMR within endothermic populations, may potentially also be attributed to variations in the physiology of the individuals caused by non-genetic factors. Such phenotypic flexibility is commonly found in living organisms [16], but it is not known whether this also would pertain to BMR. One factor which potentially could be involved in 'setting' the level of the basal metabolic rate, is the nutritional status during the early development. Both the amount and quality of food provided to avian nestlings have been shown to influence later adult body mass [17,18]. The amount of food may also influence body composition of nestlings [19,20]. Since both body mass and body composition are predictors of BMR, one could hypothesise that the level of BMR also would be influenced by early nutritional status.

In the present study, we test this possibility, by studying whether the BMR of adult Zebra finches will vary according to different nutritional status during their early growth.

2. Material and methods

The Zebra finch (*Taeniopygia guttata*) is a small finch native to the Australasia. The species will easily breed in captivity and is consequently often used in laboratory studies. We randomly assigned 15 pairs of finches to each of two large (10 m^3) walk-in aviaries. Twenty nest-boxes were placed in each aviary. These were accessible from the outside and were checked every day at around noon. All breeding birds were provided with a mixed seed diet ('Life Care'; protein-content: 10.8% of wet mass; water content: 11.7%). In one colony (low quality, LQ) this was the only food provided. In the other colony (high quality, HQ), the finches were in addition provided a commercial protein-supplement ('Eggfood Witte Molen'; protein-content: 11.3% of wet mass; water content: 9.8%) and daily fresh hard-boiled eggs (protein-content: 13.2% of wet mass; water-content: 76.4%). All types of food were provided ad libitum, as was drinking water. Ambient temperatures in the rooms with both breeding aviaries and 'holding aviaries' were kept at 24 °C and the relative humidity was kept at 40% RH. There was a light–dark regime of 12:12 h with light on at 07:00.

Breeding was recorded in both colonies from August 2001 to June 2002. All chicks produced in the two colonies were removed at an age of 6 weeks, at which time they were fully independent of their parents. After removal from the breeding colonies, they were kept in sex-specific larger holding aviaries until September 2002, when they themselves were assigned to breeding aviaries. During the 'holding period' and the subsequent breeding period, which lasted until June 2003, they all received a diet of normal 'medium' quality (NQ), consisting of the mixed seed diet and the protein-supplement. After the breeding period (in June 2003), all birds were again assigned to separate sex-specific holding aviaries and received the NQ food until September 2003, when measurements of BMR were obtained. Hence, at the time of BMR-measurements the birds were 1.5–2 years of age and the only experimental difference were in the food-quality they received during the first 6 weeks of age.

The basal metabolic rate was measured using an open-flow system. Dry air was pumped through metabolic boxes made from 1.5-l metal boxes painted flat black on the inside. Each metabolic chamber received an air flow of approximately 400 ml/min; measured accurately by a calibrated mass flowmeter (Bronkhorts). The effluent air was dried using drierite before the oxygen concentration was measured by an oxygen analyser (Servomex, two-channel analyser, type 4200). The oxygen analyser was calibrated using dry outside air (set to 20.95% oxygen) and pure stock nitrogen. Rates of oxygen consumption (VO_2) were calculated using formula 3A given by Withers [21], assuming an RQ of 0.71, and corrected for wash-out delay in the system by the method described by Niimi [22]. In this way, we obtained the instantaneous oxygen consumption rates. Birds were placed in the metabolic chamber in the evening (at about 19:00) and stayed overnight in the metabolic chamber. They were taken back to their holding aviaries at about 08:00 the next morning. An experimental set-up was constructed so that we could measure up to four birds per night. An automated valve-system switched between the four metabolic chambers, so that two chambers simultaneously were measured at a time for 26 min, interspersed between shorter periods of 4 min, during which fresh air entered the oxygen analyser. Hence, each individual was measured 26 min every hour during the night. All voltage outputs from the oxygen analyser and the mass flowmeter were stored at 30-s intervals on a datalogger (Grant Squirrel, Type 1203) and later transferred to a computer for analysis.

The lowest night-time level of VO_2, which was taken as representative of BMR, was calculated as the lowest 10-min running average of instantaneous oxygen consumption. This was usually experienced during the latter half of the night. The body mass (M_b) was measured (with an accuracy of 0.01 g) immediately before and after the experiment and a linear decrease in body mass was assumed when assessing the body mass value at the time of BMR-measurements. All measurements of BMR were conducted at an ambient temperature of 35 °C, which is within the thermoneutral zone of the Zebra finch (own unpublished results).

Before performing linear analysis on the relationship between M_b and BMR all data were log10-transformed. Linear regressions between M_b and BMR are presented as both ordinary least squares regression (OLS) as well as reduced major axes (RMA). The latter method is used because OLS might underestimate the true allometric exponent (see Pagel and Harvey [23]). The RMA-values were calculated according to Sokal and Rohlf [24]. All statistics were performed using SigmaStat ver. 3.0 (SPSS). Results are shown as mean$\pm$1 S.D.

3. Results

Food quality during the first 6 weeks of life had a distinct effect on the resultant adult body mass of Zebra finches. Hence, those individuals which were fed only seeds during early growth had an adult body mass significantly smaller that of the individuals which received a protein-rich food during early development. This was the case for both females (13.6$\pm$2.1 g for LQ-fed individuals vs. 15.5$\pm$1.1 g for HQ-fed; $t_{2,42}$=3.967, P<0.001) and for males (12.3$\pm$0.9 g for LQ-fed individuals vs. 14.5$\pm$1.5 g for HQ-fed; $t_{2,40}$=4.898, P<0.001). Within both feeding regimes, the adult body mass of the females was significantly higher than that of the males (P<0.001 for both).

In order to test for the influence of experimental group (either low-quality or high-quality food during early life) in addition to body mass and sex, which could be presumed to influence BMR, we performed a multiple linear regression with BMR (expressed as mass dependent oxygen consumption; ml O_2 h^{-1}) as the independent parameter, and group, sex and body mass as dependent parameters. Both sex and body mass were significant determinants of the variation in BMR (both P<0.001). Experimental group, however, did not contribute in explaining the BMR-variation (P=0.738). Hence, whether birds experience low- or high-quality diet during early life, will not affect their BMR later in life, despite large variation in body mass. The combined regression lines (OLS) for adults males is BMR (ml O_2 h^{-1})=10.12*$M_b^{0.504}$ (n=42, r^2=0.452, P<0.001) and for females BMR (ml O_2 h^{-1})=9.51*$M_b^{0.548}$ (n=44, r^2= 0.452, P<0.001). By using the

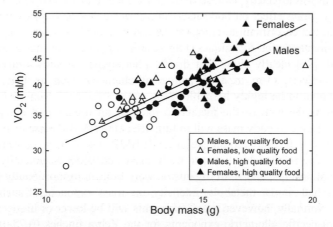

Fig. 1. Basal metabolic rate, expressed as oxygen consumption, in adult Zebra finches fed either low quality food (open symbols) or high-quality protein-rich food (filled symbols) during the first 6 weeks after hatching (circles=males, triangles=females). Regression lines (reduced major axes) are shown for males and females separately. See text for statistics.

reduced major axes method, we arrive at slightly larger exponents, the regression line being for males being BMR (ml O$_2$ h^{-1})= 5.34*$M_b^{0.749}$ and that for females BMR (ml O$_2$ h^{-1})=4.63*$M_b^{0.815}$ (Fig. 1).

4. Discussion

It is important to notice that the present study has not involved a food-deprivation experiment, since the birds in both experimental groups had free access to food at all time. Only the quality, through the protein content, were manipulated. Hence, our data are not directly comparable with the many studies showing that reduced food intake, will alter the adult morphology including body mass [18,25,26].

Our finding that food quality during early development significantly influences the adult body mass concur with the results of Boag [17] and Birkhead et al. [27] also on Zebra finches. Boag [17] likewise manipulated the protein-content of the diet given to Zebra finch nestlings and found that both the growth rate as well as the adult body mass was higher when chicks were fed high-protein food than when fed a low-protein diet. The body mass difference was found to be evident for up to one year of age. Hence, the present study supplements that of Boag [17] in that we found the diet-induced body mass difference to be present up to an age of 2 years. Other studies, in which manipulation of food quality have been performed have produced mixed results. Hochachka and Smith [28] supplemented the food of free-living Song Sparrows (*Melospiza melodia*), and in this way manipulated the food-quality of the nestlings. They also found an immediate positive effect on the growth rate in the food-supplemented nestlings. However, when measured at an age of between 56 to 108 days, there was no difference in body mass between the experimental groups. A similar lack of long-term effect on adult body mass was also reported by Ohlsson and Smith [29] after manipulation of the protein-content of the diet fed to chicks of the Ring-necked pheasants (*Phasianus colchicus*) (although in this species the tarsus length was affected). We can offer no explanation as to why food quality during early life has a strong effect on body mass in Zebra finches and apparently not in other species. It is, however, difficult to compare the results directly because they involve quite different food-manipulation techniques. Our results together with that of Boag [17] and Birkhead et al. [27] clearly show that drastic phenotypic variation can be induced by environmental effects, even in a physiological character such as body mass which generally is known to be highly heritable [30].

Since BMR is the sum of the metabolic rates of all organs and components of an organism, any change in body mass will in turn affect the BMR. Consequently, correlative relationships between body composition and BMR have been repeatably reported [19,20,31–34]. The relationship between body mass and BMR is generally described by exponential relationships, and if all organisms were built in proportionally the same way and the organs had similar metabolic intensity, the mass exponent of such relationships would be 1.0. Normally, however, mass exponents will be lower or higher than 1.0. Our finding of intraspecific allometric exponents for the Zebra finches (0.75–0.82 for RMA estimates and 0.50–0.55 for OLS estimates) is strikingly similar to what is normally found for interspecific relationships in birds [5]. In contrast, our exponents are below that normally reported for intraspecific BMR–body mass relationships in birds, where exponents well above 1.0 generally are reported (see Kvist and Lindström [35]). It is difficult to ascertain exactly why this is so, except that in contrast to most other bird species, high body mass in Zebra finches is apparently not paralleled by disproportionally larger organs having a high metabolic intensity, which have been the usual explanation for allometric exponents above 1.0. On the contrary, high body mass in Zebra finches must be paralleled by either disproportional smaller high-metabolic organs or their organs must have lower metabolic intensity. One explanation could be that heavier individuals are carrying larger amounts of fat, which has little metabolic activity compared to most other internal organs. Lindström and Rosén [36] recently showed that the accumulation of fat carried a high metabolic cost in Greenfinches (*Carduelis chloris*). However, their experiments were carried out over a very short time span (days) where such an immediate 'cost' would be eminent. Presumably, there are fewer metabolic costs involved when fat is permanently stored as in heavier vs. lighter individuals.

Irrespective of the reason for the low intraspecific allometric exponent in the Zebra finches, our study has demonstrated that despite the significant effect on body mass incurred by manipulation of the food-quality during the nestling stage, the BMR of the resultant adult birds did not differ beyond that expected based on variation in body mass alone. Hence, the early feeding regimes have apparently not induced any long-term changes in body composition or in organ metabolic intensity. Our results imply that the non-genetic phenotypic variability in body mass, which we have induced during nestling development by different feeding regimes, will not result in disproportional organ masses inducing different metabolic rates.

Acknowledgements

We thank Odd Arne Indset and Bjørn Simensen for taking daily care of our birds. The study was supported by grants from the Norwegian Science Research Council (#138698/432 and #159584/V40).

References

[1] S. Brody, Bioenergetics and Growth, Reinhold, New York, 1945.
[2] H.I. Ellis, Energetics of free-ranging seabirds, in: G.C. Whittow, H. Rahn (Eds.), Avian Energetics, Plenum Press, New York, 1984, pp. 203–234.
[3] G.W Gabrielsen, F. Mehlum, H.E. Karlsen, Thermoregulation in four species of arctic seabirds, J. Comp. Physiol. 157 (1988) 703–708.
[4] D.M. Bryant, R.W. Furness, Basal metabolic rates of north Atlantic seabirds, Ibis 137 (1995) 219–226.
[5] P.M. Bennett, P.H. Harvey, Active and resting metabolism in birds: allometry, phylogeny and ecology, J. Zool. (Lond.) 213 (1987) 327–363.
[6] M. Kersten, T. Piersma, High levels of energy expenditure in shorebirds; metabolic adaptations to an energetically expensive way of life, Ardea 75 (1987) 175–187.
[7] C.J. Hails, The metabolic rate of tropical birds, Condor 85 (1983) 61–65.
[8] T.N. Pettit, H.I. Ellis, G.C. Whittow, Basal metabolic rate in tropical seabirds, Auk 102 (1985) 172–174.
[9] B.K. Mcnab, Energy conservation and the evolution of flightlessness in birds, Am. Nat. 144 (1994) 628–642.
[10] T.L. Root, T.P. O'Connor, W.R. Dawson, Standard metabolic level and insulatory characteristics of eastern House finches, *Carpodacus mexicanus* (Müller), Physiol. Zool. 64 (1991) 1279–1295.

[11] C. Bech, I. Langseth, G.W. Gabrielsen, Repeatability of basal metabolism of breeding female kittiwakes *Rissa tridactyla*, Proc. R. Soc. Lond., B 266 (1999) 2161–2167.

[12] P. Horak, et al., Repeatability of condition indices in captive greenfinches (*Carduelis chloris*), Can. J. Zool. 80 (2002) 636–643.

[13] F. Vézina, D.W. Thomas, Social status does not affect resting metabolic rate in wintering dark-eyed Junco (*Junco hyemalis*), Physiol. Biochem. Zool. 73 (2000) 231–236.

[14] M. Wikelski, et al., Slow pace of life in tropical sedentary birds: a common-garden experiment on four stonechat population from different latitudes, Proc. R. Soc. Lond., B 270 (2003) 2383–2388.

[15] R.W. Furness, It's in the genes, Nature 425 (2003) 779–780.

[16] T. Piersma, J. Drent, Phenotypic flexibility and the evolution of organismal design, Trends Ecol. Evol. 18 (2003) 228–233.

[17] P.T. Boag, Effects of nestling diet on growth and adult size of Zebra finches (*Poephila guttata*), Auk 104 (1987) 155–166.

[18] W.A. Searcy, S. Peters, S. Nowicki, Effects of early nutrition on growth rate and adult size in song sparrows *Melospiza melodia*, J. Avian Biol. 35 (2004) 269–279.

[19] B. Moe, et al., Developmental plasticity of physiology and morphology in diet-restricted European Shag nestlings (*Phalacrocorax aristotelis*), J. Exp. Biol. 207 (2004) (in press).

[20] B. Moe, E. Stølevik, C. Bech, Ducklings exhibit substantial energy-saving mechanisms as a response to short-term food shortage, Physiol. Biochem. Zool. 78 (2005) (in press).

[21] P.C. Withers, Measurements of VO_2, VCO_2 and evaporative water loss with a flow-through mask, J. Appl. Physiol. 42 (1977) 120–123.

[22] A.J. Niimi, Lag adjustment between estimated and actual physiological responses conducted in flow-through systems, J. Fish. Res. Board Can. 35 (1978) 1265–1269.

[23] M.D. Pagel, P.H. Harvey, The taxon-level problem in the evolution of mammalian brain size: facts and artifacts, Am. Nat. 132 (1988) 344–359.

[24] R.R. Sokal, F.J. Rohlf, Biometry, 3rd ed., Freeman, New York, 1995.

[25] J. Lindström, Early development and fitness in birds and mammals, Trends Ecol. Evol. 14 (1999) 343–348.

[26] N.B. Metcalfe, P. Monaghan, Compensation for a bad start: grow now pay later? Trends Ecol. Evol. 16 (2001) 254–260.

[27] T.R. Birkhead, F. Fletcher, E.J. Pellatt, Nestling diet, secondary sexual traits and fitness in the Zebra finch, Proc. R. Soc. Lond., B 266 (1999) 385–390.

[28] W. Hochachka, J.N.M. Smith, Determinants and consequences of nestling condition in song sparrows, J. Anim. Ecol. 60 (1991) 995–1008.

[29] T. Ohlsson, H.G. Smith, Early nutrition causes persistent effects on pheasant morphology, Physiol. Biochem. Zool. 74 (2001) 212–218.

[30] A.J. Van Noordwijk, H.L. Marks, Genetic aspects of growth, in: J.M. Starch, R.E. Ricklefs (Eds.), Avian Growth and Development, Oxford University Press, New York, 1998, pp. 305–323.

[31] S. Daan, D. Masman, A. Groenewold, Avian basal metabolic rates: their association with body composition and energy expenditure in nature, Am. J. Physiol. 259 (1990) R333–R340.

[32] T. Piersma, et al., Variability in basal metabolic rate of a long-distance migrant shorebird (Red Knot, *Calidris canutus*) reflects shifts in organ sizes, Physiol. Zool. 69 (1996) 191–217.

[33] M.A. Chappell, C. Bech, W.A. Buttemer, The relationship of central and peripheral organ masses to aerobic performance variation in house sparrows, J. Exp. Biol. 202 (1999) 2269–2279.

[34] I. Langseth, et al., Flexibility of basal metabolic rate in arctic breeding kittiwakes (*Rissa tridactyla*), in: G. Heldmaier, M. Klingenspor (Eds.), Life in the Cold, Springer-Verlag, Heidelberg, 2000, pp. 471–477.

[35] A. Kvist, Å. Lindström, Basal metabolic rate in migratory waders: intra-individual, intraspecific, interspecific and seasonal variation, Funct. Ecol. 15 (2001) 465–473.

[36] Å. Lindström, M. Rosén, The cost of avian winter stores: intra-individual variation in basal metabolic rate of a wintering passerine, the greenfinch *Carduelis chloris*, Avian Sci. 2 (2002) 139–143.

International Congress Series 1275 (2004) 313–320

ELSEVIER

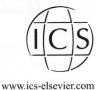

www.ics-elsevier.com

Physiological limitations of dietary specialization in herbivorous woodrats (*Neotoma* spp.)

Jennifer S. Sorensen[a,*], M. Denise Dearing[b]

[a]*School of Pharmacy, University of Tasmania, Sandy Bay, TAS, 7005, Australia*
[b]*Department of Biology, University of Utah, USA*

Abstract. For nearly three decades, a fundamental objective in the study of plant–herbivore interactions has been to understand why the consumption of a single plant species is rare in mammals, as only a handful of mammalian herbivores (<1%) are dietary specialists. Here, we provide an overview of various factors that may play a role in limiting dietary specialization. We review the energetic consequences of ingesting PSMs and the physiological tradeoffs of specialization in a juniper specialist, *Neotoma stephensi*, and generalist, *N. albigula*, woodrat. In general, the energy budgets of specialist and generalist woodrats were negatively impacted by the intake of PSMs from juniper and novel PSMs. However, juniper specialists minimized the energetic costs associated with the intake of juniper through greater energy intake and lower energy expenditure than generalists and thus had more energy for other energy-dependent activities when consuming a juniper diet. Despite the high capacity to consume juniper, juniper specialists experienced a decreased ability to consume novel PSMs, suggesting a dietary trade-off associated with specialization. These data indicate that the energetic consequences of consuming PSMs and the dietary trade-offs associated with specialization may constrain dietary specialization in herbivorous woodrats. Identifying these factors and their role in limiting and/or facilitating dietary specialization in woodrats has provided a better understanding of the foraging ecology, physiology and evolution of mammalian herbivores in general. © 2004 Published by Elsevier B.V.

Keywords: Dietary specialization; Energy budget; *Neotoma*; Plant secondary metabolite; Trade-offs

1. Background

A fundamental objective in the study of plant–herbivore interactions has been to identify factors that limit dietary specialization in mammalian herbivores. The

* Corresponding author. Tel.: +61 3 6226 2232; fax: +61 3 6226 2870.
E-mail address: jennifer.sorensen@anu.edu.au (J.S. Sorensen).

0531-5131/ © 2004 Published by Elsevier B.V.
doi:10.1016/j.ics.2004.08.070

consumption of a single plant species is rare in mammals, as only a handful of mammalian herbivores (<1%) are dietary specialists [1]. One explanation for the paucity of mammalian specialists is that mammals are limited by the quality and quantity of secondary metabolites in plants [2–5]. It is theorized that dietary specialization in mammals is limited by the physiological challenges associated with the high quantities of a limited spectrum of secondary metabolites ingested in a diet of a single plant species. The few specialists that exist are predicted to have evolved mechanisms that overcome the physiological challenges of consuming a diet of a single plant species [5]. However, the mechanisms that facilitate dietary specialization may result in an evolutionary and/or ecological trade-off [6]. Specifically, specialists may be limited in the range of secondary metabolites they can ingest, thus restricting the habitats suitable for colonization by specialists. In the subsequent sections, we review the energetic consequences of ingesting plant secondary metabolites (PSMs), mechanisms that compensate for costs and physiological tradeoffs of specialization in a juniper specialist, *Neotoma stephensi*, and generalist, *N. albigula*, woodrat. These *Neotoma* species are an ideal pair of mammalian herbivores to synthesize the constraints of PSM ingestion because they are similar in body size, share habitats, have the same ecological and evolutionary experience with many PSMs (including those in juniper) and have been well studied with respect to their foraging behavior in the field and laboratory. Moreover, recent comparative work on these species demonstrated marked differences in their energetic and physiological capacities to handle various PSMs. Descriptions of these species, their diets, experimental approach, data analysis and results that are summarized here are found in detail in Sorensen et al. [7,8].

2. Energetic consequences of PSM intake

One major physiological challenge for mammalian herbivores is the energetic cost associated with the intake of PSMs. PSMs impinge on energy availability by diluting food energy [9,10], decreasing energy absorption [11–14], increasing the excretion of endogenous energy [15–19] and increasing energy expenditure [20–22]. The energetic consequences of processing both naturally consumed and novel PSMs are substantial in woodrats. In most cases, woodrats decreased intake (dry matter/day, Fig. 1) and, therefore, energy intake (Fig. 2) when consuming PSMs compared to diets without PSMs. In addition to reduced energy intake, woodrats also increased energy excretion (Fig. 2), resulting in decreased efficiency of energy metabolism. Energy lost in the urine alone represented up to 35% of basal metabolism in woodrats. This amount is on par with costs of reproduction and thermoregulation (10% and 37% of metabolism, respectively) in golden-mantled ground squirrels [23] and growth (36% metabolism) in cotton rats [24]. The intake of PSMs typically resulted in decreased apparent metabolizable energy (AMEI, kJ/day=ingested energy not excreted in urine and feces, Fig. 1).

Moreover, the energetic costs associated with the intake of PSMs can negatively impact energy available for critical activities (Figs. 1, 2). The intake of PSMs significantly compromised energy available for energy dependent activities and body mass. Woodrats consuming PSMs reduced the distance ran on running wheels and time spent running by up to 53% [7,8]. In most cases, the intake of PSMs also compromised

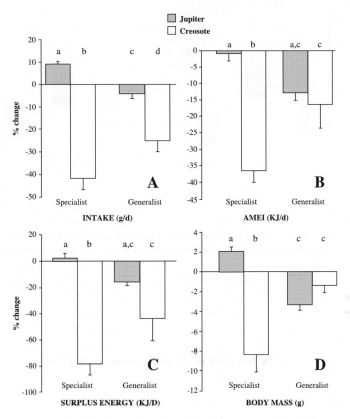

Fig. 1. Weekly percent change in (A) intake (g dry matter/day), (B) apparent metabolizable energy intake (AMEI, kJ/day=Energy intake (kJ/day)−exerted in feces (kJ/day) and urine (kJ/day)), (C) surplus energy (kJ/day=AMEI−energy spent on basal metabolic rate and voluntary wheel running) and (D) body mass for specialists and generalists on juniper and creosote diets compared to control diets. Different letters represent significant differences between means using Tukey's Honestly Significant Differences (hsd) procedure [41]. Bars are ± standard errors. Modified from Sorensen et al. [7,8].

surplus energy (i.e., ingested energy not lost in urine or feces or expended on metabolism or locomotion) needed for reproduction, thermoregulation, immunocompetency, etc. In addition, woodrats typically responded to reduced energy availability by catabolizing energy stores as indicated by loss in body mass when consuming PSMs (Fig. 1). These results highlight the substantial energetic consequence ingested PSMs can have on the overall energy budget and therefore fitness of mammalian herbivores.

3. Compensation for costs of ingested PSMs

Because energy is a limited resource, the few specialists that exist are predicted to evolve mechanisms that minimize the cost of processing PSMs and maximize energy availability. Consistent with this hypothesis, juniper specialists maintained higher surplus energy on juniper than generalists (Fig. 2). There are several factors that can contribute to maximizing surplus energy. Some specialist herbivores rely on inexpensive detoxification

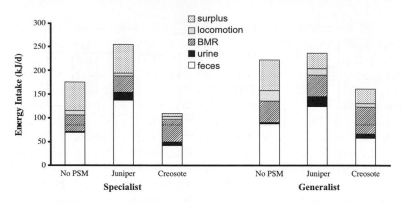

Fig. 2. Energy intake partitioned into energy exerted in feces and urine, expended on basal metabolic rate (BMR) and voluntary wheel running (locomotion) and surplus energy that could be available for reproduction, thermoregulation, immunocompetency, etc. Values are for specialists and generalists fed diets without PSMs and containing PSMs from juniper (*Juniperus monosperma*) or creosote (*Larrea tridentate*). Modified from Sorensen et al. [7,8].

pathways, such as oxidation, to a greater extent than expensive pathways, such as glucuronidation [25]. Glucuronidation results in the excretion of detoxification metabolites conjugated to glucuronic acid, a derivative of endogenous glucose. In woodrats, glucuronic acid comprised up to 12% of the urinary energy excreted on juniper diets, compared to 3% on control diets. Although both specialists and generalists increased glucuronic acid production on juniper diets, generalists excreted nearly twice the glucuronic acid per unit energy intake compared to specialists [7]. These data suggest that specialists rely on inexpensive detoxification pathways, whereas generalists utilize more expensive pathways such as glucuronidation. Although glucuronidation is one of many expensive detoxification pathways [26], reduced glucuronidation may be one physiological mechanisms that contributes to lowering the costs of processing toxins in specialists.

Increased food intake is an additional strategy that can maximize surplus energy [27–29]. However, for mammalian herbivores, greater intake of a single plant species also results in greater intake of PSMs. Compensatory feeding must therefore incorporate mechanisms that minimize the accumulation of PSMs in the body as intake of PSMs increase. Furthermore, it is predicted that dietary specialists should have adaptations for rapid elimination of PSMs and that these mechanisms will facilitate high levels of intake of PSMs from a single plant species [4,5]. In support, juniper specialists absorbed across the gut a lower proportion of ingested alpha-pinene, a predominant PSM in juniper, resulting in higher quantities of alpha-pinene excreted unchanged in the feces than generalists [30]. An enhanced capacity to eliminate ingested alpha-pinene is associated with lower blood levels of alpha-pinene per unit ingested and higher intake of juniper [31]. These data suggest that although compensatory feeding can maximize surplus energy, this strategy may be restricted to dietary specialists that possess mechanisms that effectively eliminate ingested PSMs.

Juniper specialists can further maximize energy availability by minimizing energy expenditure. Overall, specialists expended less energy on basal metabolic rate (BMR) and engaged in less locomotor activity than generalists, regardless of diet or PSM ingested

(Fig. 2, [7,8]). In addition, specialists tended to decrease BMR even further when consuming juniper diet. Data are consistent with the theory that specialization, particularly specialization on diets high in PSMs, favors reduced energy expenditure [32–34]. Data also support previous work that animals reduce metabolic rates and locomotion when costs of ingesting PSMs are high [33–36]. We propose that low BMR and PSM induced reductions in BMR in dietary specialists may be an energy compensation strategy to deal with the costs of PSM intake. Although reduced BMR and locomotor activity may compensate for energetic costs of PSM intake, there may be constraints on the ecological benefits of such a strategy. For example, low metabolism is often associated with reduced natal growth rates and fecundity in mammals [34]. Clearly, the fitness advantages and disadvantages of reduced expenditure associated with PSM intake and the role this plays in limiting dietary specialization deserve further investigation.

4. Dietary tradeoffs of specialization

Dietary tradeoffs of specialization may also limit the occurrence of mammals consuming a single species of plant. In general, specialization may be limited because specialists trade-off the ability to consume large quantities of a single plant for a reduced ability to consume novel plants [6]. The mechanisms responsible for reducing costs and enhancing excretion of secondary metabolites in the plants frequently consumed by specialists may be mechanistically and/or energetically less efficient at eliminating PSMs from novel plants. These predictions were tested by comparing the performance of juniper specialists fed juniper versus a novel plant, creosote, relative to the performance of generalists on the same diets. The phenolic resin from creosote bush (*Larrea tridentata*) contained PSMs that are novel to both specialists and generalists. Although the complete chemical profile of juniper, creosote and other plants consumed by specialists and generalists is unknown, there is strong evidence that specialists and generalists have not had evolutionary or ecological experience with the major PSMs in creosote [37–40].

The prediction that physiological trade-offs are associated with specialization was supported by studies on herbivorous woodrats. Juniper specialists were more energetically impacted by the intake of PSMs in creosote, a novel plant species, than juniper and were impacted to a greater extent than generalists (Figs. 1, 2, [8]). Juniper specialists reduced intake by 42%, AMEI by 36%, surplus energy by 79% and body mass by 8% when consuming creosote PSMs compared to diets lacking PSMs. In contrast, these parameter were not affected and often increased when specialists consumed juniper. In addition, creosote negatively impacted intake, AMEI, surplus energy and mass to a greater extent in specialists than generalists. Although generalists did reduce intake on creosote and did so to a greater degree than on juniper, reductions in AMEI, surplus energy and body mass were similar on both juniper and creosote diets. These data suggest that two distinctly different plants, one naturally consumed, one novel, each with different PSM profiles, have a similar negative effect on the performance of generalists. Data also suggest a dietary trade-off of specialization in mammalian herbivores in that juniper specialists trade-off their ability to perform well on juniper for a reduced ability to consume PSMs from a novel plant. A lower capacity to handle a wide range of plants may restrict specialization to a limited number of habitats where their preferred plant species is abundant. Furthermore, if specialists lack the capacity to exploit novel plant species they may be selected against if plant availability fluctuates.

5. Conclusion

Identifying the factors that limit and/or facilitate dietary specialization is essential to understanding the foraging ecology, distribution, physiology and evolution of mammalian herbivores. This review suggests that the energetic costs associated with consuming high quantities of a single plant species are significant and can negatively impact energy budgets. To overcome this energetic insult, mammalian herbivores may require physiological and behavioral mechanisms that mitigate the costs of processing PSMs or minimize energy expenditure. Specialization may therefore be limited by not only the costs of consuming high levels of PSMs, but also the capacity to eliminate PSMs and the consequences of reduced expenditure. In addition, once mammalian herbivores evolve to minimize costs of consuming a single plant species, they may face a dietary "dead-end", in that they have a reduced ability to consume novel species of plants. A limited ability to consume a variety of plants may make specialists less resilient to changes in their wild plant availability and restrict distributions to specific habitats. Although conclusions drawn here are restricted to a single pair of specialist and generalist mammalian herbivores and a single novel plant, this review provides a detailed overview of important factors that may limit dietary specialization in herbivorous woodrats. These data provide initial evidence that PSMs influence more than just the foraging behavior of mammalian herbivores and may also play a significant role in the physiology and evolutionary success of mammalian herbivores. However, it is essential to further test the impact of PSMs on energy budgets and the physiological tradeoffs of specialization using additional herbivores and species of plants to apply these findings to the specialists–generalist paradigm in general.

Acknowledgments

We thank B. Hudson and employees of Wupatki National Monument Visitor Center for assistance and accommodations during our trapping sessions. H. Baldwin, R. Boyle, D. Green, C. Heidelberger and S. O'Grady assisted in collecting woodrats in the field. Y. Al-Sheikh, E. van Dijk, J. Grose, E. Heward, A. Knudson, E. McLachlan, S. Rogers, L. Santos, C.A. Turnbull, A. Walters and M.Wong assisted in experimental procedures and animal husbandry and were in part supported by the University of Utah Biology Undergraduate Research Program and NSF Research Experience for Undergraduates. Research was supported by NSF IBN-0079865 and 0236402, Sigma Xi Grant-in-Aid of Research, American Society of Mammalogists Grant-in-Aid of Research and the University of Utah Graduate School Research Fellowship.

References

[1] W.J. Freeland, Plant secondary metabolites. Biochemical evolution with herbivores, in: R. Palo, C.T. Robbins (Eds.), Plant Defenses Against Mammalian Herbivory, CRC Press, Boca Raton, 1991, pp. 61–82.

[2] M.D. Dearing, A.M. Mangione, W.H. Karasov, Diet breadth of mammalian herbivores: tests of the nutrient constraints and detoxification–limitations hypotheses, Oecologia 123 (2000) 397–405.

[3] M.D. Dearing, S.J. Cork, The role of detoxification of plant secondary compounds on diet breadth in mammalian herbivores, J. Chem. Ecol. 25 (1999) 1205–1220.

[4] W.J. Foley, G.R. Iason, C. McArthur, Role of plant secondary metabolites in the nutritional ecology of mammalian herbivores: how far have we come in 25 years? in: J.G. Jung, G.C.J. Faley (Eds.), Nutritional Ecology of Herbivores: Proceedings of the 5th International Symposium of the Nutrition of Herbivores, American Society of Animal Sciences, Savoy, IL, 1999, pp. 131–209.

[5] W.J. Freeland, D.H. Janzen, Strategies in herbivory by mammals: the role of plant secondary compounds, Am. Nat. 108 (1974) 269–289.

[6] D.J. Futuyma, G. Moreno, The evolution of ecological specialization, Ann. Rev. Ecolog. Syst. 19 (1988) 207–233.

[7] J.S. Sorensen, J.D. McLister, M.D. Dearing. Plant secondary metabolites compromise the energy budgets of specialist and generalist mammalian herbivores. Ecol., in press.

[8] J.S. Sorensen, J.D. McLister, M.D. Dearing. Novel plant secondary metabolites impact dietary specialists more than generalists (*Neotoma spp*). Ecol., in press.

[9] W.J. Foley, C. McArthur, The effects and costs of allelochemicals for mammalian herbivores: an ecological perspective, in: D.J. Chivers, P. Langer (Eds.), The Digestive System in Mammals: Food, Form and Function, Cambridge Univ. Press, Cambridge, 1994, pp. 370–391.

[10] C.G. Guglielmo, W.K. Karasov, Nutritional costs of plant secondary metabolite explain selective foraging by ruffed grouse, Ecology 77 (1996) 1103–1115.

[11] F. Bozinovic, F.F. Novoa, P. Sabat, Feeding and digesting fiber and tannins by an herbivorous rodent, *Octodon degus* (Rodentia: Caviomorpha), Comp. Biochem. Physiol. 118A (1997) 625–630.

[12] C.T. Robbins, et al., Variation in mammalian physiological responses to a condensed tannin and its ecological implications, J. Mammal. 72 (1991) 480–486.

[13] L. Silverstein, B.G. Swanson, D. MOffett, Procyanldln from black beans (*Phaseolus vulgaris*) inhibits nutrient and electrolyte absorption in isolated rat ileum and induces secretion of chloride ion, J. Nutr. 126 (1996) 1688–1695.

[14] J. Song, et al., Flavonoid inhibition of sodium-dependent vitamin C transporter 1 (SVCT1) and glucose transporter isoform 2 (GLUT2), intestinal transporters for vitamin C and Glucose, J. Biol. Chem. 277 (2002) 15252–15260.

[15] S.J. Cork, Foliage of *Eucalyptus punctata* and the maintenance nitrogen requirements of koalas, *Phascolarctos cinereus*, Aust. J. Zool. 34 (1986) 17–23.

[16] J.A. Dash, Effect of dietary terpenes on glucuronic acid excretion and ascorbic acid turnover in the brushtail possum (*trichosurus vulpecula*), Comp. Biochem. Physiol. 89B (1988) 221–226.

[17] W.J. Foley, Nitrogen and energy retention and acid-base status in the common ringtail possum, Physiol. Zool. 65 (1992) 403–421.

[18] R.L. Lindroth, G.O. Batzli, Plant phenolics as chemical defenses: effects of natural phenolics on survival and growth of prairie voles (*Microtus ochrogaster*), J. Chem. Ecol. 10 (1984) 229–244.

[19] A.M. Mangione, M.D. Dearing, W.H. Karasov, Detoxification in relation to toxin tolerance in desert woodrats eating creosote bush, J. Chem. Ecol. 27 (2001) 2559–2578.

[20] F. Bozinovic, F.F. Novoa, Metabolic costs of rodents feeding on plant chemical defenses: a comparison between an herbivore and an omnivore, Comp. Biochem. Physiol. 117A (1997) 511–514.

[21] G.R. Iason, A.H. Murray, The energy costs of ingestion of naturally occurring nontannin plant phenolics by sheep, Physiol. Zool. 69 (1996) 532–546.

[22] D.W. Thomas, C. Samson, J. Bergeron, Metabolic costs associated with the ingestion of plant phenolics by *Microtus pennsylvanicus*, J. Mammal. 69 (1988) 512–515.

[23] G.J. Kenagy, S.M. Sharbaugh, K.A. Nagy, Annual cycle of energy and time expenditure in a golden-mantled ground squirrel population, Oecologia 78 (1989) 269–282.

[24] T.L. Derting, Metabolism and food availability as regulators of production in juvenile cotton rats, Ecology 70 (1989) 587–595.

[25] R. Boyle, et al., Comparative metabolism of dietary terpene, p-cymene, in generalist and specialist folivorous marsupials, J. Chem. Ecol. 25 (1999) 2109–2127.

[26] L. Casarett, et al., Casarett and Doull's Toxicology: The Basic Science of Poisons, 5th ed., McGraw-Hill, New York, 1996.

[27] K.A. Hammond, B.A. Wunder, The role of diet quality and energy need in the nutritional ecology of a small herbivore, *microtus ochrogaster*, Physiol. Zool. 64 (1991) 541–567.

[28] J.R. Speakman, J. McQueenie, Limits to sustainable metabolic rate: the link between food intake, BMR, and morphology in reproducing mice (*Mus musculus*), Physiol. Zool. 69 (1996) 746–769.

[29] M. Young Owl, G.O. Batzli, The integrated processing response of voles to fibre content of natural diets, Funct. Ecol. 12 (1998) 4–13.

[30] J.S. Sorensen, C.A. Turnbull, M.D. Dearing, A specialist herbivore (*Neotoma stephensi*) absorbs fewer plant toxins than a generalist (*Neotoma albigula*), Physiol. Biochem. Zool. 77 (2004) 139–148.

[31] J.S. Sorensen, M.D. Dearing, Elimination of plant toxins: an explanation for dietary specialization in mammalian herbivores, Oecologia 134 (2003) 88–94.

[32] R. Degabriele, T.J. Dawson, Metabolism and heat balance in an arboreal marsupial, the koala (*phascolarctos cinereus*), J. Comp. Physiol. 134 (1979) 293–301.

[33] B.K. McNab, Energy conservation in a tree-kangaroo (*Dendrolagus matschiei*) and the red panda (*Ailurus fulgens*), Physiol. Zool. 61 (1988) 280–292.

[34] B.K. McNab, in: B.K. McNab (Ed.), The Physiological Ecology of Vertebrates: A View From Energetics, Cornell University Press, Ithaca, 2002, pp. 306–389.

[35] G.L. Dasilva, The western black-and-white colobus as a low-energy strategist: activity budgets, energy expenditure and energy intake, J. Anim. Ecol. 61 (1992) 79–91.

[36] R. Boyle, M.D. Dearing, Ingestion of juniper foliage reduces metabolic rates in woodrat (*Neotoma*) herbivores, Physiol. Biochem. Zool. 106 (2003) 151–158.

[37] K.P. Dial, C.J. Czaplewski, Do packrat middens accurately represent the animals' environment or diet? The Woodhouse Mesa study, in: J.L. Bentacourt, T.R. Ven Devender, P.S. Martin (Eds.), Fossil Packrat Middins: The Last 40,000 Years of Biotic Change in the Arid West, The University of Arizona Press, Tuscon, 1990, pp. 43–58.

[38] K.P. Dial, Three sympatric species of *Neotoma*: dietary specialization and coexistence, Oecologia 76 (1988) 531–537.

[39] R.P. Adams, et al., The south-western USA and northern Mexico one-seeded junipers: their volatile oils and evolution, Biochem. Syst. Ecol. 9 (1981) 93–96.

[40] T.J. Mabry, J.E. Gill, Sesquiterpene lactones and other terpenoids, in: G.A. Rosenthal, D.H. Janzen (Eds.), Herbivores: Their Interaction With Secondary Plant Metabolites, Academic Press, New York, 1979, pp. 501–537.

[41] J.H. Zar, Biostatistical Analysis, second ed., Prentice Hall, Englewood Cliffs, NJ, 1984.

International Congress Series 1275 (2004) 321–326

ELSEVIER

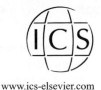

www.ics-elsevier.com

Allocation of food gains to storage versus growth in a variable environment

N. Owen-Smith*

Centre for African Ecology, School of Animal, Plant and Environmental Sciences, University of the Witwatersrand, Wits 2050, South Africa

Abstract. I address physiological connections between foraging behavior and population dynamics. How should young animals apportion the biomass gained from food consumed while foraging between growing fatter and growing bigger? Fat reserves aid survival through adverse periods, while growing faster helps animals reach reproductive size sooner. A dynamic state-dependent model enabled the optimal allocation of surplus metabolites in seasonally variable but otherwise stochastic environments to be established, with large mammalian herbivores in mind. Basic assumptions included the form of the fat-dependent and size-dependent survival functions, i.e. the state-dependence of fitness. Findings suggest that animals should store as little fat as needed as late as possible, but with the minimum need elevated by greater environmental uncertainty. Tradeoffs in allocation between growth and storage could explain why survival rates for immature animals are necessarily more variable than those of adults among large mammalian herbivores. The simple model could be expanded to establish the optimal age at first reproduction, the appropriate reproductive allocation at different ages, and tradeoffs between the metabolic costs of food processing and longevity. © 2004 Elsevier B.V. All rights reserved.

Keywords: Dynamic optimization; Fat reserves; Large herbivores; Life history; Resource allocation

1. Introduction

In this paper, I address the physiological connections between foraging behavior and population dynamics. Having foraged successfully and gained more energy and material nutrients than needed for immediate metabolic requirements, what should animals do with the surplus? Grow fatter, grow bigger, or grow babies? What are the consequences of these

---

* Tel.: +27 11 717 6454; fax: +27 11 403 1429.
E-mail address: norman@gecko.biol.wits.ac.za.

0531-5131/ © 2004 Elsevier B.V. All rights reserved.
doi:10.1016/j.ics.2004.08.079

allocations for survival chances, and reproductive success? These questions relate to the strategic issue of resource allocation to improve evolutionary fitness. But fitness defined in terms of changes in gene frequencies over generations is remote from the time frame over which physiology changes in individual organisms. How can we link physiological adaptation (or acclimation) with genetic persistence over evolutionary time? What is the appropriate proxy currency for coupling foraging success to evolutionary success? These are some of the issues I will address.

If environments remained constant, animals would have little need to store energy reserves in the form of body fat. However, animals living in seasonal environments experience times of the year when the maximum resource gains from the environment are inadequate to support nutritional requirements, with the severity of such situations varying somewhat from year to year. Thus there are periods when, rather than growing, animals lose body mass due to metabolic shortfalls, and if this loss progresses too far animals perish from starvation. To circumvent this, many animals store reserves in the form of body fat to bridge the lean period. For young, potentially growing animals, resources allocated to storage are at the expense of growth. For fully grown adults, reproductive investment rather than individual growth is traded against storage, although later the body reserves may support elevated reproductive requirements. The animals I have in mind are large mammalian herbivores, with determinate growth to some maximum body size.

How much of the surplus resources gained while foraging during the benign time of the year should be diverted to body fat, at the expense of growth? Storing as much as possible is not the best solution if there are costs to acquiring and carrying this fat. Apart from the energetic cost of carrying the additional body mass, fatter animals are likely to be less adept at escaping predators. For example, fatter birds have been shown to be slower in takeoff, and thus more likely to be grabbed when a hawk swoops [1].

Strategic "decisions" concerning resource allocation must take into account temporal variability over the course of the annual seasonal cycle, as well as uncertainty about the conditions experienced in any particular year. They must also accommodate changing stage in the life history from birth through to maturity. This requires a dynamic state-variable approach to optimization analysis.

2. Approach

Specifically, I employed stochastic dynamic programming (SDP), as outlined by Mangel and Clark [2] and Clark and Mangel [3]. At the core of the approach is a "fitness function", defining the future prospects of survival and reproduction as a function of the current state of the animal, as defined by e.g. its body size and fat reserves. The optimal solution requires maximizing this fitness function at every stage over some time horizon, dependent on the state the animal is in at that time and the result of the actions adopted from among those possible. This leads to the expected state at the next time step. In a stochastically uncertain environment, the analysis must consider all potential states that the animal could be in, as a result of chance outcomes from among the range of possibilities. The computational programming approach expedites the solution by dividing time into discrete steps, and states into discrete categories. The trick, as in all forms of dynamic optimization, is to work backwards in time from some optimal end state towards the beginning of the time period covered. The fitness function, defined most simply as probability of survival, is simply the product of the survival chances at each time step, which must be maximized through appropriate actions.

I will restrict consideration to the simplest choice, allocation to growth versus storage, avoiding the complications that arise when reproduction is considered as a third option. The state consequences entail changes in lean body size versus fat stores. Fitness increases with increasing fat reserves over some range, but then declines when the benefits of carrying such fat diminish relative to the costs. Fitness also increases with increasing body size, up to some maximum represented by the adult size, which is presumably best for balancing nutritional gains against metabolic needs given the ecological niche of the species. Furthermore, larger size brings animals sooner to the stage at which they start reproducing.

Full details of the equations, fitness functions and how the analysis was performed are presented elsewhere [4]. In this conference contribution I will simply summarize the salient findings from the modeling exercise.

3. Findings from the model

The end time for the SDP analysis is when individuals have completed body growth, and thus reached the maximum body size typical of the species. The model output indicates that fully grown, but non-reproductive animals should store as little fat as needed to get through the adverse (winter or dry) season, and deposit this fat as late as possible, so as not to carry it for longer than is necessary. The amount of fat needed is greater in more seasonally variable environments (Fig. 1a). Where there is more uncertainty in the environmental conditions likely to be experienced at any stage in the seasonal cycle, fat reserves should also be higher, built up earlier, and potentially carried for longer.

Considering growth in isolation, the optimal strategy would be to reach the size enabling reproduction as soon as possible. However, young growing animals must trade the benefits of fat stores against the costs to growth. Accordingly they are expected to have

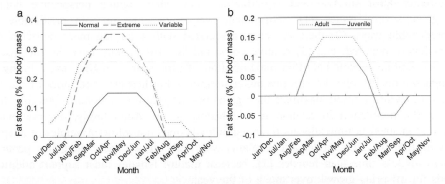

Fig. 1. Optimal fat stores for a non-growing adult over the seasonal cycle from mid-summer (June in the Northern Hemisphere, December in the Southern Hemisphere) through the adverse (winter or dry) period. (a) compares model predictions for a "normal" regime with that for an environment with more extreme seasonal contrasts, or for one that is more unpredictably variable. (b) compares the predicted pattern for a fully grown adult with that for a still-growing juvenile in the "normal" environment (modified from Owen-Smith 2002).

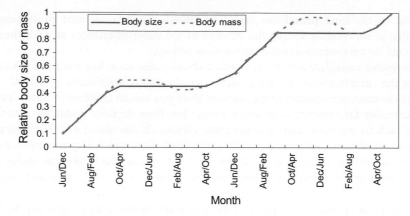

Fig. 2. Optimal growth in lean body size and in body mass (including fat stores) for a young animal from birth to adulthood, as predicted by the model. (Modified from Owen-Smith 2002).

lower fat stores, and be in poorer condition at the end of the adverse season, than fully grown animals (Fig. 1b). However, their survival prospects are likely to be poor if they have no fat, and hence growth in size (lean body mass) is restricted to a greater extent during the adverse season than if constrained by food gains alone (Fig. 2).

4. Discussion

As with many models, findings seem intuitively obvious from hindsight. However, the model provides a rigorous basis for establishing them, and for assessing more quantitatively what might underlie variation among species in observed patterns. Moreover, some implications of the model have not been so obvious to other workers.

Workers in optimal foraging theory commonly assume that animals operate as rate maximizers for energy or nutrient gains relative to the costs involved in procuring these requirements for survival and reproduction. This short-sighted perspective fails to recognize several issues: (1) environments vary over time in both predictable and unpredictable ways, (2) there are costs associated with acquiring more nutrients than immediately required, and (3) relative costs and benefits change over the life history. Hence foraging models based on maximization of time spent foraging, even during the benign season [5], rest on an erroneous assumption. Furthermore, the times of the year when individuals should maximize their gains by foraging for as along as possible differ within the population in relation to life history stage. Accordingly, observations of apparent laziness in time allocation among animals does not refute principles of adaptive optimization [6]. The model also explains why fully grown male ungulates generally forage for less time than females [7], because mature females must support additional needs for offspring growth over much of the year.

An analytical explanation for why large herbivores build up fat reserves primarily in autumn (or at the end of the wet season), shortly before resources become limiting, rather than in summer when potential foraging surpluses are greatest, seems not to have been presented previously, at least to my knowledge. It also explains why the set point for fat reserves changes seasonally and in relation to food supplies [8]. Moreover, patterns of seasonal variation in body fat can differ between males and females [9], because some of this fat is used to support the additional demands of reproduction, which for males takes place during the rut (or mating period) before or early in winter, but for females after the end of winter (or the dry season).

Tradeoffs in allocation between growth and storage also explain why survival rates for partly grown animals are necessarily lower, and also more variable between years, than those of adults, at least among large mammalian herbivores [10]. An alternative explanation of this pattern, based on canalization of life history patterns, has been proposed [11], but pays only cursory attention to the environmental constraints on resource allocation at different stages. The model also suggests that, for equivalent seasonal fluctuations in resources, animals in environments lacking effective predators should store more fat than those in environments with abundant predators. The highest body fat reserves among large mammalian herbivores are carried by reindeer inhabiting the predator-free island of Svalbard [12].

To expand the model to include resource allocation to reproduction as a third option, the fitness function must be generalized to represent not just individual survival, but the persistence of population biomass and the genes is propagates whether in the form of adults or their offspring (see Ref. [4]). Resource gains from the environment, both in the form of energy and material nutrients, convey the power to grow faster, survive better through adverse periods, and reproduce more successfully. This "biomass power" concept of fitness in physiological terms is a generalization of the energetic concept of fitness advanced by Brown et al. [13]. Although challenged, it is supported by a recent treatment of the fitness consequences for sexual selection of individual "condition", defined broadly as the amount of resources available for allocation to fitness-enhancing traits [14]. From this perspective, individual health and vigor, as well as survival prospects or that of dependent offspring, are condition-dependent. Elsewhere I have shown how the dynamic state-dependent approach can be expanded to establish the optimal age at first reproduction, the time in the seasonal cycle when reproduction should occur, the appropriate reproductive allocation at different ages, and potentially also the tradeoff between the metabolic costs of food processing and longevity [4], taking into account environmental variability.

Acknowledgments

I thank J. Burns and M. Castellini for giving me the opportunity to present this paper.

References

[1] M.S. Witter, I.C. Cuthill, R.H.C. Bonser, Experimental investigations of mass-dependent predation risk in the European starling, Anim. Behav. 48 (1994) 201–221.
[2] M. Mangel, C.W. Clark, Dynamic Modeling in Behavioral Ecology, Princeton University Press, Princeton, 1988.
[3] C.W. Clark, M. Mangel, Dynamic State Variable Models in Ecology, Oxford University Press, Oxford, 1999.
[4] N. Owen-Smith, Adaptive Herbivore Ecology. From Resources to Populations in Variable Environments, Cambridge University Press, Cambridge, 2002.

[5] G.E. Belovksy, Optimal foraging and community structure: implications for a guild of generalist grassland herbivores, Oecologia 70 (1986) 35–52.

[6] J.M. Herbers, Time resources and laziness in animals, Oecologia 49 (1981) 252–262.

[7] N. Owen-Smith, Megaherbivores. The Influence of Very Large Body Size on Ecology, Cambridge University Press, Cambridge, 1988.

[8] N. Mrosovsky, T.L. Prowley, Set points for body weight and fat, Behav. Biol. 20 (1977) 205–223.

[9] A.R.E. Sinclair, P. Duncan, Indices of condition in tropical ruminants, East Afr. Wildl. J. (1972) 143–149.

[10] J.-M. Gaillard, et al., Temporal variation in vital rates and population dynamics of large herbivores, Annu. Rev. Ecol. Syst. 31 (2000) 367–393.

[11] J.-M. Gaillard, N.G. Yoccoz, Temporal variation in survival of mammals and its impact on fitness: a case of environmental canalization? Ecology (2003) 3294–3306.

[12] N.J.C. Tyler, Body composition and energy balance of pregnant and non-pregnant Svalbard reindeer during winter, Symp. Zool. Soc. Lond. 57 (1987) 203–229.

[13] J.H. Brown, P.A. Marquet, M.L. Taper, Evolution of body size: consequences of an energetic definition of fitness, Am. Nat. 142 (1993) 573–584.

[14] J.L. Tomkins, et al., Genic capture and resolving the lek paradox, Trends Ecol. Evol. 19 (2004) 323–328.

ELSEVIER

www.ics-elsevier.com

Monitoring nutrition of a large grazer: muskoxen on the Arctic Refuge

Perry S. Barboza[a,*], Patricia E. Reynolds[b]

[a]Department of Biology and Wildlife, Institute of Arctic Biology, PO Box 757000, University of Alaska, Fairbanks, AK 99775-7000, USA
[b]United States Fish and Wildlife Service, Arctic National Wildlife Refuge, Fairbanks, AK, USA

Abstract. The number of young muskoxen (*Ovibos moschatus*) on Alaska's Arctic Refuge declined from 1986. We hypothesized that poor calf production was related to poor maternal nutrition. We analyzed samples from 40 adult females collected in 1988, 1989, 1991, 1992 and 2000. Sera and hair were depleted in N when compared with those of captive animals fed grass hay; that is, low dietary N in wild animals may result in less fractionation than in captivity. Poor nutrition in 1991 was indicated by elevation of ^{15}N in serum, low serum Cu (0.48 ± 0.05 μg mL^{-1}) and low activities of the Cu-enzyme ceruloplasmin (16 ± 1 IU.L^{-1}). Fecal enrichment of both ^{15}N and ^{13}C indicated a consistent diet based on graminoids that was similar between 1991 and 2000. Poor nutrition was probably associated with deep snow and low food abundance in 1990 or 1991. Forage abundance rather than quality may have the greatest influence on the populations dynamics of large grazers in highly seasonal environments. © 2004 Elsevier B.V. All rights reserved.

Keywords: Biomarker; Copper; Population dynamics; Ruminant; Stable isotope

1. Introduction

The nutrition of large animal populations is difficult to monitor because captures are expensive and handlings can endanger both animals and investigators. For example, the simple measurement of body mass in Arctic ungulates becomes a logistical feat when animals exceed 200 kg and when field sites can only be accessed by aircraft. Indirect measures of body condition are therefore required to monitor large animals when handling

* Corresponding author. Tel.: +1 907 474 7142; fax: +1 907 474 6967.
E-mail address: ffpsb@uaf.edu (P.S. Barboza).

0531-5131/ © 2004 Elsevier B.V. All rights reserved.
doi:10.1016/j.ics.2004.09.040

is permitted, and especially when terminal sampling is impractical for endangered or declining populations. Measures that reflect the rates of nutrient use (e.g., nitrogen recycling) are of great utility because they can be combined with measures of food selection (e.g., fecal analysis) and body reserves (e.g., body fat) to provide a dynamic index of the animal's nutrient status. Indirect measures of stored samples can therefore correlate nutrition with population dynamics of large, long-lived ungulates such as muskoxen (*Ovibos moschatus*).

Muskoxen were reintroduced into northeastern Alaska in 1969 and 1970. The population on the Arctic Refuge rapidly increased in numbers [1], as did other herds reintroduced to Canada [2]. By 1986, however, numbers of muskoxen stabilized in regions first occupied on the Arctic Refuge as mixed-sex groups dispersed into new ranges [3], as the proportion of females with calves declined and as individual females bore calves less frequently [1,4]. Several factors influence the dynamics of muskox populations, including abiotic factors, such as weather and terrain [5,6], and biotic factors, such as predation on young and adult animals [7]. Effects of weather and predation on production, survival and recruitment of young muskoxen [1] can be exacerbated by constraints on food resources that may ultimately dictate the growth and persistence of the population in an area [8,9]. Relatively sedentary populations like muskoxen, which increase rapidly in abundance, may affect forage communities in local areas [10]. The diversity and abundance of forages may therefore change in habitats occupied by muskoxen over several years [11].

We hypothesized that maternal nutrition limits calf production on the Arctic Refuge. We tested the hypothesis by analyzing blood sera, hair and feces collected from adult female muskoxen between 1988 and 2000. Isotopic measures of nitrogen (^{15}N) and carbon (^{13}C) were combined with those of copper (Cu) to monitor changes in diet and metabolism of wild females for comparison with captive muskoxen. Enrichments of N and C in feces mainly reflect changes in foods selected by herbivores [12,13], whereas those of tissues vary with both diet and metabolic processes [14]. Small deficiencies of trace minerals such as selenium and Cu can limit the reproduction of ungulates without increasing adult mortality [15]. Copper may be particularly limiting for arctic ruminants because hepatic concentrations of Cu are low in some wild populations and Cu stores may therefore limit both the reproduction and recruitment of muskoxen [16,17]. Maternal liver Cu is the principal supply of Cu for the developing fetus and for the establishment of hepatic Cu used by the young muskoxen [18,19]. Serum Cu and ceruloplasmin activities can be used as a predictor of hepatic Cu [17].

2. Methods

Seasons in the arctic are described as follows: early winter=October to January, late winter=February to April, spring and summer=May to July and autumn=August to September. These periods correspond to the annual reproductive cycle of muskoxen: breeding or rut in autumn, gestation through winter and parturition at the start of spring. Forty adult females were handled in 43 captures as follows: 8 in 1988; 11 in 1989; 11 in 1991; 7 in 1992; and 6 in 2000. Samples were collected in late winter during 1988, 1991 and 1992. Summer samples included two captures in 1998 and all collections in 1989 and 2000. Locations of capture were categorized according to Reynolds [3] in relation to the initial region of occupancy of muskoxen released into the Arctic Refuge in 1969 and 1970. Thirty-three captures were within the initial region of occupancy, with 10 captures in areas of emigration to the east (6 captures) and to the west (4 captures). Animal age was categorized as 2–4 years, 4–10 years and older than 10 years, based on the known age of previously marked individuals and estimates for unmarked animals based on horn structure [3,20].

Muskoxen were darted from a helicopter and immobilized with a mixture of carfentanyl citrate and xylazine (Cervizine, Wildlife Pharmaceuticals, Fort Collins, CO, USA). A mixture of naltrexone and yohimbine was used to reverse immobilization after sampling [3]. Guard hair was sampled from the middle of either the right or the left flank when animals were sternally recumbent. Hair was stored in sealed plastic bags at room temperature until analysis. Feces were collected from the rectum and stored in sealed plastic bags at -20 °C. Blood samples were collected from the brachial vein directly into sterile evacuated tubes without additive (Vacutainer Systems, Becton Dickinson, Franklin Lakes, NJ, USA). Sera were separated from clots by centrifugation within 4 h of collection and stored at -80 °C until analysis.

Sera, hair and feces were dried to constant mass at 55 °C before analysis for ^{13}C and ^{15}N enrichment by isotope ratio mass spectrometry (Europa Scientific 20-20 Continuous Flow IRMS, Europa Scientific, Chestershire, United Kingdom). Enrichments were expressed as δ [parts per thousand (ppt); [21]] against air (^{15}N 6.93 ± 0.19 ppt) and against peptone (^{13}C -15.87 ± 0.06; P7750 from meat; Lot 76F-0300, Sigma, St. Louis, MO). Isotopic enrichments of serum and hair were compared with samples collected in early (October) and late winter (March) from captive yearling muskoxen fed grass hay [22].

Serum ceruloplasmin was assayed by oxidase activity of o-dianisidine [16]. Acid-labile Cu that was free of protein was isolated by deproteinizing 1.0 mL of serum with 2.0 mL of 1.4 M HCl and 2.0 mL of 1.23 M tri-chloro-acetic acid. Protein was precipitated by centrifugation at $1000 \times g$ before analyzing the supernatant for Cu by atomic absorption spectrometry (324.8 nm; Model 5000, Perkin Elmer, Connecticut; [17]). Reference values for minimal concentrations of serum Cu (0.7 µg mL^{-1}) and ceruloplasmin (7.5 IU.L^{-1}) were derived from relationships with liver Cu for adult female muskoxen in the wild from Banks Island, Canada and in captivity at Fairbanks, AK [17].

We used programs in SYSTAT 10.2 (Systat Software, Richmond, CA, USA) to compare years, locations, age groups and seasons by ANOVA. Enrichments of serum, hair and feces collected from the same animals were compared with paired t-tests. Pair-wise comparisons were made with Bonferroni's adjustment.

3. Results

Measures of serum, hair and feces did not vary with age group or with location ($P > 0.05$). The nutrition of adult females were therefore similar across age groups and between areas initially and recently occupied by reintroduced muskoxen in northeastern Alaska.

Serum copper and ceruloplasmin varied with year but not with season of collection (Fig. 1). Thirty four of 43 samples were below 0.7 µg Cu mL^{-1} serum, i.e., the minimum

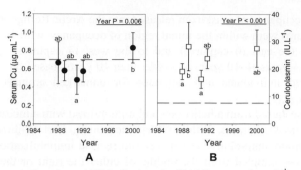

Fig. 1. (A) Serum concentrations (mean±S.D.) of unbound acid-labile copper (μg ml^{-1}) and (B) ceruloplasmin activity (IU.L^{-1}) in muskoxen captured on the Arctic Refuge from 1988 to 2000. Broken lines indicate serum concentrations of Cu (0.7μg ml^{-1}) and ceruloplasmin (7.5 IU L^{-1}) at which liver copper is predicted to be zero. Data points with different letters within each plot are significantly different ($P<0.05$).

concentration predicted for depletion of liver copper. Activities of ceruloplasmin also reflected low serum Cu, which were lowest for both measures in 1991 (Fig. 1).

Lowest indices of Cu in 1991 were associated with the highest enrichment of ^{15}N in serum. Elevated ^{15}N may indicate protein conservation and increased utilization or recycling of N from body protein ([23]; Fig. 2). Neither ^{15}N nor ^{13}C in serum varied with season, although small seasonal changes have been reported in captive animals fed consistent diets throughout the year [22]. Enrichments of serum were depleted by less than 1ppt ^{13}C and approximately 3ppt ^{15}N when compared with captive muskoxen fed grass hay (Fig. 2). The relative depletion of ^{15}N in wild animals was also apparent for hair (2.43±0.49 ppt) when compared with that of captive animals (8.21 ppt). Hair C was similarly enriched in wild and captive animals (−24.04±0.34 ppt vs. −24.28). Fecal ^{15}N (1.28±1.08 ppt) and ^{13}C (−27.81±0.66 ppt) of muskoxen on the Arctic Refuge were consistent with a graminoid diet similar to hay fed in captivity (1.05±0.52 ppt ^{15}N and −24.38±0.54 ppt ^{13}C). Isotopic enrichments of feces were similar between 1991 and 2000, suggesting a consistent diet selection between years when serum indices indicated contrasting supplies of Cu and N.

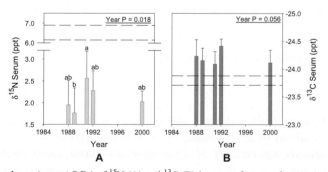

Fig. 2. Natural abundance (mean±S.D.) of ^{15}N (A) and ^{13}C (B) in serum from muskoxen captured on the Arctic Refuge from 1988 to 2000. Broken lines indicate the seasonal range in enrichments of captive muskoxen fed grass hay. Data points with different letters within each plot are significantly different ($P<0.05$).

4. Discussion

Our hypothesis that poor nutrition was associated with a decline in numbers of muskoxen was supported by the low serum Cu concentrations of adult females on the Arctic Refuge (Fig. 1). Consistent patterns between serum Cu and ceruloplasmin activity, and between patterns of serum Cu and ^{15}N enrichment suggest that nutrient supplies fluctuate annually. Indices of poor female nutrition in 1991 corresponded with low calf production and a decline in the total number of muskoxen on the Arctic Refuge from 1990 to 1992 [1,3]. Most female muskoxen on the Arctic Refuge successfully produced only one calf every three years between 1988 and 1993, whereas reproductive rates were two to three calves per three years between 1982 and 1984, when this population was growing. Reproductive rates of female muskoxen are modulated by body condition [24], such as fat reserves, as well as the dietary supply of energy and trace nutrients [25]. Serum indices of Cu, as well as hepatic concentrations of Cu, were low for female muskoxen during a decline in numbers on Banks Island, Canada [9,17]. Maternal copper can directly affect the growth of the fetus and indirectly affect the survival of young muskoxen because hepatic copper is accumulated in utero and apparently used through the first 60–100 days from birth, when the dietary supply of Cu in milk is low [19]. Poor recruitment of calves may therefore result from low immunity and growth as a consequence of poor Cu supplies from the mother, although Cu is adequate for other maternal body functions.

Supplies of N for muskoxen on the Arctic Refuge may also differ from those animals in captivity. Sera and hair of captive muskoxen were more enriched in ^{15}N than wild muskoxen, even though fecal samples indicated a similar isotopic signature in the diet. The closer correspondence between dietary ^{15}N and tissues of wild muskoxen suggests that fewer pathways are used for deposition of N than in captive animals fed abundant high-quality foods throughout the year. The highly fibrous diet of sedge and grass consumed in the wild is typically low in N and probably requires ruminal fermentation [26]. The conversion of all dietary N to microbial protein in the rumen could provide a relatively uniform isotopic signature for protein to be absorbed by the animal and a smaller number of subsequent nitrogenous transactions in the liver. These suggestions await confirmation from direct experiments on isotopic fractionation between diet, ruminal microbes and nitrogenous metabolites of muskoxen and other ruminants.

Poor nutrition of female muskoxen on the Arctic Refuge was probably not due to low concentrations of Cu or N in plants. Although forbs and woody browse generally contain more N and Cu than do the sedges and grasses consumed by muskoxen, most body mass gain and nutrient uptake by captive muskoxen is due to hyperphagia in late summer during August and September [22,27]. Seasonal movements of wild muskoxen reflect the intensity of foraging along riparian corridors in summer and residence on exposed ridges during winter [3,28]. Any deficits of Cu and N in wild muskoxen during 1991 were probably the outcome of restricted foraging opportunities due to snow cover in late winter or low abundance of foods at the end of the previous summer. Females and growing calves may be most sensitive to changes in plant production and energy demands from late summer, when young animals transition to forages [29], and when females regain body mass [30]. Changes in weather or climate that attenuate the season of plant growth or restrict mobility through late summer may adversely affect the growth and reproduction of muskoxen [31] in a similar fashion to other ungulates at high latitudes [32,33]. Adverse weather conditions can exacerbate calf mortalities by increasing energy demands for thermoregulation and movement, which may diminish the ability to escape predation or resist disease. The combined effects of constrained nutrition and increasing predation by bears may therefore continue to limit the numbers of muskoxen on the Arctic Refuge. Muskoxen in expanded range to the east and west of this region should be monitored to assess any effects of animal density on nutrition of females and their young.

Acknowledgements

This work was partially supported by a grant to P.S. Barboza from the Alaska Science and Technology Foundation (#98-4-128). Technical assistance was expertly provided by H. Reynolds, K. Budsberg, T. Howe, N. Haubenstock and T. Lackey.

References

[1] P.E. Reynolds, K.J. Wilson, D.R. Klein, in: D.C. Douglas, P.E. Reynolds, E.B. Rhode (Eds.), Arctic Refuge Coastal Plain Terrestrial Wildlife Research Summaries, U.S. Geological Survey, Biological Resources Division, Reston VA, 2002, pp. 54–64.

[2] D. Le Henaff, M. Crete, Introduction of muskoxen in northern Quebec: the demographic explosion of a colonizing herbivore, Canadian Journal of Zoology 67 (1989) 1102–1105.

[3] P.E. Reynolds, Dynamics and range expansion of a reestablished muskox population, Journal of Wildlife Management 62 (1998) 734–744.

[4] P.E. Reynolds, Reproductive patterns of female muskoxen in northeastern Alaska, Alces 37 (2001) 403–410.

[5] M. Forchhammer, D. Boertmann, The muskoxen *Ovibos moschatus* in north and northeast Greenland: population trends and the influence of abiotic parameters on population dynamics, Ecography 16 (1993) 299–308.

[6] C. Nellemann, P.E. Reynolds, Predicting late winter distribution of muskoxen using an index of terrain ruggedness, Arctic and Alpine Research 29 (1997) 334–338.

[7] P.E. Reynolds, H.V. Reynolds, R.T. Shideler, Predation and multiple kills of muskoxen by grizzly bears, URSUS 13 (2002) 79–84.

[8] C.R. Olesen, H. Thing, P. Aastrup, Growth of wild muskoxen under two nutritional regimes in Greenland, Rangifer 14 (1994) 3–10.

[9] N.C. Larter, J.A. Nagy, Calf production, calf survival, and recruitment of muskoxen on Banks Island during a period of changing population density from 1986–99, Arctic 54 (2001) 394–406.

[10] C.P.H. Mulder, R. Harmsen, The effect of muskox herbivory on growth and reproduction in an arctic legume, Arctic and Alpine Research 27 (1995) 44–53.

[11] M. Raillard, J. Svoboda, High grazing impact, selectivity, and local density of muskoxen in Central Ellesmere Island, Canadian High Arctic, Arctic, Antarctic, and Alpine Research 32 (2000) 278–285.

[12] D.M. Post, et al., Sexual segregation results in differences in content and quality of bison (*Bos bison*) diets, Journal of Mammalogy 82 (2001) 407–413.

[13] M. Sponheimer, et al., An experimental test of carbon-isotope fractionation between diet, hair, and feces of mammalian herbivores, Canadian Journal of Zoology 81 (2003) 871–876.

[14] J.F. Kelly, Stable isotopes of carbon and nitrogen in the study of avian and mammalian trophic ecology, Canadian Journal of Zoology 78 (2000) 1–27.

[15] W.T. Flueck, Effect of trace elements on population dynamics: selenium deficiency in free-ranging black-tailed deer, Ecology 75 (1994) 807–812.

[16] P.S. Barboza, J.E. Blake, Ceruloplasmin as an indicator of copper reserves in wild ruminants at high latitudes, Journal of Wildlife Diseases 37 (2001) 324–331.

[17] P.S. Barboza, et al., Copper status of muskoxen: a comparison of wild and captive populations, Journal of Wildlife Diseases 39 (2003) 610–619.

[18] E.P. Rombach, P.S. Barboza, J.E. Blake, Trace mineral reserves of muskoxen during gestation: copper, ceruloplasmin, and metallothionein, Comparative Biochemistry and Physiology 134C (2002) 157–168.

[19] E.P. Rombach, P.S. Barboza, J.E. Blake, Utilization of copper during lactation and neonatal development in muskoxen, Canadian Journal of Zoology 80 (2002) 1460–1469.

[20] C.R. Olesen, H. Thing, Guide to field classification by sex and age of the muskox, Canadian Journal of Zoology 67 (1989) 1116–1119.

[21] R.R. Wolfe, Radioactive and Stable Isotope Tracers in Biomedicine: Principles and Practice of Kinetic Analysis, Wiley-Liss, New York, 1992.

[22] T.C. Peltier, P.S. Barboza, Growth in an arctic grazer: effects of sex and dietary protein on yearling muskoxen, Journal of Mammalogy 84 (2003) 915–925.

[23] K.L. Parker, P.S. Barboza, T.R. Stephenson, Protein conservation in female caribou (*Rangifer tarandus*): effects of decreasing diet quality during winter, Journal of Mammalogy (2004) in press.

[24] J.Z. Adamczewski, et al., The influence of fatness on the likelihood of early-winter pregnancy in muskoxen (*Ovibos moschatus*), Theriogenology 50 (1998) 605–614.

[25] R.G. White, J.E. Rowell, W.E. Hauer, The role of nutrition, body condition and lactation on calving success in muskoxen, Journal of Zoology, London 243 (1997) 13–20.

[26] N.C. Larter, J.A. Nagy, Peary caribou, muskoxen and Banks Island forage: assessing seasonal diet similarities, Rangifer 17 (1997) 9–16.

[27] T.C. Peltier, P.S. Barboza, J.E. Blake, Seasonal hyperphagia does not reduce digestive efficiency in an arctic grazer, Physiological and Biochemical Zoology 76 (2003) 471–483.

[28] J.A. Schaefer, F. Messier, Winter activity of muskoxen in relation to foraging conditions, Ecoscience 3 (1996) 147–153.

[29] K.K. Knott, P.S. Barboza, R.T. Bowyer, Postnatal development and organ maturation in *Rangifer tarandus* and *Ovibos moschatus*, Journal of Mammalogy (2004) (In press).

[30] R.G. White, D.F. Holleman, B.A. Tiplady, Seasonal body weight, body condition, and lactational trends in muskoxen, Canadian Journal of Zoology 67 (1989) 1125–1133.

[31] L.D. Mech, Lack of reproduction in muskoxen and arctic hares caused by early winter? Arctic 53 (2000) 69–71.

[32] B. Griffith, et al., in: D.C. Douglas, P.E. Reynolds, E.B. Rhode (Eds.), The Porcupine caribou herd, Arctic Refuge Coastal Plain Terrestrial Wildlife Research Summaries, U.S. Geological Survey, Biological Resources Division, Reston VA, 2002, pp. 8–37.

[33] E. Post, N.C. Stenseth, Climatic variability, plant phenology, and northern ungulates, Ecology 80 (1999) 1322–1339.

International Congress Series 1275 (2004) 334–340

www.ics-elsevier.com

Red blood cell metabolism shows major anomalies in Rhinocerotidae and Equidae, suggesting a novel role in general antioxidant metabolism

E.H. Harley[a],*, M. Matshikiza[a], P. Robson[b], B. Weber[a]

[a]Department of Clinical Laboratory Sciences, University of Cape Town, Cape Town, 7925 Observatory, South Africa
[b]Department of Physiological Sciences, University of Stellenbosch, South Africa

Abstract. The black rhinoceros, *Diceros bicornis*, shows some striking anomalies in red cell biochemistry compared with humans: many enzyme levels are grossly different, ATP levels are very low, and the red cells contain very high levels of free tyrosine. On exposure to oxidative stress dityrosine, a substance never previously described in free form in cells can be detected. Uric acid, another soluble free radical scavenger, can also on occasions be readily demonstrable, often at very high concentrations, in rhinoceros and equine red cells. Assays for oxygen radical absorptive capacity (ORAC) in intact red cells, and in cell free preparations containing tyrosine or urate, give results consistent with a role for tyrosine and purine derivatives as additional defence mechanisms against reactive oxygen intermediates. The integration of these in vitro and in vivo analyses reveals insights and mechanisms which should be exploitable for the development of preventative or therapeutic measures against hemolytic and other free radical-induced disorders in both rhinoceros and other mammals, including man. © 2004 Elsevier B.V. All rights reserved.

Keywords: Rhinoceros; Horse; Tyrosine; Uric acid; Erythrocyte; Antioxidant; Free radical

1. Introduction

Over the past three decades, habitat encroachment and poaching have progressively reduced the worldwide population of African black rhinoceroses (*Diceros bicornis*) from more than 60,000 to approximately 2500, less than 5% of which currently reside under captive conditions. This captive population has been threatened by several disease

* Corresponding author. Tel.: +47 21 406 6222; fax: +47 21 448 8150.
 E-mail address: harley@chempath.uct.ac.za (E.H. Harley).

0531-5131/ © 2004 Elsevier B.V. All rights reserved.
doi:10.1016/j.ics.2004.08.062

syndromes, including acute hemolytic anaemia which is one of the most common causes of death in captivity. Despite extensive haematological investigation [1], the causes of this remained uncertain. However, the black rhinoceros does show some striking peculiarities in respect to its normal red cell biochemistry: many enzyme activities are very different, catalase especially being only about 2% of levels in human red cells, and ATP levels are remarkably low relative to other mammals [2,3].

We have also demonstrated diminished erythrocyte glycolysis through the hexose monophosphate shunt [4], and this, together with the presence of Heinz bodies in erythrocytes of normal individual rhinoceroses [2], suggests that impairments in antioxidant capacity may contribute to the hemolytic tendency.

2. Materials and methods

Blood samples were obtained opportunistically from apparently healthy wild black and white rhinoceroses immobilised for translocation, radio-collaring, or other purposes, in the Kruger National Park, Hluhluwe-Umfolozi Park, and Addo Elephant National Park, South Africa. Red blood cells were either used fresh or were frozen as droplets into liquid nitrogen [5] for later analysis or experimentation.

Analysis of acid extracts of red cells by HPLC and identification of metabolites are as described previously [6].

Dityrosine was synthesised in vitro from unlabelled or ^{14}C-labelled tyrosine using horseradish peroxidase [7].

Oxygen radical absorptive capacity (ORAC) was assayed according to Cao et al. [8], where the prevention of fluorescent decay of 0.04 µM oxidant-sensitive β-phycoerythrin in the presence of 40 mM of the free-radical generator 2,2′-Azobis(2-amidinopropane) dihydrochloride (AAPH) (Sigma-Aldrich) by either a standard scavenger (Trolox) or the test solution of tyrosine, urate, plasma, or cell extract was followed at 5-min intervals in an Aminco SPF 500 fluorimeter at an emission of 565 nm and an excitation of 540 nm.

3. Results

Whilst investigating nucleotide profiles of acid-extracted rhinoceros red blood cells using anion-exchange and reversed-phase HPLC, and confirming that all rhinoceros species show very low ATP levels, we observed a major U/V absorbing peak with a distinctive 260/280 ratio. Comparisons with other U/V absorbing metabolites showed the elution positions, and 260/280 ratio of this substance to correspond to the amino-acid tyrosine. Confirmation of this identity was provided by the characteristic absorption profile given by diode array scan, the retention time and ninhydrin positivity on cation-exchange amino acid analysis, the excitation and emission properties on fluorescence spectrometry and mass number identity with tyrosine on mass spectrometry.

Eight fresh red blood cell specimens taken from free-ranging black rhinoceroses gave a mean intracellular concentration of tyrosine of 0.78 ± 0.11 mM, levels which are at least 50-fold greater than those found in normal human red cells. Despite this, plasma levels of tyrosine were far lower, and similar to those found in human plasma. Examination of human, canine, feline, lepine, and bovine erythrocytes showed no detectable tyrosine on

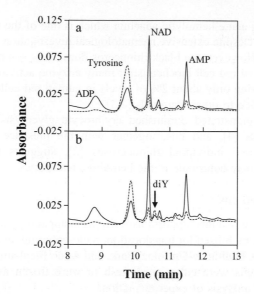

Fig. 1. Reversed-phase chromatography of neutralised acid-soluble extracts of rhinoceros red cells. Red cells were incubated for 30 min at 37 °C with either (a) Hank's balanced salt solution with no additions, or (b) with the addition of 2 mM H_2O_2; diY, dityrosine.

HPLC analysis, but equine erythrocytes from both horse and Plains zebra showed tyrosine at about one tenth of the levels found in rhinoceros.

Protein-bound dityrosine is known to form nonenzymatically from interactions between H_2O_2 and hemoglobin [9], but free dityrosine production has not been documented as a biological process. We therefore undertook to see whether we could identify free dityrosine after exposure of rhinoceros red cells to H_2O_2, and detected a novel UV absorbing species (Fig. 1) on reversed-phase HPLC with the known fluorescent properties of dityrosine [7]. Although this was readily detected in both black and white rhinoceros

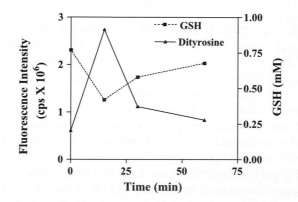

Fig. 2. Variation in levels of dityrosine and GSH over time after treatment of rhinoceros red cells incubated at 37 °C in Hank's balanced salt solution after addition of H_2O_2 to a final concentration of 2 mM at time 0. Each point shows the mean of duplicate measurements.

Table 1
In vitro studies using dialysed cell-free preparations (DCFP)

Additions	Dityrosine detected (μM)
Tyrosine+H_2O_2	no (<0.5)
Tyrosine+H_2O_2+DCFP	yes (4.1)
Tyrosine+H_2O_2+DCFP+GSH	no (<0.5)
Tyrosine+H_2O_2+heated DCFP	yes (149.3)
Tyrosine+H_2O_2+Fe^{++}	no (<0.5)
Tyrosine+H_2O_2+hemoglobin	yes (20.5)
Tyrosine+H_2O_2+hemin	yes (49.5)

Tyrosine (0.5 mM) and H_2O_2 (2 mM) were incubated with heat-inactivated or non-heat-inactivated dialysed cell-free preparations (DCFP) of rhinoceros red cell lysates at 37 °C for 0, 15, 30, 60, and 90 min before quantitation of dityrosine production by fluorescence spectroscopy. Results are the mean of duplicate assays at the time of maximum dityrosine accumulation. Additions were 0.5 mM GSH, 0.1 mM ferrous sulfate (BDH), or 10 μM bovine hemin.

red cells, it was not detected in human erythrocytes identically treated. Confirmation of the identity of this species as o,o'dityrosine was provided by fluorescence properties, U/V absorbance properties, co-elution with synthetic dityrosine, and mass spectrometry. This increase in H_2O_2-induced dityrosine production coincided with a decrease in reduced glutathione (GSH) concentrations (Fig. 2), with GSH concentrations rising again as dityrosine levels fell during the recovery phase.

In order to determine whether the dityrosine production was an enzyme-catalysed process, dialysed cell free lysates were incubated with tyrosine, H_2O_2, and other additions (Table 1). Dityrosine could be easily detected with unheated and, more surprisingly, also with heated cell extracts. Dissecting the components of the cell extract showed then that the presence of either hemoglobin or heme was sufficient for dityrosine production, indicating that the heme ring alone could provide catalysis.

During the course of these experiments, an additional U/V absorbing species was intermittently encountered in some rhinoceros and some equine red cell extracts and sometimes it was the most prominent of the U/V absorbing species. Its absorption characteristics, elution positions on anion-exchange and reversed-phase HPLC, and disappearance from HPLC analyses after uricase treatment identified the species as uric acid. The puzzling quantitative variability compromised adequate investigation until a series of eight horses undertaking an endurance race were studied (Table 2), when the results suggested that red cell urate levels were strongly influenced by intense muscular activity. Complementary in vitro studies indicated that although red cell urate levels were not stable over periods in excess of a few hours at body or room temperature, transport in or

Table 2
Levels of intracellular red cell urate (μM)

	A	B	C	D	F	G	H	J
Twenty-four hours before exercise	56.4	0.0	0.0	0.0	67.6	0.0	0.0	1.7
Immediately after exercise	118.4	0.0	422.0	7.6	0.0	0.0	0.0	2.0
One hour after exercise	108.8	0.0	824.0	35.2	157.6	0.0	32.4	35.5

Urate was measured in red cell extracts from eight horses (A–J). Blood was taken before and after undergoing an endurance exercise of 80 km, with a mean duration for the exercise of 5.1 h.

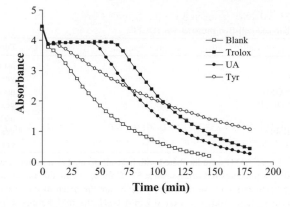

Fig. 3. ORAC of urate and tyrosine: time-dependent fluorescence decay of β-phycoerythrin after addition of AAPH in the presence of: Blank, no additions; Trolox, 5 μM Trolox; UA, 12.5 μM urate; Tyr, 12.5 μM tyrosine.

out of the red cell was slow and inadequate to explain the rapid increase or decrease in levels over the short-term in vivo, suggesting that the urate was being synthesised and destroyed within the red cell, perhaps by oxidative processes.

Since we had shown heme to catalyse oxidation of tyrosine in vitro, a similar test was tried with urate. Urate incubated with either heme or H_2O_2 alone gave no change, but all three together resulted in rapid urate degradation. Since urate is well-known as an effective scavenger of oxygen free radicals, and since tyrosine has also been proposed to serve as an antioxidant in seminal fluid [10] we compared the oxygen radical absorptive capacities (ORAC) of urate and tyrosine, and found that both exhibited similar antioxidant capacities, with ORAC values of 14550 and 12680 mmol/l for 5 mmol/l solutions of tyrosine and uric acid, respectively, although kinetics differed, with urate showing higher affinity for the oxidant (Fig. 3). Plasma extracts of both rhino and human samples showed ORAC kinetics similar to that of free tyrosine, probably due to the tyrosine in serum proteins. We then

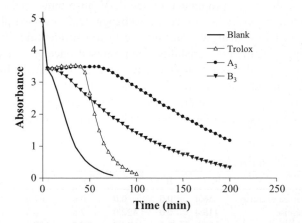

Fig. 4. ORAC of horse red cell extracts either lacking or containing urate, together with a blank and a Trolox control. A_3 is a high urate containing sample from horse A (see Table 2) and B_3 is a sample lacking detectable urate from horse B, both at 1 h after exercise.

compared the ORAC of two horse red cell extracts (Fig. 4), one with no detectable urate (horse B one h after exercise) and the other with high urate levels (horse A, one h after exercise, with 108 μM urate) demonstrating the markedly increased ORAC of the urate containing sample.

4. Discussion

The finding of high levels of tyrosine in mammalian red cells is unprecedented and its presence in both rhinocerotidae and equidae implies a long evolutionary history and presumably a useful physiological role. During an inflammatory response, activated macrophages produce myeloperoxidase and H_2O_2. The latter can then form the antimicrobial agents hypochlorous acid (HOCl) and peroxynitrite, as a consequence of which tyrosine in the vicinity can be converted to tyrosine chloramine, and nitrotyrosine, in reactions in which the tyrosyl radical is proposed to play a central role.

The amino-acid taurine is found in human neutrophils and epithelial cells and is assumed to have a role in protecting cellular components from strong oxidants such as the HOCl produced during phagocytic killing of microorganisms by the myeloperoxidase system [11]. It is possible that the physiological elevation of tyrosine in red blood cells in rhinoceroses might have an analogous role, and complements the similar protective role of urate. The generation of urate in red cells, as well as its removal, have at present no straightforward explanation, but it is possible that free-radical processes are involved in both formation of urate from, for example, hypoxanthine, and in the degradation to substances such as allantoin; both these pathways occur normally in some mammalian tissues, and both can be oxidative processes, the former catalysed by xanthine oxidase, and the latter by uricase. The (presumed) absence of both these enzymatic processes in red cells may be offset by the results of the in vitro experiments reported here which imply that heme may catalyse similar reactions in the presence of strong oxidants, analogous to the way heme can catalyse the oxidation of tyrosine.

It has recently been shown [12] that black rhinoceroses in the USA become progressively iron overloaded with time in captivity. The iron overload is likely to arise from the change from a natural diet (browse) rich in powerful iron-binding substances, for which the black rhinoceros would have had to have evolved equally powerful iron-absorptive mechanisms, to a captive diet of available fodder items unlikely to restrict iron availability to the same extent. Iron catalyses free radical production by the Fenton and Haber–Weiss reactions, so the cause of the hemolytic anaemia in these individuals may well be a decompensation of red cell antioxidant mechanisms in red cells with unusual antioxidant defences in the face of excess iron-induced free radical production. A feature of this idea is that it suggests novel therapeutic or preventative approaches such as reintroduction of more natural browse or addition of iron chelators to the diet.

These results leave a number of unresolved problems, including (1) how does tyrosine accumulate in rhinoceros red cells?, (2) what is the physiological role of heme with respect to oxidant production or removal?, (3) what is the explanation for the unusual dynamics of red cell urate production and destruction, and (4) do levels of red cell tyrosine, urate (and ORAC) vary under different dietary or exercise regimes, or in response to antioxidant treatments?

These results also, however, provide some intriguing new insights and suggestions for new physiological processes and mechanisms. These are: (1) Comparative studies on mammalian red blood cells can demonstrate novel, and generally unpredictable, physiological phenomena. (2) Tyrosine and uric acid in red blood cells both have the capability of scavenging oxidants and/or oxygen free radicals. (3) Given the magnitude and variety of antioxidant mechanisms in red blood cells, the question arises as to whether these mechanisms are primarily there to protect the red blood cell itself, or is their main purpose the provision of a convenient "package" of scavengers and enzymes for delivery to other tissues where free radicals need to be removed? If the latter were correct, then it would define a new pathophysiological role for the red blood cell of general relevance to veterinary and perhaps human medicine.

Acknowledgements

These studies were supported by grants from the International Rhino Foundation, the National Research Foundation, and the Medical Research Council of South Africa. The authors are grateful to D. Grobler, P. Morkel, P. Rogers, R. Cherry, and J. Raath for procuring rhinoceros blood samples, and to I. Baumgarten for technical assistance.

References

[1] D.E. Paglia, et al., Acute intravascular hemolysis in the black rhinoceros: erythrocyte enzymes and metabolic intermediates, Am. J. Vet. Res. 47 (1986) 1321–1325.

[2] D.E. Paglia, Acute episodic hemolysis in the African black rhinoceros as an analogue of human glucose-6-phosphate dehydrogenase deficiency, Am. J. Hematol. 42 (1993) 36–45.

[3] D.E. Paglia, R.E. Miller, Erythrocyte ATP deficiency and acatalasemia in the black rhinoceros (*Diceros bicornis*) and their pathogenic roles in acute episodic hemolysis and mucocutaneous ulcerations, Proc. Joint Conference, American Associations of Zoo and Wildlife Veterinarians, Oakland, CA, 1992, pp. 217–219.

[4] D.E. Paglia, et al., Radiometric assessment of hexose monophosphate shunt capacity in erythrocytes of rhinoceroses, Am. J. Vet. Res. 62 (2001) 1113–1117.

[5] P.D. Issitt, Methods for Preserving Small Quantities of Red Cells in the Frozen State, Applied Blood Group Serology, 3rd ed., Montgomery Scientific Publications, 1985, p. 65.

[6] B.W. Weber, D.E. Paglia, E.H. Harley, Elevated free tyrosine in rhinoceros erythrocytes, Comp. Biochem. Physiol. 138 (2004) 105–109.

[7] C. Giulivi, K.J.A. Davies, Dityrosine: a marker for oxidatively modified proteins and selective proteolysis, Methods Enzymol. 233 (1994) 363–371.

[8] G. Cao, H.M. Alessio, R.G. Cutler, Oxygen-radical absorbance capacity assay for antioxidants, Free Radic. Biol. Med. 14 (1993) 303–311.

[9] C. Giulivi, K.J.A. Davies, Dityrosine and tyrosine oxidation products are endogenous markers for the selective proteolysis of oxidatively modified red blood cell hemoglobin by (the 19S) proteasome, J. Biol. Chem. 268 (1993) 8752–8759.

[10] F.W. van Overveld, et al., Tyrosine as important contributor to the antioxidant capacity of seminal plasma, Chem. Biol. Interact. 127 (2000) 151–161.

[11] M.B. Grisham, et al., Chlorination of endogenous amines by isolated neutrophils. Ammonia-dependent bactericidal, cytotoxic, and cytolytic activities of the chloramines, J. Biol. Chem. 259 (1984) 10404–10413.

[12] D.E. Paglia, et al., Role of excessive maternal iron in the pathogenesis of congenital leukoencephalomalacia in captive black rhinoceroses (*Diceros bicornis*), Am. J. Vet. Res. 62 (2001) 343–349.

International Congress Series 1275 (2004) 341–350

www.ics-elsevier.com

The impact of lactation strategy on physiological development of juvenile marine mammals: implications for the transition to independent foraging

Jennifer M. Burns*, Cheryl A. Clark, Julie P. Richmond

Department of Biological Sciences, University of Alaska Anchorage, 99508, USA

Abstract. Lactating marine mammals provision their offspring either by providing large amounts of lipid-rich milk over a short period during which females fast (capital provisioning), or smaller amounts of less energetically dense milk over an extended period during which females forage (income provisioning). While it has long been recognized that these two strategies carry different costs for the female, the effect of these two strategies on the physiological status of newly weaned pups has rarely been considered. Recent comparative studies on the development of diving capacity, as assessed by measuring total body oxygen stores, have demonstrated that the provisioning strategy does affect pup development. Phocid pups, which grow rapidly during their brief nursing period undergo a strong post-parturition anemia and are weaned with relatively immature oxygen stores, possibly due to limited iron intake. Otariid pups, which grow at a slower pace over a longer period, are weaned with body oxygen stores that are significantly more mature. This suggests that newly independent phocid pups must quickly develop foraging skills in order to acquire the nutrients necessary to mature physiologically. In contrast, newly weaned otariids have more mature oxygen stores, and may have previous foraging experience, which may allow for increased behavioral flexibility. © 2004 Elsevier B.V. All rights reserved.

Keywords: Lactation strategy; Harbour seal (*Phoca vitulina*); Steller sea lion (*Eumetopias jubatus*); Diving physiology; Development

* Corresponding author. Tel.: +1 907 786 1527; fax: +1 907 786 4607.
  E-mail address: jburns@uaa.alaska.edu (J.M. Burns).

0531-5131/ © 2004 Elsevier B.V. All rights reserved.
doi:10.1016/j.ics.2004.09.032

1. Introduction

Within the pinniped lineage, there are two main strategies used by females to provision their dependent offspring. Females either utilize a capital investment strategy, whereby most, if not all of the energy provided to the pup comes from the female's endogenous reserves, or an income-based strategy, whereby females provision their offspring initially from endogenous reserves that are later supplemented by periodic foraging trips [1]. All Otariidae and Odobenidae demonstrate the income provisioning strategy, while most Phocidae utilize the capital provisioning strategy [2,3]. Due to their small size, some phocids such as harbour and ringed seals, cannot store enough energy to provision their offspring without supplemental foraging [4]. That the maternal strategy used has a large impact on the growth and condition of the pups is clear. Phocid pups are provisioned with energy-rich milk, and as a result grow quickly and accumulate large lipid reserves during the short lactation period [5]. In contrast, otariid pups are suckled on less energetically dense milk, grow more slowly, and rarely show the large variation in body composition seen in phocid pups [2,6,7]. In addition to impacting growth rates, the lactation strategy may also impact physiological development during the dependent period. While physiological development takes many forms, for the purpose of this paper, we will focus on the development of body oxygen stores, as these are critical for sustaining diving and foraging activity in newly weaned and independent pups [8,9]. In addition, there is growing evidence that juvenile diving activities can be limited due to their smaller size and reduced mass-specific oxygen stores, as compared to adults [10–13]. Therefore, if the developmental patterns of capital and income provisioned pups differ, this may also affect how they interact with their environment in the weeks and months postweaning.

To determine if lactation strategy influences the pattern of physiological development, we compare the ontogeny of body oxygen stores in a phocid, the harbour seal (*Phoca vitulina*), and an otariid, the Steller sea lion (*Eumetopias jubatus*). Following a review of our work on age-related changes in haematology and body oxygen stores, we then present preliminary data on the iron status of juvenile and adult harbour seals. Limitations in iron intake have been implicated in developmental anaemia in terrestrial species that subsist on iron-poor milks [14,15]. Since heme levels strongly influence body oxygen stores, iron kinetics may also influence pinniped development [16,17]. We recognize that female harbour seals forage during the lactation period [4], and that this reduces the strength of our comparisons. However, because harbour seal pups demonstrate the rapid growth, large accumulations of lipid, and a short dependent period characteristic of most capital provisioned pups, we believe that the presented comparisons are valid.

2. Methods

2.1. Animal handling and oxygen store development

Data for harbour seals comes from work conducted in Monterey Bay, California from September 1997 through June 2000 (*n*=109) and Prince William Sound, Alaska in June 1998 and 1999 (*n*=113) [18], and 167 animals captured in Mont Joli, Quebec, Canada in the summers of 2000–2002 [16]. Steller sea lions (*n*=365) were captured throughout

Alaska in collaboration with Alaska Department of Fish and Game and the National Marine Mammal Laboratory [17]. At capture, all seals were weighed, sexed, and aged, and a subset of harbour seals handled in California ($n=63$) and Alaska ($n=58$) had their body composition determined by deuterium dilution [19]. To determine total body oxygen stores, an initial blood sample was collected from which haematocrit (HCT) and haemoglobin (Hb) were determined. Plasma volume was measured using the Evan's blue dye method [20], and blood volume (BV) was determined by dividing plasma volume by the measured HCT. Both blood and plasma volumes are reported on both an absolute and lean body mass-specific basis as available. Blood oxygen stores were determined following [21], using the individually measured HCT, Hb, and plasma volume. Muscle myoglobin content was determined from biopsy samples (<0.2 g) [22]. Total body oxygen stores were determined by adding the stores in lung, muscle and blood [21]. Further details on the capture and handling techniques, the methods used to measure body oxygen stores, and the statistical results are reported in the original publications from which this review is drawn [16–18].

2.2. Iron analyses

Iron status was determined for 73 harbour seals captured in Canada. Serum iron levels and total iron binding capacity (TIBC) were determined coulometrically using an ESA ferrochem II iron analyser [23]. Percent saturation was calculated as serum iron/TIBC. Serum ferritin concentration was measured by ELISA [24]. All iron assays were carried out at the Kansas State University College of Veterinary Medicine. General linear models were used to test for the effect of age and sex, and significant differences ($p<0.05$) identified by Bonferroni post hoc comparisons. To determine if iron status had a significant impact on blood oxygen stores, iron values were added as covariates to GLM models of age effects on oxygen stores. Prior to all analyses data normality was assessed using probability plots, and data transformed as necessary.

3. Results

3.1. Animal handling and oxygen store development

As expected, the growth rates and age-related changes in body composition differed between the two species. Harbour seals grew rapidly (0.56 ± 0.01 kg day^{-1}) over the ~25-day lactation period and body condition increased from 10% at birth to 39.4 ± 0.1% at weaning, before falling to an average value of 25.1 ± 1.3% in yearling and adults [18,25,26]. In contrast, Steller sea lions grew at a slower rate (as determined from average mass values for each age class) of 0.3 kg day^{-1} between 1 and 9 months of age, and 0.12 kg day^{-1} between 9 and 21 months of age [17].

As results from the development of oxygen stores in each of these groups have previously been presented [16–18], data are only summarized here. Typically, neonates had elevated HCT and Hb values, which declined in the first days (harbour seals) to weeks (Steller sea lions) of life, then increased later in the nursing period (Fig. 1). For harbour seals, this drop in HCT and Hb caused a decline in mass-specific blood oxygen stores during the lactation period, as all age classes except the relatively hydrated neonates had similar plasma volumes [16,18]. The decline in mass-specific blood oxygen stores could

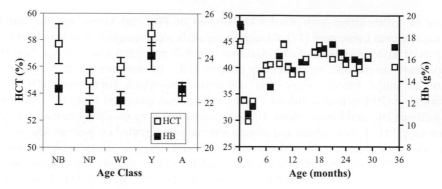

Fig. 1. Age-related changes in mean haematocrit (HCT) and haemoglobin (Hb) content in harbour seals from California [18], and Steller sea lions from Alaska ([17]; neonatal values from [28]). Harbour seal age categories are newborn (NB), nursing pup (NP), weaned (WP), yearling (Y), and adult (A).

not be attributed solely to age-related changes in body condition, as it persisted when stores were scaled to lean body mass [18]. Nor was there any effect of body composition on blood oxygen stores within any age class. In contrast, while Steller sea lions also showed elevated HCT, Hb, and plasma volumes in neonates [27,28], there was a gradual decline in mass-specific plasma volume over the first 21 months of life [17]. However, because HCT and Hb increased rapidly from 1 to 10 months (Fig. 1), blood oxygen stores were similar to those of adults by the end of the first year of life [17].

In harbour seals, muscle myoglobin concentration did not increase until after weaning, but reached adult values by the end of the first year of life [18]. There was no effect of body condition on muscle myoglobin concentration in any age class [18]. In contrast, average myoglobin levels increased gradually with age in nursing Steller sea lions, but did not reach adult levels until after the end of the second year [17].

Total body oxygen stores integrate all measured stores, and therefore also varied with age (Fig. 2). In harbour seals, total body oxygen stores declined with age from neonates through to weaning, and then increased in yearlings and adults, when measured on a mass-specific basis [16,18]. However, stores increased from birth to adulthood when measured

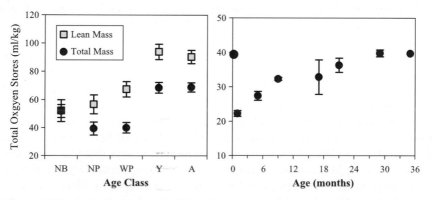

Fig. 2. Mean (±S.E.) total body oxygen stores for harbour seals, scaled to total and lean body mass [18], and Steller sea lions [14]. Neonatal Steller sea lion values taken from Ref. [27]. Age categories as in Fig. 1.

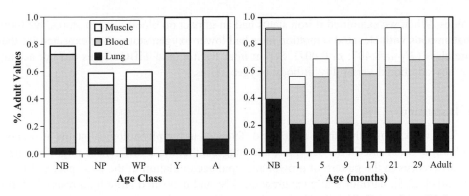

Fig. 3. Total body oxygen stores, as a percent of adult values, for harbour seals and Steller sea lions. Total stores are subdivided to show the relative contribution of lung, blood, and muscle oxygen stores. Age categories as in Fig. 1.

on a lean-body-mass basis [18]. In contrast, Steller sea lion total oxygen stores declined during the first month of life, but increased consistently after that, and reached adult values by the time juveniles were 21 months of age [17]. In both cases, the initial decline in oxygen stores was due to the early drop in HCT and Hb.

When the relative maturity of oxygen stores at different stages was compared between Steller sea lions and harbour seals, it was clear that while both species showed an initial decline in oxygen stores, harbour seals were not able to recover during the short nursing period, and so were weaned with oxygen stores that were small (52–60%) relative to those of adults [16,18]. In contrast, mass-specific oxygen stores increased during the lactation period in Steller sea lions, such that pups were weaned with stores very similar to those of adults (80–90%, depending on weaning age) (Fig. 3).

3.2. Iron status

There were significant age-related changes in serum iron, ferritin, and TIBC values with age, but no age-related differences in the percent saturation (Table 1). Serum iron and TIBC increased from neonates through early lactation, then declined to low values in weaned pups and adults (serum iron $F_{4,72}$=5.076, p=0.001, TIBC $F_{4,72}$=20.975, p<0.001). In contrast, serum ferritin levels were lowest in neonates, increased during lactation, and were highest in adults ($F_{4,72}$=13.728, p<0.001). In no case did sex influence parameter

Table 1
Mean (±S.E.) serum iron, ferritin, TIBC, and saturation values for harbour seals captured in Mont Joli, Canada in 2000 and 2001

Age class	n	Serum iron (μg dl^{-1})	Serum ferritin (ng ml^{-1})	TIBC (μg dl^{-1})	Saturation (%)
Neonates	15	369±37[a,b]	14±6[a]	572±19[a]	65.1±6.0
Early lactation	15	497±36[b]	35±6[b]	599±19[a]	80.6±6.0
Late lactation	14	475±38[b]	29±7[b]	582±20[a]	81.7±6.2
Weaned pups	13	311±40[a]	22±7[a,b]	442±21[b]	69.0±6.4
Adult females	13	260±38[a,b]	70±7	357±21[b]	68.9±6.4

Superscripts indicate that values were similar between age classes.

values. When we examined if iron status had an impact on blood oxygen stores, we found that animals with elevated saturation rates had lower oxygen stores than expected for their age class ($F_{1,39}=8.407$, $p=0.007$). Serum iron, ferritin, and TIBC values did not account for any additional variability in body oxygen stores.

4. Discussion

This work shows that there are clear differences in the physiological status at weaning of harbour seals and Steller sea lions, and suggests that these differences might be caused by differences in the pattern of growth and lipid accumulation in the two species. Like all phocids [1,2,5], harbour seal pups grew quickly, and deposited large lipid reserves during their short lactation period. Their rapid growth in body mass appears to outpace the development of new red cells, and as a result, oxygen storage capacity in the blood declines throughout the lactation period, when measured on both a lean and total body mass basis [16,18]. That this reduction in storage capacity is due to lagging red cell production rather than a decline in fluid volume is highlighted by the fact that plasma volume is similar in all age classes except the relatively hydrated neonates [16,18]. Since muscle oxygen stores do not increase during lactation, harbour seals are therefore weaned with oxygen stores that are less than 60% those of adult animals. Research on the physiological development of other phocid species has produced similar results: at the end of the postweaning fast, Weddell seals have oxygen stores that are 64% those of adults [11], Northern elephant seals (*Mirounga angust irotris*) 66% [9], hooded seals (*Cystophora cristata*) 62% [29], and grey seals (*Halichoerus gypus*) 67% [30]. The similarity of these values is remarkable, particularly given the large difference in the time between birth and independent foraging in these same species (32–82 days). We conclude that the pattern of physiological development reported here for harbour seals is a trait shared by all phocids, and therefore reflects constraints due to the capital provisioning strategy employed by most phocid females [1,2,31].

In contrast, Steller sea lions pups, like other otariids [3], grew more slowly over a much longer period of time, and deposited smaller lipid reserves than phocids [32]. Despite their slower growth rate, sea lions also showed a strong post-parturition anaemia, that was not relieved until 5 months of age, when pups swimming and diving activity increased [17,33,34]. As a result, blood volume and oxygen stores were relatively constant with age. This, in combination with increasing muscle oxygen stores, allowed juvenile Steller sea lions to increase their total body oxygen stores during the lactation period, so that oxygen stores were 69% those of adults when they began to dive, and 80–90% those of adults at weaning [17]. Data from other otariids suggest that the developmental pattern seen in Steller sea lions is characteristic of the group, and that most otariids are weaned with oxygen stores more similar to those of adults than seen in phocids [35–38].

Despite different patterns of physiological development, both harbour seals and Steller sea lions showed a strong early anaemia that coincided with the period of rapid growth and large gains in mass and lipid reserves. Developmental anaemia has been observed in many terrestrial species, and for rapidly growing neonates is typically attributed to an iron-poor milk diet [14,15]. Our examination of the iron status of harbour seal pups suggested their haematological development was also constrained by rates of iron intake during the period of most rapid growth. Iron stores (as indexed by serum ferritin) were low, and both TIBC and saturation levels were high in pups, as expected under conditions where iron is in high demand, but poorly available [39,40]. The similarly elevated saturation rates in lactating adult females may reflect the transfer of iron from tissue stores to milk. The remarkably high saturation rates (typical mammalian values are 20–30% [39,40]), and the negative correlation between saturation rates and oxygen stores further suggests that young juveniles may be constrained by both iron availability and the rate at which transport proteins can be produced [39,40]. While we do not yet have information on iron status in juvenile sea lions, northern fur seal (*Callorhinus ursinus*) pups have lower ferritin and higher TIBC values than do older animals [41], suggesting that the iron limitation observed in harbour seals may also exist in otariids. If iron limitation does contribute to the observed anaemia, then the postweaning increase in oxygen stores in harbour seals may result from intake of iron-rich prey items [15]. Similarly, supplemental foraging early in the lactation period may ameliorate early anaemia in Steller sea lions [33,34], just as it does in terrestrial species.

If iron kinetics influence oxygen store development, then it may also play a role in the postweaning fasts of phocid pups, a feature absent from the life history strategy of otariids [3]. Following weaning, many phocids fast on land for a period of days to weeks, and even those that do begin diving during lactation, such as harbour [42] and Weddell seals [43], apparently do not forage immediately upon weaning. Several studies have demonstrated that this fasting period is critical to proper physiological development, as body oxygen stores and the ability to regulate metabolic processes increase during the fast [9,30,44,45]. While increases in body oxygen stores during a period of fasting and mass loss are initially perplexing, we believe that this pattern can be explained by iron recycling. The majority (>80%) of a body's iron is stored in the erythron [46], and therefore changes in the size of the red cell pool has the potential to dramatically alter iron status. Because plasma volume is a constant proportion of body mass [16,18], as pups lose mass during the postweaning fast, absolute plasma volume drops. If red cells are not destroyed but retained in circulation, this will lead to an increase in HCT and blood volume, without any need for new cell production. For example, a 20% decline in the mass of harbour seal pups, as occurs in the weeks postweaning [42], would bring weaned pup HCT values to levels higher than those of adults, and increase blood volume from 12% to 14% of body mass. In addition, because iron is highly conserved [47], if some red cells are destroyed, their iron would then be available to support increases in muscle myoglobin content, as has been observed in fasting Northern elephant seal pups and emperor penguins [9,48].

Thus, the postweaning fast may allow phocid pups that rapidly gained mass (and blood volume) during the brief lactation period to reallocate iron stores, so that they can increase the size of oxygen stores relative to adult values during a period of mass loss. The similarity in relative maturity at the onset of foraging (~2/3 adult stores) across all phocids studied to date, suggests that there is a minimum threshold of maturity, below which foraging cannot be efficiently sustained. Since final completion of development only occurs postweaning, it likely requires additional nutritional input. Otariids, with their longer lactation period and slower growth rates are much more physiologically mature at weaning, and therefore may not require additional time to complete their physiological development.

Acknowledgements

The authors would like to thank the many people that made this research possible, in particular Dan Costa, Kathy Frost, Mike Hammill, Jim Harvey, Lorrie Rea, and Jason Schreer. Funding for harbour seal research in Canada was provided by the Department of Fisheries and Oceans, Canada, the Natural Sciences and Engineering Research Council of Canada, and NSF grant #EPS-0092040. Work in California and Alaska was funded by the University of California Office of the President and Institute of Marine Science. Sea lion research was funded by CIFAR (NA17RJ1224) and co-operative agreement with NOAA and ADFG (NA17FX1079). Work was carried out under Marine Mammal Protect Act permits 974, 2000, 358–1564, 782–1532, and 1003–1646. All protocols were reviewed and approved by the Institutional Animal Care and Use committees at UAA, UCSC, ADFG and DFO.

References

[1] I.L. Boyd, Time and energy constraints in pinniped lactation, Am. Nat. 152 (5) (1998) 717–728.
[2] K.M. Kovacs, D.M. Lavigne, Maternal investment and neonatal growth in phocid seals, J. Anim. Ecol. 55 (1986) 1035–1051.
[3] K.M. Kovacs, D.M. Lavigne, Maternal investment in otariid seals and walrus, Can. J. Zool. 70 (1992) 1953–1964.
[4] D.J. Boness, W.D. Bowen, O.T. Oftedal, Evidence of a maternal foraging cycle resembling that of otariid seals in a small phocid, the harbor seal, Behav. Ecol. Sociobiol. 34 (1994) 95–104.
[5] S.H. Ridgeway, et al., Diving and blood oxygen in the white whale, Can. J. Zool. 62 (1984) 2349–2351.
[6] D.J. Boness, W.D. Bowen, The evolution of maternal care in pinnipeds, Bioscience 46 (9) (1996) 645–654.
[7] T.M. Schulz, W.D. Bowen, Pinniped lactation strategies: evaluation of data on maternal and offspring life history traits, Mar. Mamm. Sci. 20 (1) (2004) 86–114.
[8] J.M. Burns, The development of diving behavior in juvenile Weddell seals: pushing physiological limits in order to survive, Can. J. Zool. 77 (1999) 773–783.
[9] P.H. Thorson, Development of diving in the northern elephant seal. PhD thesis University of California Santa Cruz, 1993.
[10] K.J. Frost, M.A. Simpkins, L.F. Lowry, Diving behavior of subadult and adult harbor seals in Prince William Sound, Alaska, Mar. Mamm. Sci. 17 (4) (2001) 813–834.
[11] J.M. Burns, M.A. Castellini, Physiological and behavioral determinants of the aerobic dive limit in Weddell seal (*Leptonychotes weddellii*) pups, J. Comp. Physiol. 166 (1996) 473–483.
[12] L. Irvine, et al., The influence of body size on dive duration of underyearling southern elephant seals (*Mirounga leonina*), J. Zool. Lond. 251 (2000) 463–471.
[13] M. Horning, F. Trillmich, Ontogeny of diving behavior in the Galapagos fur seal, Behaviorology 134 (15) (1997) 1211–1257.
[14] M.E. Fowler, Zoo and Wild Animal Medicine, 2nd ed., W.B. Saunders, Philadelphia, PA, 1986.
[15] K. Halvorsen, S. Halvorsen, The "early anemia": its relation to postnatal growth rate, milk feeding, and iron availability: experimental study in rabbits, Arch. Dis. Child. 48 (1973) 842–849.
[16] C.A. Clark, Tracking changes: postnatal blood and muscle oxygen store development in harbor seals (*Phoca vitulina*). MSc thesis University of Alaska Anchorage, 2004.
[17] J.P. Richmond, Ontogeny of total body oxygen stores and aerobic dive potential in the Steller sea lion (*Eumetopias jubatus*). MSc thesis University of Alaska Anchorage, 2004.
[18] J.M. Burns, et al., Development of body oxygen stores in harbor seals: effects of age, mass, and body composition, Physiol. Biochem. Zool. (2004), submitted.
[19] W.D. Bowen, S.J. Iverson, Estimation of total body water in pinnipeds using hydrogen-isotope dilution, Physiol. Zool. 71 (3) (1998) 329–332.

[20] N. Foldager, C.G. Blomqvist, Repeated plasma volume determination with the Evans blue dye dilution technique: the method and the computer program, Comput. Biol. Med. 21 (1/2) (1991) 35–41.

[21] G.L. Kooyman, et al., Aerobic diving limits of immature Weddell seals, J. Comp. Physiol. 151 (1983) 171–174.

[22] B. Reynafarje, Simplified method for the determination of myoglobin, J. Lab. Clin. Med. 61 (1963) 138–145.

[23] J.E. Smith, K. Moore, D. Schoneweis, Coulometric technique for iron determinations, Am. J. Vet. Res. 42 (1981) 1084–1087.

[24] G.A. Andrews, et al., Enzyme-linked immunosorbent assay to quantitate serum ferritin in the northern fur seal (*Callorhinus ursinus*), Zoo Biology 23 (2004) 79–84.

[25] Y. Dubé, M.O. Hammill, C. Barrette, Pup development and timing of pupping in harbour seals (*Phoca vitulina*) in the St. Lawrence River estuary, Canada, Can. J. Zool. 81 (2003) 188–194.

[26] W.D. Bowen, D.J. Boness, S.J. Iverson, Estimation of total body water in Harbor seals: how useful is bioelectrical impedance analysis? Mar. Mamm. Sci. 14 (4) (1998) 765–777.

[27] C. Lenfant, K. Johansen, J.D. Torrance, Gas transport and oxygen storage capacity in some pinnipeds and the sea otter, Respir. Physiol. 9 (1970) 277–286.

[28] L.D. Rea, et al., Health status of young Alaska Steller sea lion pups (*Eumetopias jubatus*) as indicated by blood chemistry and hematology, Comp. Biochem. Physiol. 120A (1998) 617–623.

[29] J.M. Burns, A.S. Blix, L.P. Folkow, Physiological constraint and diving ability: a test in hooded seals, *Cystophora cristata*, FASEB J. 14 (4) (2000) A440.

[30] S.R. Noren, et-al., The development of blood oxygen stores from birth through the postweaning fast of grey seal (*Halichoerus grypus*) pups: should they fast or forage? 15th Biennial Conference on the Biology of Marine Mammals, Greensboro, NC, USA 119, 2003.

[31] W.N. Bonner, Lactation strategies in pinnipeds: problems for a marine mammalian group, Symp. Zool. Soc. Lond. 51 (1984) 253–272.

[32] L.D. Rea, et-al., Percent total body lipid content increases in Steller sea lion (*Eumetopias jubatus*) pups throughout the first year of life in a similar pattern to other otariid pups. 15th Biennial Conference on the Biology of Marine Mammals, Greensboro, NC, USA, 2003, pp. 135.

[33] K.L. Raum-Suryan, et al., Dispersal, rookery fidelity, and metapopulation structure of Steller sea lions (*Eumetopias jubatus*) in an increasing and a decreasing population in Alaska, Mar. Mamm. Sci. 183 (3) (2002) 746–764.

[34] R.L. Merrick, T.R. Loughlin, Foraging behavior of adult female and young-of-the-year Steller sea lions in Alaskan waters, Can. J. Zool. 75 (5) (1997) 776–786.

[35] M.J. Donohue, Energetics and development of northern fur seal, *Callorhinus ursinus*, pups. PhD thesis, University of California Santa Cruz, 1998.

[36] M. Horning, F. Trillmich, Development of hemoglobin, hematocrit, and erythrocyte values in Galapagos fur seals, Mar. Mamm. Sci. 13 (1) (1997) 100–113.

[37] S.L. Fowler, D.P. Costa, Foraging in a nutrient-limited environment: development of diving in the threatened Australian sea lion, *Neophoca cinerea*. 15th Biennial Conference on the Biology of Marine Mammals, Greensboro, NC, USA 54, 2003.

[38] J.P.Y. Arnould, et-al., Lean and fast, fat and slow: the comparative growth strategies of sympatric Antarctic and subantarctic fur seal pups, Crozet Archipelago.15th Biennial Conference on the Biology of Marine Mammals, Greensboro, NC, USA 8, 2003.

[39] P. Ponka, Regulation of heme biosynthesis: distinct control mechanisms in erythroid cells, Blood 89 (1) (1997) 1–25.

[40] C.A. Finch, H. Huebers, Perspectives in iron metabolism, N. Engl. J. Med. 306 (25) (1982) 1520–1528.

[41] L.M. Mazzaro, et al., Serum indices of body stores of iron in Northern fur seals (*Callorhinus urisnus*) and their relationship to hemochromatosis, Zoobiology 23 (2004) 205–218.

[42] M.M.C. Muelbert, W.D. Bowen, Duration of lactation and postweaning changes in mass and body composition of harbour seal, *Phoca vitulina*, pups, Can. J. Zool. 71 (1993) 1405–1414.

[43] J.M. Burns, J.W. Testa, Developmental changes and diurnal and seasonal influences on the diving behavior of Weddell seal (*Leptonychotes weddellii*) pups, in: B. Battaglia, J. Valencia, D.W.H. Walton (Eds.), Antarctic Communities, Cambridge University Press, Cambridge, 1997, pp. 328–334.

[44] S. Kohin, Respiratory physiology of northern elephant seal pups: adaptations for hypoxia, hypercapnia and hypometabolism. PhD thesis, University of California Santa Cruz, 1998.

[45] T. Zenteno-Savin, Physiology of the endocrine, cardiorespiratory and nervous systems in pinnipeds. Integrative approach and biomedical considerations. PhD thesis University of Alaska Fairbanks, 1997.

[46] H.G. van Eijk, G. de Jong, The physiology of iron, transferrin, and ferritin, Biol. Trace Elem. Res. 35 (1992) 13–24.

[47] J.H. Jandl, J.H. Katz, The plasma-to-cell cycle of transferrin, J. Clin. Invest. 42 (1963) 314.

[48] P.J. Ponganis, et al., Development of diving capacity in emperor penguins, J. Exp. Biol. 202 (1999) 781–786.

International Congress Series 1275 (2004) 351–358

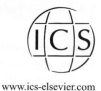

www.ics-elsevier.com

The energetics of foraging in large mammals: a comparison of marine and terrestrial predators

Terrie M. Williams*, Laura Yeates

Department of Ecology and Evolutionary Biology, Center for Ocean Health-Long Marine Laboratory, 100 Shaffer Road, University of California at Santa Cruz, Santa Cruz, CA 95060, USA

Abstract. The combination of large body size, carnivory and endothermic costs leads to high caloric demands in many mammalian predators. Tactics used to capture prey to meet these demands vary among mammals, and ranges from prolonged tracking to high-speed chases. Furthermore, accessibility to air differs for species that hunt in water or on land. To determine the behavioral and energetic consequences of these different foraging methods and habitats, we measured the energetic cost of hunting, energy acquired from ingested prey, and patterns of energy acquisition in free-ranging Weddell seals (body mass=461 kg) and sea otters (mass=25 kg). The values were then compared to terrestrial predators ranging in mass from 25 to 170 kg. We found that foraging dive duration was 2.4±0.4 min for otters and 16.3±0.6 min for seals, and that dives were interspersed with short to moderate duration rest periods. In contrast, large terrestrial mammals hunted in one to two sessions per day that lasted several hours. The efficiency of an individual hunting event ranged from 3.8 in the sea otter to 10.2 for Weddell seals. This compared to 2.2 for African wild dogs and 3.8 for African lions feeding on ungulates. In general, adaptations for marine living including elevated basal metabolic rates and the dive response represent major influences on hunting efficiency that is further modified by the energetic cost of specific hunting tactics. © 2004 Elsevier B.V. All rights reserved.

Keywords: Foraging; Energetics; Carnivore; Marine mammal; Hunting efficiency

1. Introduction

Survival by large carnivorous mammals requires a continuous balance between energy expended in daily living and energy acquired by hunting [1]. To accomplish the latter,

---

* Corresponding author. Tel.: +1 831 459 5123; fax: +1 831 459 3383.
E-mail address: williams@biology.ucsc.edu (T.M. Williams).

0531-5131/ © 2004 Elsevier B.V. All rights reserved.
doi:10.1016/j.ics.2004.08.069

mammalian predators display a wide range of techniques for locating, capturing and killing prey. In the terrestrial environment, hunting behaviours range from the cautious stalk and ambush of leopards [2] to the high-speed chases of cheetahs [3]. Among the large canids and felids, hunting can be a coordinated group activity as exemplified by African wild dogs and African lions [4,5] or solitary forays as typically displayed by cheetahs [3], leopards [4] and many species of foxes [2]. Depending on the size of the predator and hunting style, numerous small prey or single large prey items may be taken to satisfy daily energy needs.

Many of the same hunting strategies can be found among marine mammal predators. Seals may use high-speed chases after locating prey [6], while mysticete whales slowly sieve through swarms of krill [7]. Like terrestrial carnivores, marine mammals have been observed to forage in cooperative units [8] as well as acting as solitary hunters [6].

Although large terrestrial and marine predators display many similar hunting tactics, the constraints on acquiring prey differ markedly. Sensory modalities used to detect prey, and thermal and locomotor costs differ due to the unique physical characteristics of air and water [9]. Perhaps, the most obvious difference between these two hunting environments is the accessibility to air. Unlike terrestrial mammals, aquatic mammals must shuttle between two important resources when hunting, oxygen in air above the water surface and the prey located at depth. The result is a marked effect on foraging behaviour and economics [10–12].

In view of the diverse methods of hunting and the constraints imposed by different habitats, we would expect that energetic costs and benefits associated with foraging differ for marine and terrestrial carnivores. To address this, we determined the cost of hunting for two species of marine mammal, the Weddell seal (*Leptonychotes weddellii*) and sea otter (*Enhydra lutris*) representing large and small species with different foraging styles. Energetic cost of hunting dives, energy acquired from ingested prey, and patterns of energy acquisition determined from daily activity budgets were assessed. Results for the marine mammals were compared to the published values for terrestrial mammals including the African wild dog (*Lycaon pictus*) and African lion (*Panthera leo*). We found that the cost of hunting differed between the two marine mammals as well as between marine and terrestrial carnivores. Moreover, daily energetic balance depended on whether the mammal hunted on land or in water.

2. Materials and methods

2.1. Animals

Four adult female Weddell seals (body mass=461.3±36.1 kg) and one adult female sea otter (estimated body mass=25.0 kg) were used in the behavioural field studies. The seals were captured with a purse-string net on the sea ice near Ross Island (McMurdo Sound, Antarctica) in November and December of 2002. After a 24- to 48-h holding period, the animals were instrumented with a video-data recording system and swimming stroke monitor as described in Davis et al. [6] and Williams et al. [13]. Following instrumentation, the animals were released into a diving hole in the ice and were free to forage, move throughout the Sound, and dive to the ocean bottom at approximately 585 m in depth. After 4–8 days, the instruments were removed for data and video retrieval. The sea otter used in this study was 1 of 45 study animals captured with diver-held Wilson traps along the coast of San Simeon, CA during October 2001–2003. All otters were surgically implanted with a calibrated temperature-sensitive VHF radio transmitter (Advanced Telemetry Systems, Isanti, MN) and provided with a color-coded flipper tag according to Tinker [14]. Following instrumentation, the otters were immediately released at the point of capture. Behaviour of free-ranging sea otters was monitored over a 2-year period following instrumentation.

In addition to the behavioral studies, the energetic cost of diving was determined for nine wild, adult Weddell seals (1 female, 8 males; body mass=387.4±6.6 kg) diving from an isolated hole in McMurdo Sound [15], and for two captive, adult male sea otters (body mass=26.0±1.0 kg) diving in a 9.1 m deep water tower. The sea otters were maintained in outdoor fiberglass holding pools (4.2 m diameter, 1.2 m deep; 6.0 m diameter, 1.5 m deep) at the California Department of Fish and Game (Santa Cruz, CA) and fed a mixed invertebrate diet. Fresh seawater was continuously added to the pools at ambient ocean temperatures. On test days, the otters were moved to the diving tower for approximately 1 h metabolic trials.

2.2. Oxygen consumption during diving

The energetic cost of diving was determined from the difference between resting and recovery oxygen consumption of Weddell seals and sea otters immediately following individual dives. Details of the open flow respirometry system, experimental protocol, and analysis for Weddell seals have been presented in Williams et al. [13]. An identical respirometry system was used for sea otters trained to dive in a seawater storage tower (6.0 m diameter, 9.1 m deep, UCSC). Measurements were made on post-absorptive animals as confirmed by video recordings (Weddell seals) or by a 12-h overnight fast (trained sea otters). Breathing by all diving animals was limited to a Plexiglas dome mounted at water level over the isolated ice hole or water tower. Subsamples of the dome exhaust were dried (Drierite, Hammond Drierite, OH) and scrubbed of carbon dioxide (Sodasorb, Chemetron, MO) before entering an oxygen analyzer (model FC1-B, Sable Systems, Henderson, NV). Air was pulled through the domes at 80–510 l min^{-1} using a vacuum pump (Sears Wet/Dry Vac, Chicago, IL) or mass flow meter (Sable Systems, Henderson, NV). Oxygen content of the samples was logged every 0.5–1.0 s on a laptop computer and the rate of oxygen consumption calculated using the equations of Davis et al. [16]. All values were corrected to STPD and each system was calibrated daily with nitrogen and standard gases according to Fedak et al. [17].

2.3. Hunting behaviour and activity budgets

Underwater behaviours of the Weddell seals were monitored continuously using a video-data logging system carried by the animal as it dove below the sea ice. Details of the instrumentation, attachment procedures, and analyses have been described previously [6,13,18]. A low light-sensitive camera with an array of near-infrared LEDs was mounted on a neoprene patch that was glued on the fur of the head. The camera provided a view of the seal's eyes and muzzle, and of the water for approximately 70 cm in front of the nose. Video images were recorded and synchronized in real time with dive depth that was monitored with a pressure transducer. All videos were screened for encounters with prey. Mouth movements were not in the field of view; therefore, we used visual detection of prey within 10 cm of the Weddell seal's muzzle and coincident head movements to denote fish ingestion. Daily activity budgets of the Weddell seals were reconstructed from the video recordings and divided into dive and rest periods. Because the animals rested submerged, on the water surface and lying on the ice, rest periods included all quiescent times when the seals were hauled out or at <50 m in depth. Only dives in which seals fed exclusively on Antarctic silverfish (*Pleuragramma antarcticum*) were analysed in this study.

Daily activity pattern and prey consumption of sea otters were determined by 24 h observation sessions using a 30× spotting scope (Questar, Isanti, MN) following the methods of Ralls and Siniff [19]. Surface and submerged activities were determined from changes in the character of the transmitted radio signals (i.e. interrupted signals represented diving bouts), making it possible to measure activity patterns and time budgets during the hours of darkness. Parameters recorded included behaviour (rest, grooming, swimming, diving and feeding), duration of surface and submerged intervals, and size and identification of prey species ingested. These data were correlated to time, location, and weather conditions. Prey identification during daylight hours was facilitated by the surface feeding behaviour of sea otters and their coastal location. For this study, we assumed that prey specialists did not change the type of prey consumed during the night, and estimated nocturnal prey ingestion according to Ralls et al. [20].

2.4. Hunting efficiency

The efficiency of hunting was defined as the ratio of energy acquired from the ingestion of prey to the energy expended during a single hunting event. Hunting events for marine mammals were delimited by individual dives in which prey were encountered (seals) or brought to the water surface (otters). For Weddell seals, the energy acquired was determined from the average number of fish ingested on a foraging dive and an average caloric content of 78 kcal (325 kJ) per fish [21]. The energy expended for hunting was calculated from the average duration of individual foraging dives and the relationship between oxygen consumption and dive duration (Eq. (3) in Ref. [13]). Similarly, the energy acquired by sea otters eating turban snails (*Tegula* spp.) was calculated from the average number of snails obtained on an individual dive with a caloric value of 2 kcal (8.3 kJ) per g snail [22]. The energy expended for hunting was calculated as for seals using the average duration of foraging dives and the rate of oxygen consumption measured for the same dive duration in the water tower.

Comparative values for hunting efficiency by African hunting dogs and African lions were calculated from published values for daily prey ingestion rates and energetic costs of hunting. These species were chosen due to their body size, carnivorous diet, and availability of data. Ingested energy from prey was calculated from the average mass and caloric content of prey consumed during individual hunting events. On average, food intake by wild dogs is approximately 3.5 kg meat per day [23] generally made in two separate kills [4]. We assumed that 75% of the intake was lean meat at 193 kcal 100 g^{-1} (808 kJ 100 g^{-1}) and 25% was viscera at 130 kcal 100 g^{-1} (544 kJ 100 g^{-1}) [24]. The energetic cost of hunting for wild dogs taken from Gorman et al. [23] was divided into two hunting periods per day. For lions, we used an average gorging of 7–11 kg of meat and viscera from a single kill in the evening [4] with the same caloric values as above. Energetic cost of the hunt by lions was calculated from activity budgets of nomadic males from Schaller [4] assuming that resting periods constituted basal metabolic rate (BMR) levels. BMR was determined from the regression for vertebrate eaters from McNab [25] using an average body mass of 170 kg. The difference between daily field metabolic rate (10,549 kcal day^{-1} or 511 W; Williams, unpublished data) and energy utilized for resting periods (5485 kcal day^{-1} or 266 W) represents the energy available for walking, killing and feeding. Because actual hunting periods for lions are difficult to define [4], we used the entire difference to represent the cost of hunting; that is, when the lions were not resting they were conducting activities associated with hunting. All values for hunting efficiency represent total energy utilization and acquisition, and do not include corrections for assimilation efficiency.

3. Results

3.1. Hunting behaviour and activity budgets

Despite differences in predatory tactics, the pattern of hunting and prey acquisition showed many similarities for Weddell seals and sea otters (Fig. 1; Table 1). For both marine mammals, foraging dives were interspersed with short to intermediate duration rest periods on the water surface. For example, one free-ranging seal foraging in McMurdo Sound during the austral summer made 25 dives during a 24-h period of which 24 involved encounters with Antarctic silverfish. Total time for deep (>50 m) foraging dives was 471 min. This

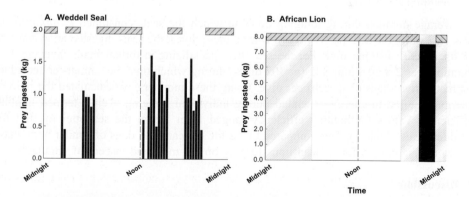

Fig. 1. Feeding patterns for large marine and terrestrial mammals. Daily activity pattern and prey ingestion during a hunting day are compared for an adult Weddell seal feeding on Antarctic silverfish (A) and for a nomadic African lion feeding on ungulates (B). Vertical bars represent the timing and mass of fish consumed for individual dives by the seal, and timing and mass of meat eaten in a single day by the lion. Rest periods are denoted by the horizontal, hatched grey bars at the top of each figure. Data for the seal is from the present study and for the lion is from Schaller [4]. Periods of darkness are shown by the shaded areas. Note that during the austral summer in McMurdo Sound, there is constant sunlight.

Table 1
Hunting efficiency of marine and terrestrial carnivores

	Hunt duration (min)	Hunt cost (ml O_2 kg^{-1})	kcal expended	kcal ingested	Efficiency
Marine					
Sea otter (25 kg)	2.4±0.4	45.4	5	19	3.8
Weddell seal (461 kg)	16.3±0.6	69.2±3.1	137±7	1397±77	10.2±0.7
Terrestrial					
Wild dog (25 kg)	104	–	1288	2836	2.2
African lion (170 kg)	180	–	5062	19,498	3.8

For marine mammals a hunting event is defined as a single dive.
A hunting event by terrestrial mammals is defined by the period to bring down a single prey item. Values are shown as mean±S.E. n=37 dives for four Weddell seals feeding on Antarctic silverfish and n=302 dives for one sea otter specializing on turban snails. Values for African wild dogs were derived from Gorman et al. [23] and for African lions from Schaller [4] as described in the text.

compares with 969 min spent in shallow water or resting on the surface in periods ranging from approximately 20 min to two longer periods exceeding 9 h each (Fig. 1). Overall, the seal spent 41.1% feeding and the remainder of the time resting or at shallow depths.

Similarly, sea otters interspersed foraging bouts with resting and grooming periods of 20–310 min. Because sea otters showed considerable individual preferences for specific prey, we will focus the remainder of the discussion on one specialist feeding on turban snails, a common prey item for this species [14]. This otter preformed nearly continuous 2.4 min dives (Table 1) during 60–200 min foraging bouts that occurred day and night, only taking the time to consume the prey between dives. Overall, the otter spent 50.4% of the day diving for snails, 31.5% resting on the water surface, and 18.1% in other activities including grooming and surface swimming.

3.2. Hunting efficiency

Average duration during foraging dives in which the seals consumed *P. antarcticum* was 16.3 min±0.6 S.E. (n=37 dives). During these dives, the seals ingested an average of 18.0±1.0 S.E. fish per dive. For the sea otter specializing in turban snails, average dive duration was 2.4±0.4 min S.E. (n=302 dives) during which time the animals collected an estimated five snails (3 g each) per dive. Using these numbers, we calculated the ratio of energy acquired to energy expended during individual foraging events, termed hunting efficiency. Values for hunting efficiency ranged from 3.8 in the sea otter to 10.2 for Weddell seals (Table 1). This compared to 2.2 for African wild dogs of similar body mass to sea otters, and 3.8 for African lions feeding on the meat and viscera of ungulates.

4. Discussion

A major difference in foraging behaviour between marine and terrestrial carnivores is the duration of individual hunting or predation events (Fig. 1). Due to constraints associated with access to air during predation, marine mammals must acquire prey in relatively short forays [10–12]. Thus, the duration of individual foraging dives was only 2.4–16.3 min in sea otters and Weddell seals. This compares with hunting events that often last several hours in large terrestrial carnivores depending on the size of the prey taken [4].

Such an intermittent style of energy acquisition, while disruptive to rest periods, did not necessarily result in low hunting efficiencies for marine mammals. Rather, the energy expended relative to the energy gained per hunting event was equal to or greater in marine mammals than in the terrestrial mammals examined here (Table 1).

The highest hunting efficiency for an individual predation event was observed for Weddell seals and exceeded those of sea otters, wild dogs, and lions by nearly threefold. This could be attributed to the exceptionally low energetic cost of individual dives by the seals, which were associated with metabolic responses occurring with prolonged submergence [26]. Because hunting efficiency depends on the time scale examined, differences between terrestrial and marine carnivores was altered and become less distinct when examined for a 24-h period. For example, the 391 kg Weddell seal in Fig. 1 performed 24 foraging dives resulting in a daily energy expenditure for hunting of 3295 kcal (13,807 kJ). The resulting daily hunting efficiency of 5.1 for Weddell seals was only 34% higher than for African lions.

These results only apply to hunting days, which differ in the pattern of occurrence for the species examined. Sea otters [19], African wild dogs [23], and lions [4] generally hunt daily or within a few days after feeding. These three species generally take in sufficient calories to in a single hunting day to meet the metabolic needs of the animal for 1–3 days. Thus, the snail hunting sea otter in this study obtained 5647 kcal (23,663 kJ) in 302 dives to support a daily field energy requirement (based on time energy budgets) of 4887 kcal (20,478 kJ). Observations showed that this animal fed daily. In comparison, the terrestrial species take in enough food to support the animals for several days. The unusual species in this regard was the Weddell seal. With the energetic cost of a foraging dive averaging 137 kcal (575 kJ, Table 1) and each fish representing 78 kcal (325 kJ), an adult Weddell seal would need to consume 2 fish to remain in caloric balance [21]. However, once in an aggregation of silverfish, Weddell seals will consume 18–20 fish (approximately 900–1000 g) before terminating a foraging dive, and then continue to ingest fish at this rate on several subsequent dives (Fig. 1). On any individual foraging dive, Weddell seals will consume 11 times the calories required to account for the cost of hunting, or 2 times its daily caloric demands.

Based on these results, we find that a marine lifestyle represents a major influence on hunting behaviour and efficiency in large mammals. For both marine and terrestrial species, hunting efficiency and the resultant daily caloric balance is further modified by the energetic cost of specific hunting tactics. Admittedly, the cost of locating prey, the predictability and abundance of prey, and the number of successful and unsuccessful capture attempts will impact hunting efficiency, especially as marine and terrestrial habitats are altered. In view of this, further investigation concerning the relationship between energy resources provided by the environment and the physiological capabilities and limitations of energy acquisition in large predators is warranted.

Acknowledgements

This research was supported by grants from the National Science Foundation (Office of Polar Programs) and Minerals Management Service. Special thanks to L. Fuiman for insightful comments on the manuscript, W. Hagey (Pisces Designs) and R. Davis for the development of the video and data recorders for the seals, and M. Rutishauser, T. Fink, B.

Long, and J. Gafney for assistance with the otters. All experimental procedures followed NIH guidelines and were evaluated and approved by institutional Animal Use Committees.

References

[1] D.W. Stephens, J.R. Krebs, Foraging Theory, Princeton University Press, Princeton, 1986.

[2] R.D. Estes, Behavior Guide to African Mammals, University of California Press, Berkeley, 1991.

[3] T.M. Caro, Cheetahs of the Serengeti Plains, The University of Chicago Press, Chicago, 1994.

[4] G.B. Schaller, The Serengeti Lion, The University of Chicago Press, Chicago, 1972.

[5] C. Packer, D. Scheel, A.E. Pusey, Why lions form groups: food is not enough, Am. Nat. 136 (1) (1990) 1–19.

[6] R.W. Davis, et al., Hunting behavior of a marine mammal beneath the Antarctic fast ice, Science 283 (1999) 993–996.

[7] A. Acevedo-Gutierrez, D.A. Croll, B.R. Tershy, High feeding costs limit dive time in the largest whales, J. Exp. Biol. 205 (2002) 1747–1753.

[8] R.W. Baird, H. Whitehead, Social organization of mammal-eating killer whales: group stability and dispersal patterns, Can. J. Zool. 78 (2000) 2096–2105.

[9] P. Dejours, Water and air physical characteristics, in: P. Dejours, L. Bolis, C.R. Taylor, E.R. Weibel (Eds.), Comparative Physiology: Life in Water and on Land, Springer Fidia Research Series, New York, 1987, pp. 3–11.

[10] N. Dunstone, R.J. O'Connor, Optimal foraging in an amphibious mammal: I. The aqualung effect, Anim. Behav. 27 (1979) 1182–1194.

[11] N. Dunstone, R.J. O'Connor, Optimal foraging in an amphibious mammal: II. A study using principal component analysis, Anim. Behav. 27 (1979) 1195–1201.

[12] D.L. Kramer, The behavioral ecology of air breathing by aquatic animals, Can. J. Zool. 66 (1988) 89–94.

[13] T.M. Williams, et al., The cost of foraging by a marine predator, the Weddell seal Leptonychotes weddellii: pricing by the stroke, J. Exp. Biol. 207 (6) (2004) 973–982.

[14] M.T. Tinker, Sources of variation in the foraging behavior and demography of the sea otter, Enhydra lutris. PhD thesis, University of California, Santa Cruz, 2004.

[15] G.L. Kooyman, et al., Pulmonary gas exchange in freely diving Weddell seals, Res. Physiol. 17 (1977) 283–290.

[16] R.W. Davis, T.M. Williams, G.L. Kooyman, Swimming metabolism of yearling and adult harbor seals Phoca vitulina, Physiol. Zool. 58 (1985) 590–596.

[17] M.A. Fedak, L. Rome, H.J. Seeherman, One-step N_2 dilution technique for calibrating open-circuit O_2 measuring systems, J. Appl. Physiol. 51 (1981) 772–776.

[18] L.A. Fuiman, R.W. Davis, T.M. Williams, Behavior of midwater fishes under the Antarctic ice: observations by a predator, Mar. Biol. 140 (2002) 815–822.

[19] K. Ralls, D.B. Siniff, Time budgets and activity patterns in California sea otters, J. Wildl. Manage. 54 (1990) 251–259.

[20] K. Ralls, B.B. Hatfield, D.B. Siniff, Foraging patterns of California sea otters as indicated by telemetry, Can. J. Zool.-Rev. Can. Zool. 73 (1995) 523–531.

[21] M.A. Castellini, R.W. Davis, G.L. Kooyman, Annual Cycles of Diving Behavior and Ecology of the Weddell Seal, Bulletin of the Scripps Institution of Oceanography, University of California, San Diego, vol. 28, University of California Press, Berkeley, 1992.

[22] E.R. Farout, J.A. Ames, D.P. Costa, Analysis of sea otter (Enhydra lutris) scats collected from a California haulout site, Mar. Mamm. Sci. 2 (1986) 223–227.

[23] M.L. Gorman, et al., High hunting costs make African wild dogs vulnerable to kleptoparasitism by hyaenas, Nature 391 (1998) 479–481.

[24] Geigy Scientific Tables, Units of measurement, body fluids, composition of the body, nutrition, vol. 1, CIBA-GEIGY, Basle, 1981.

[25] B.K. McNab, Complications inherent in scaling the basal rate of metabolism in mammals, Q. Rev. Biol. 63 (1) (1988) 25–54.

[26] G.L. Kooyman, Diverse Divers, Springer-Verlag, Berlin, 1989.

International Congress Series 1275 (2004) 359–366

www.ics-elsevier.com

When does physiology limit the foraging behaviour of freely diving mammals?

Daniel P. Costa[a,*], Carey E. Kuhn[a], Michael J. Weise[a], Scott A. Shaffer[a], John P.Y. Arnould[b]

[a]Department of Ecology and Evolutionary Biology, University of California, 100 Shaffer Road, Santa Cruz, CA 95060-5730, USA
[b]School of Biological and Chemical Sciences, Deakin University, Burwood, VIC 3125, Australia

Abstract. Diving animals offer a unique opportunity to study the importance of physiological constraint and the limitation it can impose on animal's behaviour in nature. This paper examines the interaction between physiology and behaviour and its impact on the diving capability of five eared seal species (Family Otariidae; three sea lions and two fur seals). An important physiological component of diving marine mammals is the aerobic dive limit (ADL). The ADL of these five seal species was estimated from measurements of their total body oxygen stores, coupled with estimates of their metabolic rate while diving. The tendency of each species to exceed its calculated ADL was compared relative to its diving behaviour. Overall, our analyses reveal that seals which forage benthically (i.e. on the sea floor) have a greater tendency to approach or exceed their ADL compared to seals that forage epipelagically (i.e. near the sea surface). Furthermore, the marked differences in foraging behaviour and physiology appear to be coupled with a species demography. For example, benthic foraging species have smaller populations and lower growth rates compared to seal species that forage epipelagically. These patterns are relevant to the conservation and management of diving vertebrates. © 2004 Published by Elsevier B.V.

Keywords: Aerobic dive limit; Diving; Foraging; Physiological constraint; Pinnipeds

1. Introduction

While comparative physiology documents the range of physiological variation across organisms, field physiology provides insight into the homeostatic mechanisms that animals

---

* Corresponding author. Tel.: +1 831 459 2786; fax: +1 831 459 3383.
E-mail address: costa@biology.ucsc.edu (D.P. Costa).

0531-5131/ © 2004 Published by Elsevier B.V.
doi:10.1016/j.ics.2004.08.058

actually employ in nature. In addition, understanding an animal's natural history is a prerequisite for designing meaningful field investigations that integrate physiology with behaviour and ecology [1]. In this context, pinnipeds (seals and sea lions) provide a unique system to study the role of physiology and its impact or constraint on the foraging ecology and behaviour of diving vertebrates. Pinnipeds are tractable study organisms because they have an amphibious life style so they can be captured on shore multiple times to deploy and recover instrumentation to study their behaviour at sea as well as to collect measurements for physiological evaluation [2–4]. Consequently, there is a reasonable understanding of the basic physiological processes that occur when animals dive. We know that the ultimate constraint on diving ability is determined by an animal's physiological performance. However, within these limits, the range of diving behaviour is determined by ecological factors such as the distribution, abundance, depth, and energy content of prey [5]. Technological developments over the last two decades have significantly increased our ability to study the behaviour of diving animals in nature [6–8]. These studies as well as many others have recorded a wide range of behavioural patterns, and have implicated physiology as a limiting or enabling feature of a species performance [3,6,7,9,10].

The diving capability of a marine mammal is determined by its available oxygen and fuel stores and the rate they are consumed by metabolic processes [6]. The quantity of oxygen and metabolic fuels stored in tissues can differ substantially among marine mammals, but their consumption occurs via aerobic or anaerobic pathways [6]. The time required to consume fuels aerobically while diving is thought to be the major determinant of diving performance [3,4,6,7,10]. Hence, the aerobic dive limit (ADL) has been experimentally defined as the dive duration beyond which blood lactate levels increase above resting levels due to anaerobic metabolism [3]. When Weddell seals (*Leptonychotes weddelli*) exceed the aerobic threshold, the post-dive surface interval increases disproportionately faster than dive duration [3,11]. An increased surface interval is required to clear lactic acid accumulated during the previous dive. One of the disadvantages of exceeding the ADL is that, while a diver may increase the duration of a single dive, the total accumulated time spent underwater in a bout of dives is reduced because more time at the surface is required to clear lactic acid. Although the relationship between physiology and behaviour is fairly well documented for Weddell seals, the relationship is far less clear among other pinniped species.

In this paper, we extend our earlier examination [12] of this relationship between aerobic dive limit and foraging behaviour to include new information on other species of otariids (i.e. eared seals). More importantly, we review our analyses in light of both ecological and demographic implications. In total, our analyses include data for five otariid species that represent the extremes of diving behaviours reported for otariids. The Antarctic fur seal (*Arctocephalus gazella*) makes short shallow dives, while the Australian (*Neophoca cinerea*) and New Zealand (*Phocarctos hookeri*) sea lions and the Australian fur seal (*A. pusillus doriferus*) make deep prolonged dives to the benthos [13–17]. We also include data from California sea lions (*Zalophus californianus*) foraging off the California coast where they dive epipelagically [18], and from the Sea of Cortez where they forage quite deep on mesopelagic prey [Kuhn, Aurioles-Gamboa, Costa unpublished]. Like our earlier study [12], we compare the differences in diving behaviour and calculated aerobic dive limit (cADL) between individual animals. In this way, we elucidate intra- and interspecific variation in the tendency of individuals to reach or exceed their cADLs and, thus, gain insight into the diving performance of free-ranging animals in nature.

2. Methods and materials

Individual specific cADL for adult females of 11 Australian sea lions, 11 New Zealand sea lions, 10 California sea lions, 9 Australian fur seals and 15 Antarctic fur seals were determined by dividing each animal's total available oxygen stores by its specific diving metabolic rate (DMR). DMR was assumed to be equivalent to the at-sea field metabolic rate (FMR), which can be measured by oxygen-18 doubly labelled water [19]. It is important to note that at-sea FMR integrates the costs of highly variable surface swimming, diving and resting. Therefore, true DMR could be higher or lower. Nevertheless, DMR estimated in our analyses should reflect relative differences in metabolic effort between individuals. Furthermore, no measures of blood lactate were collected to confirm the true ADL of our study animals so we refer to our estimates as cADL.

The total available oxygen store of each animal was calculated following methods described elsewhere [20,21] with the incorporation of data on blood volume [22] [Weise, Arnould, Shaffer and Costa unpublished data] and muscle myoglobin [23], [Costa, Gales, Weise, Arnould, Shaffer, Crocker and Burns, unpublished data] content for each species (Table 1).

The data on diving behaviour of Antarctic and Australian fur seals, and Australian and New Zealand sea lions were taken from published reports on each species [14–17]. Information on the diving behaviour of California sea lions comes from recently acquired unpublished data from six females at San Nicolas Island, Channel Islands, California, and from four females at Los Islotes Island, Bay of La Paz, Baja California [Kuhn, Aurioles-Gamboa, and Costa unpublished data]. Measurements of metabolic rate and diving behaviour for Australian and New Zealand sea lion, and Antarctic fur seals were collected concurrently on the same individuals [14–16]. DMR of California sea lions were obtained from previously published FMR data [5] and DMR for Australian fur seals were derived from FMRs acquired on Antarctic fur seals normalized for differences in body mass [24].

Table 1
The summary of parameters used to determine cADL of otariids

Species	Mass (kg)	Diving behaviour		O$_2$ stores (ml O$_2$ kg^{-1})	FMR (kJ kg^{-1} min^{-1})	cADL (min)
		Depth (m)	Duration (min)			
Epi/Mesopelagic						
Antarctic fur seal	41.8	23	1.16	38.1	29.6	1.6
California sea lion	85.3	42.2	1.93	42.7	15.6	2.7
Mesopelagic						
California sea lion	102.0	125	4.18	58.6	15.6	3.8
Benthic						
Australian fur seal	77.7	64	3.20	49.9	29.6	1.7
Australian sea lion	79.2	59	3.21	41.9	22.0	2.3
New Zealand sea lion	112.5	124	3.40	45.7	20.2	2.3

3. Results

The results show that oxygen storage capacity differs between each species of otariid (Table 1). As oxygen storage capacity increases among species, there is a significant increase in dive duration (Fig. 1). Concomitantly, all five species exhibit differences in their tendency to exceed the cADL according to their foraging mode (Fig. 2). That is, otariid species that forage benthically appear to operate well above the cADL whereas the species that forage epipelagically appear to operate well within the cADL. Furthermore, our data not only support this general pattern but also they shows that diving performance varies within a species, reflecting the different environments that these animals forage within. For example, California sea lions foraging off the Southern California coast (i.e. San Nicolas Island) routinely make relatively short shallow (epipelagic) dives and forage on surface prey [25], whereas sea lions foraging off Los Islotes consistently make deeper, longer dives to feed on mesopelagic prey (Fig. 2 and Ref. [26]).

4. Discussion

Our data support the hypothesis that there is significant inter- and intra-specific variation in the tendency of otariids to reach their maximum physiological capability while diving. Interestingly, the different responses of the five species relate more to their very different diving patterns and foraging ecologies than their phylogenies (i.e. fur seals versus sea lions; Fig. 2). Our data exemplify the pattern that benthic hunters maximize the time they spend at the benthos (Fig. 3). When foraging in deep water, benthic hunters may operate at levels closer to their maximum physiological capacity than epipelagic foragers. Unlike epipelagic or near-surface feeders, benthic foragers must have enough oxygen to get to the bottom of a dive as well as to search for prey once there. The deeper the dive, the longer the time spent in transit with proportionately less time available to search for prey [27].

Animals that operate at or near their maximum physiological performance are less likely to have the capacity to increase their foraging effort in response to reductions in

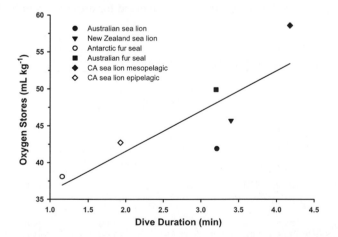

Fig. 1. Relationship between oxygen storage capacity and dive duration in five species of otariids. Open symbols are for epipelagic (near surface) foragers and solid symbols for benthic or mesopelagic foragers. $R^2 = 0.68$.

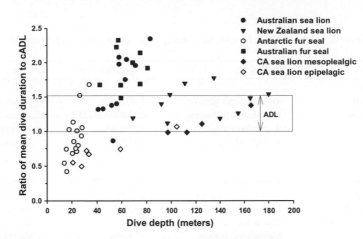

Fig. 2. Dive performance defined as the ratio between average dive duration and the predicted aerobic dive limit as a function of dive depth in five pinnipeds species. Open symbols are for epipelagic (near surface) foragers and solid symbols for benthic or mesopelagic foragers. Range of cADL outlined by the box is the cADL plus 50% to account for the variability in FMR estimates.

food availability whether due to environmental changes, fishery related activities, or both. However benthic prey are a more predictable resource that are less influenced by oceanographic perturbations such as El Niños compared to epipelagic prey. Animals that operate within their physiological capacity would be able to draw upon a greater energy reserve to pursue prey at deeper depths. Moreover, they could dive longer than normal if need be, or forage for longer periods, to accommodate the variability in prey resources [12,16].

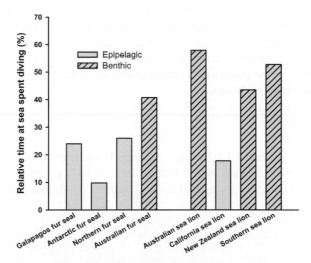

Fig. 3. The relative time spent diving while at sea compared across otariid species. Data for Galapagos fur seals (*Arctocephalus galapagoensis*) are from Ref. [28]; data for Northern fur seals (*Callorhinus ursinus*) are from Ref. [29], data for California sea lions are from Ref. [18]; and data for Southern sea lion (*Otaria flavescens*) are from Ref. [30].

Table 2
Pinniped population numbers and trends for epipelagic, mesopelagic, and benthic foraging species (see Ref. [34] for review)

Common name	Species	Population size	Trend
Epi/Mesopelagic			
Antarctic fur seal	*Arctocephalus gazella*	1,600,000	increasing
California sea lion	*Zalophus californianus*	237,000–244,000	increasing
Cape fur seal	*A. pusillus pusillus*	1,700,000	increasing
Subantarctic fur seal	*A. tropicalis*	>310,000	increasing
Benthic			
Australian sea lion	*Neophoca cinerea*	9300–11,700	stable or increasing
Australian fur seal	*A. pusillus doriferus*	60,000	slowly increasing
New Zealand sea lion	*Phocarctos hookeri*	13,000	stable
South American sea lion	*Otaria flavenscens*	275,000	decreasing
Steller sea lion	*Eumatopias jubatus*	<75,000	decreasing[a]

[a] Stock specific.

Other data on diving behavior further this argument. Benthic foragers, whether fur seal or sea lion, expend more effort foraging by spending >40% of their time at sea underwater compared to epipelagic species that spend <30% of their time at sea underwater (Fig. 3). These findings may explain why many fur seal species (and the epipelagic foraging California sea lion) have experienced substantial population growth. In contrast, all the sea lion species that feed on or near the sea bottom (e.g. Steller, *Eumetopias jubatus*; Australian; southern, *Otaria byronia*; and New Zealand sea lion) and the Australian fur seal (a benthic forager), have stable or declining populations [31–33], and (Table 2) despite the fact that many sympatrically breed with near-surface feeding fur seals [16].

A further compounding dilemma for benthic foragers is the possibility that juvenile animals may experience lower survival than adults. Given that adults operate at or near their physiological limit, juveniles who have less physiological capabilities than adults due to their small body size and inexperience would have an even harder time foraging benthically. If correct, juvenile survival would be reduced in these species and thus, decrease recruitment in the population. These patterns are relevant to the conservation and management of diving vertebrates.

Acknowledgements

This work was supported by National Science Foundation Grant # OPP-9981683, Office of Naval Research grant N00014-02-1-1012, NOAA award NA16OC2936, UC Mexus Program SC-03-15 and was carried out as part of the Tagging of Pacific Pelagics Program, TOPP.

References

[1] G.A. Bartholomew, The role of natural history in contemporary biology, Bioscience 36 (5) (1986) 324–329.
[2] R.D. Hill, et al., Heart rate and body temperature during free diving of Weddell seals, Am. J. Physiol. 253 (1987) R344–R351.

[3] G.L. Kooyman, et al., Aerobic and anaerobic metabolism during voluntary diving in Weddell seals: evidence of preferred pathways from blood chemistry and behavior, J. Comp. Physiol., B 138 (1980) 335–346.

[4] P.J. Ponganis, M.A. Kooyman, M.A. Castellini, Determinants of the aerobic dive limits of weddell seals: analysis of diving metabolic rates, postdive end tidal PO_2's, and blood and muscle oxygen stores, Physiol. Zool. 66 (5) (1993) 732–749.

[5] D.P. Costa, Reproductive and Foraging energetics of pinnipeds: implications for life history patterns, in: D. Renouf (Ed.), Behaviour of Pinnipeds, Chapman and Hall, London, 1991, pp. 300–344.

[6] G.L. Kooyman, Diverse Divers: Physiology and Behavior, Springer-Verlag, Berlin, 1989.

[7] D.P. Costa, The secret life of marine mammals: novel tools for studying their behavior and biology at sea, Oceanography 6 (3) (1993) 120–128.

[8] B.A. Block, et al., Revealing pelagic habitat use: the tagging of Pacific pelagics program, Oceanol. Acta 25 (2003) 255–266.

[9] D.P. Costa, Reproductive and foraging energetics of high latitude penguins, albatrosses, and pinnipeds: implications for life history patterns, Am. Zool. 31 (1991) 111–130.

[10] I.L. Boyd, J.P. Croxall, Dive durations in pinnipeds and seabirds, Can. J. Zool. 74 (1996) 1696–1705.

[11] G.L. Kooyman, et al., Aerobic dive limits of immature Weddell seals, J. Comp. Physiol., B 151 (1983) 171–174.

[12] D.P. Costa, N.J. Gales, M.E. Goebel, Aerobic dive limit: how often does it occur in nature? Comp. Biochem. Physiol. 129A (2001) 771–783.

[13] I.L. Boyd, N.J. Lunn, T. Barton, Time budgets and foraging characteristics of lactating Antarctic fur seals, J. Anim. Ecol. 60 (1991) 577–592.

[14] D.P. Costa, M.E. Goebel, J.T. Sterling, Foraging energetics and diving behavior of the Antarctic fur seal, *Arctocephalus gazella* at Cape Shirreff, Livingston Island, in: C. Davidson, C. Howard-Williams, P. Broady (Eds.), Antarctic Ecosystems: Models for wider ecological understanding, The Caxton Press, Christchurch, NZ, 2000, pp. 77–84.

[15] D.P. Costa, N.J. Gales, Foraging energetics and diving behaviour of lactating New Zealand seal lions, *Phocarctos hookeri*, J. Exp. Biol. 203 (2000) 3655–3665.

[16] D.P. Costa, N.J. Gales, Energetics of a benthic diver: seasonal foraging ecology of the Australian sea lion, *Neophoca cinerea*, Ecol. Monogr. 73 (1) (2003) 27–43.

[17] J.P.Y. Arnould, M.A. Hindell, Dive behavior, foraging locations, and maternal attendance patterns of Australian fur seals (*Arctocephalus pusillus doriferus*), Can. J. Zool. 79 (2001) 35–48.

[18] S.D. Feldkamp, R.L. DeLong, G.A. Antonelis, Diving patterns of California sea lions, *Zalophus Californianus*, Can. J. Zool. 67 (1989) 872–883.

[19] N. Lifson, R. McClintock, Theory of use of the turnover rates of body water for measuring energy and material balance, J. Theor. Biol. 12 (1966) 46–74.

[20] R.W. Davis, S. Kanatous, Convective oxygen transport and tissue oxygen consumption in Weddell seals during aerobic dives, J. Exp. Biol. 202 (1999) 1091–1113.

[21] R.L. Gentry, et al., Synthesis and conclusions, in: R.L. Gentry, G.L. Kooyman (Eds.), Fur Seals: Maternal Strategies on Land and at Sea, Princeton University Press, Princeton, 1986, pp. 220–264.

[22] D.P. Costa, N.J. Gales, D.E. Crocker, Blood volume and diving ability of the New Zealand sea lion, *Phocarctos hookeri*, Physiol. Zool. 71 (2) (1998) 208–213.

[23] J.Z. Reed, P.J. Butler, M.A. Fedak, The metabolic characteristics of the locomotory muscles of Grey seals (*Halichoerus grypus*), Harbour seals (*Phoca vitulina*), and Antarctic Fur seals (*Arctocephalus gazella*), J. Exp. Biol. 194 (1994 Sep.) 33–46.

[24] D.P. Costa, J.P. Croxall, C.D. Duck, Foraging energetics of Antarctic Fur Seals in relation to changes in prey availability, Ecology 70 (3) (1989) 596–606.

[25] M.S. Lowry, et al., Seasonal and annual variability in the diet of California sea lion *Zalophus califorianus* at San Nicholas Island, California, 1981–86, Fish Bull. 89 (1991) 331–336.

[26] D. Aurioles-Gamboa, A. Zavala-Gonzalez, Ecological factors that determine distribution and abundance of the California sea lion *Zalophus californianus* in the Gulf of California, Cienc. Mar. 20 (1994) 535–553.

[27] D.P. Costa, T.M. Williams, Marine mammal energetics, in: J. Reynolds, S. Rommel (Eds.), The Biology of Marine Mammals, Simthsonian Institution Press, Washington, DC, 2000, pp. 176–217.

[28] G.L. Kooyman, F. Trillmich, Diving behavior of Galapagos Fur Seals, in: R.L. Gentry, G.L. Kooyman (Eds.), Fur Seals: Maternal Strategies on Land and at Sea, Princeton University Press, Princeton, 1986, pp. 186–195.

[29] R.L. Gentry, G.L. Kooyman, M.E. Goebel, Feeding and Diving behavior of the Northern Fur Seal, in: R.L. Gentry, G.L. Kooyman (Eds.), Fur Seals: Maternal Strategies on Land and at Sea, Princeton University Press, Princeton, 1986, pp. 60–78.

[30] C. Campagna, et al., Movements and location at sea of the South American sea lions (*Otaria flavescens*), J. Zool., Lond. 257 (2001) 205–230.

[31] I.L. Boyd, et al., Population demography of Antarctic fur seals—the costs of reproduction and implications for life-histories, J. Anim. Ecol. 64 (1995) 505–518.

[32] N.J. Gales, D.J. Fletcher, Abundance, distribution and status of the New Zealand sea lion, *Phocarctos hookeri*, Wildl. Res. 26 (1999) 35–52.

[33] N.J. Gales, P.D. Shaughnessy, T.E. Dennis, Distribution, abundance and breeding cycle of the Australian sea lion, *Neophoca cinerea* (Mammalia: Pinnipedia), J. Zool., Lond. 234 (1994) 353–370.

[34] D.P. Costa, M.J. Weise, J.P.Y. Arnould, Worldwide pinniped population status and trends, in: J. Estes (Ed.), Whales, Whaling, and Ocean Ecosystems, 2004, in press.

International Congress Series 1275 (2004) 367–374

ELSEVIER

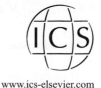

www.ics-elsevier.com

Energetics of cooperative breeding in meerkats
Suricata Suricatta

M. Scantlebury[a,*], T.H. Clutton-Brock[b], J.R. Speakman[c,d]

[a]*Mammal Research Institute, Department of Zoology and Entomology, University of Pretoria, Pretoria 0002, South Africa*
[b]*Department of Zoology, University of Cambridge, UK*
[c]*Aberdeen Centre for Energy regulation and Obesity (ACERO), University of Aberdeen, School of Biological Sciences, Aberdeen, UK*
[d]*ACERO, Division of Energy Balance and Obesity, Rowett Research Institute, Aberdeen, UK*

Abstract. We investigate whether energetic constraints play a role in determining social structure in cooperatively breeding meerkats *Suricata suricatta*. Energetics may be important at various stages of the reproductive cycle. Peak lactation and peak pup feeding are potentially the most energetically stressful periods for lactating mothers and subordinate helpers, respectively. Here, we review current data on lactation and present additional information on helping behaviour. Daily energy expenditure (DEE) of dominant females, subordinate helpers and pups were not particularly high during peak lactation. However, metabolisable energy intakes of lactating mothers (calculated from isotope-based estimates of offspring milk energy intake) were not significantly different from maximal suggested limits (at around seven times resting metabolic rate). DEEs of lactating mothers also increased with litter size, but decreased with group size. By comparison, during peak pup feeding, DEE values of helpers were not greater than those measured prior to breeding. Nor was there any apparent difference in DEE between "keen" and "lazy" helpers, suggesting that helping may not be energetically costly. These results confirm hypotheses that, in cooperatively breeding societies, breeders have high energy costs, which can be reduced by helpers. However, they do not support the notion that helpers incur substantial energetic costs in raising young. © 2004 Elsevier B.V. All rights reserved.

Keywords: Doubly labelled water; Energy expenditure; Lactation; Carnivore; Evolution

---

* Corresponding author. Tel.: +27 12 420 4872; fax: +27 12 362 5242.
E-mail address: m.scantlebury@zoology.up.ac.za (M. Scantlebury).

0531-5131/ © 2004 Elsevier B.V. All rights reserved.
doi:10.1016/j.ics.2004.08.063

1. Introduction

Research into the evolution of cooperative breeding has focused on three main questions [1,2]: Why do helpers remain in their natal group after reaching sexual maturity? Why do they not breed? And why do they assist other individuals to rear their young? Usual answers include that dispersal and reproduction have high costs in young animals, and, that non-breeding individuals can gain increments to the indirect component of their inclusive fitness that are sufficient to offset the marginal fitness costs of helping. While previous studies have outlined the probable answers to these questions, we still lack the understanding required to explain the processes involved.

Energetic constraints have previously been suggested to play a key role in limiting the capacity of females to breed successfully without helpers [3–5]. They may limit offspring survival [6] as well as prevent or delay independent breeding of subordinates [7–9]. In some cooperative breeders, for example, the development of feeding skills appears to be unusually slow, providing a plausible explanation of why younger individuals do not attempt to disperse or breed until their feeding skills (and therefore energy intake) approach that of adults [10]. However, few studies have directly examined the importance of energy in cooperative breeding systems. Studies of birds have shown that helping may be energetically costly and incur a delayed mortality cost to the donor [11,12], but may also increase growth rates of offspring [13]. Other studies have shown that helpers may have positive effects on breeders by reducing their energy expenditure [3,5] or thermoregulatory costs [14,15]. Therefore, to understand the evolution of cooperative breeding in mammals, it is important to determine whether energetics may also have played a role.

In some cooperative societies, parents are capable of breeding without helpers, but in a few, breeding is typically unsuccessful in the absence of helpers. One suggestion is that high reproductive skew may evolve in tandem with high energetic costs of reproduction. Hence, one hypothesis for the occurrence of obligate cooperative breeding is that, following the evolution of cooperation, selection for female fecundity (and hence the energy required for reproduction) has increased such that breeders are unable to raise their young unassisted [4]. This hypothesis predicts that: (i) the daily energy expenditure (DEE) of breeding females is high, (ii) helpers invest substantial amounts of energy in raising young, and, (iii) the presence of multiple helpers reduces the energy costs to breeding females.

Meerkats are a classic example of an obligate cooperatively breeding mammal. They are small (<0.9 kg), diurnal carnivores that live in groups of 2–40, accompanied by dependent offspring. Groups typically include a single dominant pair and a variable number of helpers of both sexes. The dominant female may breed up to four times per year and is responsible for 80% of the litters born in her group. Subordinates of both sexes assist in raising young (0–4 weeks of age) by guarding pups at the natal burrow ("babysitting"), feeding them (1–3 months of age) after they start to move with the group ("pup-feeding") and acting as sentinels while the group is foraging ("guarding") [16,17]. Subordinate females breed occasionally, either in synchrony with the dominant female or at other times [18]. In addition, in up to 20% of litters, subordinate females may lactate to the dominant female's pups, even if they have not bred themselves ("allo-lactators"). The number of allo-lactators varies, usually between 0 and 2, and is correlated with the total number of female helpers in the group [19]. When mixed litters do occur, it is unclear whether subordinates lactate principally to their own offspring or indeed whether they produce milk that is of the same energy content as that of the dominant female.

In contrast to the observed helping behaviours and the mutualistic benefits individuals may derive from increasing by their presence the size of the group they live in [20], both dominant and subordinate females are commonly infanticidal (towards pups of their own group) [21]. This suggests that there may be possible bottlenecks on energy provisioning to offspring at some stage in reproduction. Therefore, it may be to a mother's benefit to try to make sure that her own pups are the ones to pass through this bottleneck.

Energetics may be important at various stages of the reproductive cycle. In meerkats, two periods are likely to be of primary concern: peak lactation and peak pup feeding. Studies of female mammals show that food intake generally increases throughout gestation and lactation and reaches a maximum during peak lactation [22]; the female must provide sufficient milk for offspring that are large but still dependent on her for all their nutritional requirements. Therefore, peak lactation is likely to be a key period as it defines the time that is potentially the most energetically stressful for the mother. By comparison, during peak pup feeding, offspring are dependent on helpers who must forage to meet both their own increased energy demands and those of the growing offspring. Therefore, this period is potentially the most energetically stressful for helpers.

2. Discussion

2.1. Energy costs of reproduction: peak lactation

DEE of dominant lactating females, dominant males, subordinate females, subordinate males, allo-lactating subordinate females and pups were measured using the doubly labelled water technique [19,23,24]. We calculated metabolisable energy intake (MEI) of lactating females from isotope-based estimates of milk energy intake of offspring [25]. DEE of dominant lactating females was higher than other categories of animals but was not significantly high compared with allometric predictions of same-size free-ranging eutherians [26]. However, MEI was not significantly different from allometric values for maximal energy intake of 1601 kJ day^{-1} [27], equating to a sustained energy intake of about seven times resting metabolic rate (RMR) (using a mean value of 241 kJ day^{-1} for RMR, Scantlebury et al., unpublished data). This indicates that mothers were indeed energetically stressed in an attempt to produce enough milk for their growing offspring.

By comparison, the DEE and MEI values of non-lactating helpers were not high compared with allometric predictions (Fig. 1). For example, the predicted values of maximal MEI for subordinate males and females were 1390 and 1318 kJ day^{-1}; measured values were about half this prediction. Hence, helpers were not energetically stressed during peak lactation. Allo-lactating subordinate females were the only category of animals that lost weight during the measurement period. This mass loss was likely to have supported the energy costs of their lactation [19].

We also found that the presence of helpers affected the DEE of dominant lactating females: DEE was positively correlated with litter size and negatively correlated with the number of helpers (Fig. 2). In contrast, there was no relationship between litter size and the

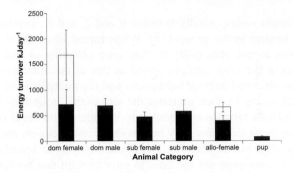

Fig. 1. Filled bars denote measured DEE values of dominant lactating females, dominant males, subordinate non-breeding females, subordinate males, allo-lactating females and pups during peak lactation. Open areas above bars show calculated extra energy turnovers of dominant females and allo-lactating females (milk production) and pups (growth).

number of helpers with the DEE of helpers. This indicates that non-lactating helpers serve to reduce the DEE of the lactating mother. This suggestion is supported by the fact that increased numbers of helpers do not significantly affect pup mass around the time of weaning, but do influence maternal mass around the time of the mothers' subsequent conception [28]. Non-lactating helpers, therefore, allow dominant females to channel more of their resources into milk. This may have been achieved by relieving dominant females from babysitting duties [29], by improving their foraging efficiency [30] or perhaps by reducing thermoregulatory costs at night [31].

Using a larger data set collected from the same site and on the same groups but over a greater time period (1996–2001 inclusive), we found that the body mass of helpers generally decreased during the babysitting period as a whole (pups aged 0–24 days) with the magnitude of the mass loss positively related to the amount of time spent babysitting [29,32]. However, there were no significant differences between the DEE of helpers during lactation and non-breeding times, or between the DEE of males and females (Fig. 3). Data were collected from ~300 individual meerkats from 14 different groups and analysed for 22,082 morning, pre-foraging weights during non-breeding periods, 14,128 during babysitting periods and 24,060 during pup feeding [32].

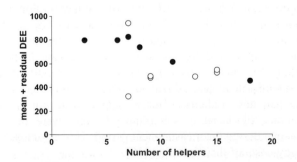

Fig. 2. Mean plus residual DEE (kJ day^{-1}) against the number of helpers. Open and filled circles denote dominant and subordinate females respectively. DEE of dominant lactating females decreased with the number of helpers whereas the DEE of helpers did not [19].

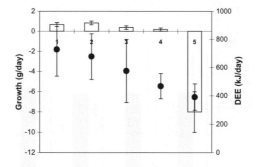

Fig. 3. Body mass change (g day^{-1}) of (1) subordinate male helpers during non-breeding times, (2) subordinate female helpers during non-breeding times, (3) subordinate males during lactation, (4) subordinate (non-breeding) females during lactation and (5) subordinate allo-lactating females; denoted by bars. Mass loss of allo-lactating females is shown for the period of peak lactation, whereas growth of other categories of animals is integrated over the entire babysitting period. Closed symbols denote measured DEE values (kJ day^{-1}) of the same categories of animals.

2.2. Energy costs of reproduction: peak pup feeding

During pup feeding, offspring are wholly dependent on helpers to provision them with food (dominant individuals hardly ever feed young). Therefore, the period when the pups demand the maximum rate of feeding (when they are approximately 50–60 days old) is potentially energetically stressful for helpers. There is a strong evidence to suggest that helpers do indeed invest substantial amounts of resources in raising young. For example, increases in litter size are positively associated with increases in the proportion of food items that helpers give away. Furthermore, when groups are manipulated to decrease the ratio of helpers to pups (either by cross-fostering pups or by temporarily removing helpers), helpers have reduced rates of daily weight gain [32]. However, we do not know whether these apparent costs translate into actual differences in the energy costs of the various activities, and whether any particular activity (such as pup feeding) is limited, for example, by the rate of energy expenditure or the rate of energy collection, that an individual helper can sustain [33], as has suggested to be important in birds [8,34]. Presumably, it may be worthwhile foraging to feed pups at a high rate, as a small drop in foraging effort might produce a significant increase in mortality risk of offspring [30].

In an initial investigation, we measured the DEE values of subordinate males during peak pup feeding and compared these values with those obtained during peak lactation and non-breeding periods. Subordinate males were measured because subordinate females have a high likelihood of becoming evicted at breeding times [21]. Male helpers varied in the total amount of food items that they provisioned to pups. In some individuals, more than 30% of prey items found were offered to pups, whereas in others, less than 5% of items were given away (Scantlebury et al., unpublished data). There was no overall significant difference in the DEE of "keen" and "lazy" helpers at peak pup feeding or between these values and those measured previously prior to breeding ($F=3.51$, $P=0.053$) (Fig. 4). Therefore, it is not the case that DEE of helpers is particularly high during peak pup feeding, or that they forage particularly hard to meet energy demands. The fact that no significant differences in the DEE of keen and

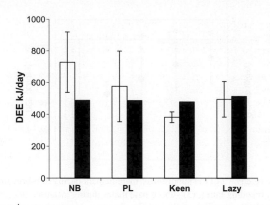

Fig. 4. DEE values (kJ day^{-1}) of subordinate males during times of non-breeding (NB) (n=6), peak lactation (PL) (n=6) and during peak pup feeding for "keen" (n=3) and "lazy" (n=3) individuals. Open bars denote measured values; filled bars denote allometrically predicted values (log$_e$ FMR=1.929+0.650log$_e$ body mass (g)) [26].

lazy helpers were observed could be a result of the few numbers of individuals that have been measured to date, but, importantly these data suggest that the costs of helping per se may not be as high as previously thought. However, these results must also be interpreted with some caution as our impressions of animals' helping activity may be based on a small sample of the total duration over which the DEE measurement is integrated, and therefore observations may not be truly representative of differences in helping behaviour. Alternatively, keen helpers may not increase their foraging efforts during pup feeding, but they may bear the costs of helping by drawing on their own body reserves, which they may then recuperate during subsequent non-breeding periods [32].

In summary, reproduction is energetically costly for dominant lactating females, who are energetically stressed in an attempt to eat enough to provide enough milk for their growing offspring. The concurrent energy throughput of helpers is significantly lower. Non-breeding helpers do, however, allow mothers to reduce their DEE during lactation, either by increasing their foraging efficiency or perhaps by increasing their thermoregulatory costs at night. In contrast to predictions from behavioural observations [32], during peak pup feeding, we did not find that subordinate helpers significantly increased their DEE, or that there was any difference in the DEE between keen and lazy helpers.

Acknowledgements

We thank Mr. and Mrs. H. Kotzee and the Northern Cape Conservation Authority for their permission to work at Rus en Vrede. The research was financed by the Natural Environment Research Council and the Biotechnology and Biological Science Research Council, UK.

References

[1] S.T. Emlen, The evolution of cooperative breeding in birds, in: JR Krebs, NB Davies (Eds.), Behavioural Ecology: An Evolutionary Approach, Blackwell Scientific publications, 1978, pp. 245–281.

[2] S.T. Emlen, Predicting family dynamics in social vertebrates, in: JR Krebs, NB Davies (Eds.), Behavioural Ecology: An Evolutionary Approach, Blackwell Scientific publications, 1997, pp. 228–253.

[3] H.U. Reyer, K. Westerterp, Parental energy expenditure: a proximate cause of helper recruitment in the pied kingfisher (*Ceryle rudis*), Behav. Ecol. Sociobiol. 17 (1985) 363–369.

[4] S.R. Creel, N.M. Creel, Energetics, reproductive suppression and obligate communal breeding in carnivores, Behav. Ecol. Sociobiol. 28 (1991) 263–270.

[5] A. Anava, et al., Effect of group size on field metabolic rate of Arabian babblers provisioning nestlings, Condor 103 (2001) 376–380.

[6] R.J. Boland, R. Heinson, A. Cockburn, Experimental manipulation of brood reduction and parental care in cooperatively breeding white-winged choughs, J. Anim. Ecol. 66 (1997) 683–690.

[7] R.G. Heinsohn, Slow learning of foraging skills and extended parental care in cooperatively breeding white-winged choughs, Am. Nat. 137 (6) (1991) 864–881.

[8] R.G. Heinsohn, A. Cockburn, Helping is costly to young birds in cooperatively breeding white-winged choughs, Proc. R. Soc. Lond., B 256 (1994) 293–298.

[9] A. Cockburn, Evolution of helping behaviour in cooperatively breeding birds, Ann. Rev. Ecolog. Syst. 29 (1998) 141–177.

[10] J.L. Brown, Helping and Communal Breeding in Birds, Princeton University Press, 1987.

[11] K.N. Rabenold, in: P.B. Stacey, W.D. Koenig (Eds.), Cooperative Breeding in Birds, Cambridge University Press, 1990, pp. 159–196. Ch. 6.

[12] H.U. Reyer, in: P.B. Stacey, W.D. Koenig (Eds.), Cooperative Breeding in Birds, Cambridge University Press, 1990, pp. 590–599. Ch. 17.

[13] A. Anava, et al., Growth rate and energetics of Arabian babbler (*Turdoides squamiceps*) nestlings, AUK 118 (2) (2001) 519–524.

[14] J.B. Williams, M.A. DuPlessis, Field metabolism and water flux of sociable weavers *Philetairus socius* in the Kalahari Desert, Ibis 138 (2) (1996) 168–171.

[15] C. Boix-Hinzen, B.G. Lovegrove, Circadian metabolic and thermoregulatory patterns of red-billed woodhoopoes (*Phoeniculus purpureus*): the influence of huddling, J. Zool. (Lond.) 244 (1998) 33–41.

[16] T.H. Clutton-Brock, et al., Individual contributions to babysitting in a cooperative mongoose, *Suricata suricatta*, Proc. R. Soc. Lond., B 267 (2000) 301–305.

[17] T.H. Clutton-Brock, et al., Contributions to cooperative rearing in meerkats, Anim. Behav. 61 (2001) 705–710.

[18] T.H. Clutton-Brock, et al., Cooperation, control and concession in meerkat groups, Science 291 (2001) 48–481.

[19] M. Scantlebury, et al., Energetics of lactation in cooperatively breeding meerkats *Suricata suricatta*, Proc. R. Soc. Lond., B 269 (2002) 2147–2153.

[20] H. Kokko, R.A. Johnstone, T.H. Clutton-Brock, The evolution of cooperative breeding through group augmentation, Proc. R. Soc. Lond., B 268 (2001) 187–196.

[21] T.H. Clutton-Brock, et al., Infanticide and expulsion of females in a cooperative mammal, Proc. R. Soc. Lond., B 265 (1998) 2291–2295.

[22] J.L. Gittleman, S.D. Thompson, Energy allocation in mammalian reproduction, Am. Zool. 28 (1988) 863–875.

[23] N. Lifson, R. McClintock, Theory of the turnover rates of body water for measuring energy and material balance, J. Theor. Biol. 12 (1966) 46–74.

[24] J.R. Speakman, The Doubly Labelled Water Technique: Theory and Practice, Chapman and Hall, London, 1997.

[25] O.T. Oftedal, S.J. Iverson, Hydrogen isotope methodology for the measurement of milk intake and the energetics of growth in suckling young, in: A.C. Huntly (Ed.), Marine Mammal Energetics, Society for Marine Mammalogy: Special Publications, vol. 1, 1987, pp. 67–96.

[26] J.R. Speakman, The cost of living: field metabolic rates of small mammals, in: A.H. Fitter, D.G. Rafaelli (Eds.), Advances in Ecological Research, Academic Press, London, 2000.

[27] J. Weiner, Physiological limits to sustainable energy budgets in birds and mammals: ecological implications, TREE 7 (11) (1992) 384–388.

[28] A.F. Russell, et al., Breeding success in cooperative meerkats: effect of helper number and maternal state, Behav. Ecol. 14 (2003) 486–492.

[29] T.H. Clutton-Brock, et al., Costs of cooperative behaviour in suricates, *Suricata suricatta*, Proc. R. Soc. Lond., B 265 (1998) 185–190.

[30] T.H. Clutton-Brock, et al., Predation, group size and mortality in a cooperative mongoose, *Suricata suricatta*, J. Anim. Ecol. 68 (1999) 672–683.

[31] A.F. Russell, Factors affecting pup growth and survival in cooperatively breeding meerkats *Suricata suricatta*, J. Anim. Ecol. 71 (2002) 700–709.

[32] A.F. Russell, Cost minimisation by helpers in cooperative vertebrates, PNAS 100 (6) (2003) 3333–3338.

[33] K.A. Hammond, J. Diamond, Maximal sustained energy budgets in humans and animals, Nature 386 (1997) 457–462.

[34] R. Drent, S. Daan, The prudent parent: energetic adjustments in avian breeding, Ardea 68 (1980) 225–252.

Author index

Keyword index